Policing and the Mentally Ill

International Perspectives

Duncan Chappell

Advances in Police Theory and Practice Series

Series Editor: Dilip K. Das

Policing and the Mentally Ill: International Perspectives
Duncan Chappell

Security Governance, Policing, and Local Capacity
Kam C. Wong

Policing in Hong Kong: History and Reform
Jan Froestad with Clifford D. Shearing

Police Performance Appraisals: A Comparative Perspective
Serdar Kenan Gul and Paul O'Connell

Police Reform in The New Democratic South Africa
Moses Montesh and Vinesh Basdeo

Los Angeles Police Department Meltdown: The Fall of the Professional-Reform
Model of Policing
James Lasley

Financial Crimes: A Global Threat
Maximillian Edelbacher, Peter Kratcoski, and Michael Theil

Police Integrity Management in Australia: Global Lessons for Combating
Police Misconduct
Louise Porter and Tim Prenzler

The Crime Numbers Game: Management by Manipulation
John A. Eterno and Eli B. Silverman

The International Trafficking of Human Organs: A Multidisciplinary Perspective
Leonard Territo and Rande Matteson

Police Reform in China
Kam C. Wong

Mission-Based Policing
John P. Crank, Dawn M. Irlbeck, Rebecca K. Murray, and Mark Sundermeier

The New Khaki: The Evolving Nature of Policing in India
Arvind Verma

Cold Cases: An Evaluation Model with Follow-up Strategies for Investigators
James M. Adcock and Sarah L. Stein

Policing Organized Crime: Intelligence Strategy Implementation
Petter Gottschalk

Security in Post-Conflict Africa: The Role of Nonstate Policing
Bruce Baker

Policing and the Mentally Ill
International Perspectives

Edited by
Duncan Chappell

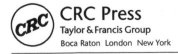

CRC Press
Taylor & Francis Group
Boca Raton London New York

CRC Press is an imprint of the
Taylor & Francis Group, an **informa** business

CRC Press
Taylor & Francis Group
6000 Broken Sound Parkway NW, Suite 300
Boca Raton, FL 33487-2742

First issued in paperback 2019

ISBN-13: 978-1-4398-8116-3 (hbk)
ISBN-13: 978-0-367-86673-0 (pbk)

Library of Congress Cataloging-in-Publication Data

Policing and the mentally ill : international perspectives / editor, Duncan Chappell.
  pages cm
  Includes bibliographical references and index.
  ISBN 978-1-4398-8116-3 (hbk. : alk. paper)
  1. Mentally ill offenders. 2. Mental illness. 3. Police services for the mentally ill. 4. Law enforcement. I. Chappell, Duncan.

HV6133.P65 2013
364.3'8--dc23   2012043756

Visit the Taylor & Francis Web site at
http://www.taylorandfrancis.com

and the CRC Press Web site at
http://www.crcpress.com

Contents

Series Preface

Although the literature on police and allied subjects is growing exponentially, its impact upon day-to-day policing remains small. The two worlds of research and practise of policing remain disconnected even though cooperation between the two is growing. A major reason is that the two groups speak in different languages. The research work is published in hard-to-access journals and presented in a manner that is difficult to comprehend for a layperson. On the other hand, police practitioners tend not to mix with researchers and remain secretive about their work. Consequently, there is little dialogue between the two, and almost no attempt to learn from one another. Dialogue across the globe, among researchers and practitioners situated in different continents, is of course even more limited.

I attempted to address this problem by starting the IPES (www.ipes.info), where a common platform has brought the two together. IPES is now in its 15th year. The annual meetings that constitute most of the major events of the organisation have been hosted in all parts of the world. Several publications have come out of these deliberations, and a new collaborative community of scholars and police officers has been created whose membership runs into several hundreds.

Another attempt was to begin a new journal, aptly called *Police Practice and Research: An International Journal* (PPR), that has opened the gate to practitioners to share their work and experiences. The journal has attempted to focus upon issues that help bring the two on a single platform. PPR completed its 13th year in 2012. It is certainly evidence of growing collaboration between police research and practise that PPR, which began with four issues a year, expanded into five issues in its fourth year, and now it is issued six times a year.

Clearly, these attempts, despite their success, remain limited. Conferences and journal publications do help create a body of knowledge and an association of police activists but cannot address substantial issues in depth. The limitations of time and space preclude larger discussions and more authoritative expositions that can provide stronger and broader linkages between the two worlds.

It is this realisation of the increasing dialogue between police research and practise that has encouraged many of us—my close colleagues and

I connected closely with IPES and PPR across the world—to conceive and implement a new attempt in this direction. I am now embarking on a book series, *Advances in Police Theory and Practice*, that seeks to attract writers from all parts of the world. Further, the attempt is to find practitioner contributors. The objective is to make the series a serious contribution to our knowledge of the police as well as to improve police practises. The focus is not only on work that describes the best and successful police practises, but also one that challenges current paradigms and breaks new ground to prepare police for this century. The series seeks comparative analysis that highlights achievements in distant parts of the world as well as encourages an in-depth examination of specific problems confronting a particular police force.

The present book in this series is concerned with interactions between police and persons with mental illnesses. According to the World Health Organisation, during their lifetime more than one quarter of all individuals will develop one or more mental or behavioural disorders. Given prevalence data like this, it is not surprising that wherever they reside on the planet, many persons suffering from a mental disorder, or, as is more commonly termed in popular parlance, a mental illness, are likely to come into contact with police at some stage in their lives. Indeed, research conducted in a number of countries suggests that about 10% of all community police work involves some form of interaction with a person with a mental illness. From a police perspective, these encounters are not only frequent but also often sensitive and challenging.

Despite the difficulties associated with this important aspect of community policing, surprisingly scant attention has been given to the development of empirically tested and established best practise approaches to managing police interactions with persons with mental illnesses. The literature that does exist is principally derived from North American sources, although more recent and interesting developments have been reported in Australia and parts of Europe. Beyond these areas of the developed world, little is known and even less published on this topic. In part this dearth of literature, and attendant research, is also a reflection of the fear and stigma that continue to be attached to mental illness and those who suffer from it in many societies across the globe.

The principal aim of this book is to seek to reduce this gap in the literature by providing an international overview of the latest research and policy developments in the field, and the challenges still to be confronted in many places in overcoming cultural and associated barriers to protecting the rights of the mentally ill, including the provision of adequate treatment and related health services.

It is hoped that through this series it will be possible to accelerate the process of building knowledge about policing and help bridge the gap between the two worlds—the worlds of police research and police practise. This is an invitation to police scholars and practitioners across the world to come and join in this venture.

Dilip K. Das, Ph.D.

Founding President, International
Police Executive Symposium (IPES)
www.ipes.info

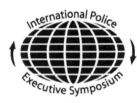 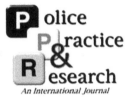

Founding Editor-in-Chief,
Police Practise and Research:
An International Journal (PPR)
www.tandf.co.uk/journals

Preface

The original idea for this book came to me from organising a number of panels on the topic of policing and persons with mental illnesses for the International Academy of Law and Mental Health (IALMH) 32nd International Congress on Law and Mental Health held at Humboldt University in Berlin, Germany, in July 2011. With the nucleus of a book being available from the various papers presented at this congress, a proposal was made to CRC Press for this book to be published as a volume in the Advances in Police Theory and Practice Series, under the general editorship of Dr. Dilip Das. To my delight the proposal was accepted and the project has since moved to a successful conclusion, with the 16 invited chapters in this book offering a wide range of cross-cultural perspectives on an aspect of policing that all too often in the past has not received the attention and priority it deserves.

It is particularly pleasing that so many policing practitioners have chosen to contribute to this book. As readers will discover, although the book does not seek in any way to provide an exhaustive account of contemporary developments in any single country or region, the principal focus is on Australia, where local law enforcement agencies have displayed a remarkable enthusiasm for and commitment to change in their management of interactions with citizens with mental illnesses. The specialised police responses (SPRs) that have emerged in the Australian states of New South Wales (NSW) and Queensland are described in some detail in separate chapters of the book. I am extremely grateful to the staff of the Mental Health Intervention Team (MHIT) in NSW and the Mental Health Intervention Program (MHIP) in Queensland for their personal support and encouragement in making these contributions possible. I was also able to participate in person in the MHIT four-day intensive training programme and am now a proud MHIT graduate.

Initiatives like the MHIT and MHIP that are occurring in Australia are in many ways unique, and certainly worthy of further study and possible replication in other parts of the world since they have taken a concept that was really designed for much smaller urban-based law enforcement agencies in North America and applied it to very large police forces with mandates to deliver services across huge geographic areas, and in rural and remote communities as well as in densely populated cities. When launching these initiatives, there has also been a willingness among Australian police practitioners to engage in the evaluation of outcomes and to rely on evidence-based

information when setting policies and directions. Close research relationships have been established between academia and the Australian police
community, especially through the activities of the Australian Research
Council Centre of Excellence in Policing and Security (CEPS), a largely feder-
ally funded programme designed to support applied and theoretical research
of national significance and importance. CEPS and its director, Professor
Simon Bronitt, have been very supportive of the activities surrounding the
preparation of this book, and I express my gratitude for this assistance.

I also express my warm thanks to all of the authors mentioned in the list
of contributors. They have displayed great patience and understanding over
the many months that it has taken to gather, review, and ultimately deliver to
the publisher the 16 chapters contained in the book. These warm thanks also
extend to Carolyn Spence and Kathryn Younce at CRC Press, and Dilip Das
as the series editor, all of whom have willingly granted me several extensions
of time to complete the project.

Duncan Chappell
Sydney, Australia

Introduction

Genesis and Structure

The genesis of this book is to be found in a number of places, but as its content will reveal, it reflects primarily a growing acknowledgement and recognition in many parts of the world that interactions between police and persons with mental illnesses comprise an important and sensitive aspect of everyday community policing. The way in which these interactions are handled can have a profound impact on the lives of all involved. In countries possessing democratic traditions and committed to the rule of law, these interactions will usually be guided by legislative mandates that give police wide discretion in the way they act. Thus, for the mentally ill, encounters with police may result in their referral for assistance and treatment by trained mental health professionals, or their return to family members committed to their care. However, as will become clear from what follows, all too frequently the outcome of these interactions is far less therapeutic and leads instead to a cycle of arrests and ineffective treatment referrals that may ultimately result in incarceration in a correctional rather than health facility (see Chapters 10 and 11). In extreme cases it may also lead to a fatal outcome since, as will be seen, a significant proportion of police use of deadly force incidents involve persons with mental illnesses (see Chapters 8 and 9).

Linked closely to the acknowledgement and recognition of the importance of this policing function has been the growth of an informal movement, usually involving police working in collaboration with mental health and other emergency services workers, committed to the development of better ways of managing interactions with persons with mental illnesses. It is generally agreed that this movement had its origins in the U.S. state of Tennessee in the late 1980s when, following a tragic deadly force incident involving a mentally ill person in the city of Memphis, it was decided to establish crisis intervention teams (CITs) in this quite small municipal law enforcement agency. These specialised police teams, designed around a volunteer group of officers trained to identify the signs and symptoms of mental illness, were tasked with attending crisis incidents with mentally ill persons, de-escalating the situation, and referring those involved for treatment (see Chapters 1 and 4).

The perceived success of this CIT venture in Memphis has led to its subsequent adoption in numerous police departments across the United States and Canada over the past two decades. Around the same time, a variation of this Memphis model arose in the state of California, where the Los Angeles City and County law enforcement agencies became concerned with the frequency with which persons with mental illnesses who inter-acted with them failed to become engaged with mental health services, even when referred to them by police. As a result of this concern, the agencies decided to establish, in cooperation with community-based mental health services, co-responder teams (CRTs). These CRTs paired police with mental health staff who responded to incidents involving a person in mental health crisis (see Chapters 1 and 4). These North American developments have since spread internationally, and especially across the Pacific to Australia, where variants of the CIT and CRT models are to be found in several jurisdictions (see Chapters 4–6).

In the chapters that follow, a description is provided of the way in which this Memphis and related seed has been transplanted and prospered in for-eign climes. An account is also given of the many challenges that remain in responding to the needs of mentally ill persons. Many of these challenges are not ones that can be resolved by the police alone, and involve complex interactions between and assistance from health, welfare, housing, and allied services in the community. These challenges are also far more intense and far-reaching in countries that lack the various social welfare services and resources located in the developed nations of the world.

The book is structured in three parts. In Section I attention is devoted to developments in North America and Europe, which traditionally have been the loci of much of the innovation and change experienced in policing and related areas. However, while a substantial literature, much of it research based, now exists in North America on this subject, the same is not so true of Europe, where, as Rhonda Moore indicates in her review of the relevant literature (Chapter 3), a number of European countries have only begun recently to recognise this as a priority issue for policing, and those that have do not seem to have committed significant research resources to testing the effectiveness of different approaches to managing police interactions with the mentally ill. It should be acknowledged, however, that it is quite possible that there are more interesting and innovative approaches occurring in areas of Europe that fail to be recognised because of language and related barriers.

Section II of the book, which contains the bulk of the content, is devoted entirely to developments in Australia. More will be said about these devel-opments below, but they reflect a substantial and continuing professional commitment by a number of large police agencies in Australia to initiating major changes in the management of this aspect of their work. Two of the chapters are in fact contributed by these agencies: New South Wales (NSW) (Chapter 4) and Queensland (Chapter 5). These police initiatives have been matched in a number of cases by a willingness to expose their outcomes to independent external review. The use of evidence-based policing concepts has taken hold and been applied successfully.

In Section III the particular challenges of providing humane and effective policing for persons with mental illnesses in parts of the developing world are examined. These challenges often involve dealing with entrenched cultural beliefs and practices that are based on superstition, fear, and prejudice regarding persons thought to be mentally ill.

A brief review is now provided of some of the major themes and issues that arise from the contributions contained in each part of the book.

Section I: North America and Europe

Melissa Reuland, Laura Draper, and Blake Norton (Chapter 1) provide an account of the continuing spread of the Memphis-related seed across the United States. Given the remarkable diversity and fragmentation of policing in the United States, with about 18,000 state and local law enforcement agencies, half of which possess fewer than 10 sworn personnel, it is not surprising that state-based specialised police response (SPR) programmes have emerged to deliver the types of service provided by CIT and CRT SPRs in larger agencies. Based on the analysis described in the chapter, Reuland and her colleagues report a quite favourable outcome for these state-based programmes, although there remain some questions about their longer-term viability and possible replacement, in certain cases, by regional initiatives.

In Chapter 2 Dorothy Cotton and Terry Coleman consider contemporary developments in Canada designed to improve relationships between police and people with mental illnesses. Canada, too, has a quite diverse and fragmented law enforcement structure, although not in any sense equating to that found south of the border. Canada has also initiated numbers of SPR programmes with widespread coverage. These programmes include dedicated staff and in-service training and education of police personnel, together with memoranda of understanding (MOUs) between the police and mental health service agencies. Important landmark research has also been undertaken in Canada examining the experiences of people with mental illnesses who have been in contact with police. This research suggests that this consumer group in general has more positive than negative views about these interactions, although they remain somewhat ambivalent about aspects of this relationship.

Cotton and Coleman point to the data deficiencies that still exist in regard to many aspects of the interface between police and persons with mental illnesses. These include an absence of any national standards for the collection of information about this interface as well as data concerning the victimisation experiences of persons with mental illnesses. The lack of data of this type makes it very difficult to conduct any systematic evaluation of the effectiveness and efficiency of individual SPRs in this area. It should be noted that these observations undoubtedly have relevance and import well beyond the borders of Canada. So, too, do the rhetorical questions raised in the concluding section of Cotton and Coleman's chapter when they ask: "Are police–mental health liaison initiatives an indication of a failure on the part of the health care system—or a legitimate and appropriate police activity? Are these initiatives addressing a fundamental problem or merely serving as a stopgap measure to address a symptom?"

As already noted, Rhonda Moore's contribution in Chapter 3 deals with developments in Europe. Her chapter comprises an update of an earlier literature review she conducted of the same topic covering a period up to 2009. In the succeeding three years, new literature has emerged in English from jurisdictions other than the United Kingdom. Thus, in Denmark, France, and the Netherlands there is now evidence of SPRs being developed for police interactions with mentally ill persons. In Denmark the local initiative, following testing, has been launched on a country-wide basis with legislative backing, while in the Netherlands collaborative efforts between police and other agencies, including health, to improve service delivery to persons with mental illnesses seem well established. In France the SPRs identified appear less extensive in their ambitions and reach. Clearly there is scope for much more extensive developments to take place in other European countries, together with academic input in the form of testing and evaluation of new SPRs. At present, and unlike the situation described here in North America and Australia, there seems to be a lack of academic attention to or interest in this area of policing.

Section II: Developments in Australia

New South Wales

The Memphis-related seeds that have reached Australia over recent years have borne good fruit, as, in particular, Chapters 4 and 5 demonstrate. David Donohue and Gina Andrews describe in their chapter the developments that have occurred in NSW, Australia's most populous state, with the largest police force. Like both the United States and Canada, Australia has a federal system of government, but under the country's constitution the delivery of both police and health services is vested largely in the six states and two territories that make up the federation. The NSW Police Force (NSWPF), with an authorised strength of about 16,000 personnel, is responsible for providing police services over a geographic area the size of the state of Texas in the United States. The distances involved in undertaking this service delivery represent one of the major challenges for the NSWPF, as they do as well for most of its law enforcement counterparts in the other states and territories.

Donohue and Andrews give an account of the factors that led to the decision by the NSWPF to initiate its own SPR for interactions between police and persons with mental illnesses in the form of the Mental Health Intervention Team (MHIT) approach. This approach was strongly influenced by the experience observed of the CIT SPR conducted by police in the city of Chicago in the United States. However, it is an approach that is also tailored to the specific needs of a law enforcement agency operating over a vastly larger area than that of the city of Chicago, and with a very different structure and size. In fact, the NSWPF's MHIT initiative is unique in many ways, not the least of which being that it is based on an evidence-tested design, and an intensive and premium training programme.

Apart from the training programme, the MHIT objectives set by the NSWPF are all intended to minimise police involvement with mental health consumers in the belief that such contact stigmatises the individuals involved and criminalises what should really be seen as another facet of health care delivery. In accord with these principles, the NSWPF has taken measures to limit or end its role of transporting persons with mental illnesses to or between mental health treatment facilities. Only when there is high risk of violence or danger involved with such transport are police to be called upon to ensure the safe and humane carriage of the individual concerned.

Donohue and Andrews indicate, in a candid manner, some of the key internal challenges that have arisen in seeking to give effect to these MHIT objectives. These include ongoing cynicism among operational police about mental health concerns. It has been found that older and more experienced officers appreciate that mental health training is of direct assistance in managing the day-to-day complexities of community policing. There are now plans to undertake a one-day training programme for all members of the NSWPF, in addition to the MHIT programme, which aims to ensure that about 10% of the force will have participated in this resource-intensive and costly training by 2015.

Despite these challenges, the NSWPF MHIT has attracted widespread national attention among Australian law enforcement agencies, and a number are now considering adopting it as a model for their own SPRs as well as sending staff to participate in the MHIT training. Law enforcement interest in the MHIT has also come from New Zealand and several countries in the Asia Pacific region.

Queensland

Chapter 5 has been contributed by the Queensland Police Service (QPS) and describes the SPR relating to persons with mental illnesses that has been put in place in that jurisdiction. Queensland is one of the most decentralised states in Australia and covers an area two and a half times the size of the state of Texas, or more than seven times the size of the United Kingdom. It has a police force of more than 10,500 officers.

As the QPS indicates, the decision to introduce what is now termed the Mental Health Intervention Program (MHIP) arose from the collaborative activities of QPS and Queensland Health (QH). Like the NSW MHIT, the QPS model drew upon the experience of Memphis, although in a more direct fashion than was the case with the NSWPF. In 2002, after conducting a successful pilot training programme and evaluation based on the Memphis experience, QPS and QH sponsored a conference on policing and mental health best practise, to which were invited representatives from the Memphis police as well as other overseas experts. Following this meeting, steps were taken to put in place a statewide MHIP over the period 2006–2009. The MHIP involves a tri-agency partnership between QPS, QH, and the Queensland Ambulance Service (QAS), bolstered by MOUs. The three main components of the programme comprise targeted and, where appropriate, joint training for personnel, the appointment of district MHIP coordinators in each agency, and information sharing between QPS and QH. The latter arrangement allows QH to provide confidential information about a mental health consumer where there is a serious risk to life, health, or safety.

New measures have also been put in place by QPS to enhance the capturing of information about mental health incidents in QPRIME, the police computerised operational database. This enhancement has, among other things, facilitated the provision of much more accurate and helpful statistical information about the nature and scope of the QPS engagement with mental health consumers. Even so, no formal independent evaluation has yet been conducted of MHIP, although it has now become a permanent QPS programme, and one that is believed to have had very positive benefits for both mental health consumers and police involved in crisis situations. These achievements have resulted in moves to expand the MHIP to other vulnerable individuals, including those with intellectual disabilities, and in the area of suicide intervention and prevention.

Victoria

Victoria Police, a law enforcement agency with more than 12,000 sworn personnel responsible for policing Australia's second most populous state, are not among the contributors to this book, but like their counterparts in

NSW and Queensland, they have been involved in important initiatives in the area of mental health and policing. In Chapters 6–8, each contributed by researchers affiliated with Monash University located in Melbourne, the capital city of the state of Victoria, mention is made of these initiatives in tandem with a contemporary review of a relevant range of both local Australian and overseas policing research.

Stuart Thomas, in Chapter 6, offers some views on the core requirements of a best practise model for police encounters with people with mental illnesses, based on the findings from an extensive research programme conducted with Victoria Police. As Thomas explains, Victoria Police have opted for a SPR that seems to be modelled on the Los Angeles CRT programme described earlier. In Victoria Police, ambulance and mental health crisis assessment and treatment teams have collaborated to provide an emergency response to attend crisis situations where mental health issues are suspected. Known as the PACER programme, it involves the dispatch to such crisis situations of a unit staffed by a uniformed police officer and a mental health clinician.

Thomas highlights a number of research-determined practical markers for change in the policing environment surrounding interactions with the mentally ill, foremost of which is that police need to consider that these interactions are in fact the norm rather than the exception. As a large-scale survey of operational police across Victoria revealed, officers reported that they were interacting with a person experiencing mental illness on a frequent basis. Survey respondents estimated that approximately one-fifth of the people whom they came in contact with in a week were mentally ill, and these contacts were consuming a significant amount of their time and resources. Findings like these, says Thomas, need to be taken into consideration when designing best practise approaches that reflect policing realities rather than abstract concepts. They also point to the need for adequate mental health services to be available in the community to support a programme like PACER.

Tamsin Short, in Chapter 7, explores the research literature relating to two areas of police interactions with mentally ill persons: criminal offending and crime victimisation. Short concentrates on severe mental illnesses, and specifically, major psychotic and mood disorders. Fewer than 1 in 100 individuals can expect to be diagnosed during their lifetime with a severe mental disorder, yet it is this group who accounts for the consumption of the vast majority of public mental health services. People with severe mental illness are also overrepresented in the criminal justice system as both perpetrators and victims of violent crime.

Short emphasises the importance of ensuring that police training, together with public education, incorporates an appropriate understanding of the risks of violence associated with severe mental disorders. Thus, the existence of a violence risk factor does not result inevitably in a violent outcome. It can be said, however, that people with severe mental disorders are statistically more likely to engage in violent crime than others in the community, especially if they have a co-morbid history of substance misuse, offending behaviour, or crime victimisation. However, contrary to community perceptions, it is family members and carers of such persons rather than strangers who are most at risk of becoming the victims of this violence.

Short's analysis of the research literature also indicates that persons with severe mental illnesses are a vulnerable group who are likely to experience higher levels of violent victimisation than the general population. Despite this victimisation, which can be both chronic and severe in nature, much of it goes undetected and unreported because of reluctance by persons with severe mental illnesses to report crimes to the police. This reluctance can stem from a number of factors, including fear and paranoia arising from their mental illness, or from prior negative experiences with police. Again, these are all findings that should be considered when designing police training and associated programmes.

Use of Force

Dragana Kesic, in Chapter 8, and Katrina Clifford, in Chapter 9, address the issues surrounding police use of force during interactions with people with mental illnesses. As both authors indicate, this is an area where controversy often arises, and especially so when the outcome is the death of an individual. It is an unfortunate reality that in Australia, as has been the case elsewhere, such deaths do occur, as Clifford shows in her overview of fatal mental health crisis interventions in Australia. Although fatal outcomes remain relatively rare, what is troubling is the proportion of these critical incidents that involve mentally ill individuals. The Australian trends are consistent with international research, which shows that such individuals are four times more likely to be killed by the police in crisis situations. A further disturbing trend in Australia, at least in the past, has been the disproportionate number of these fatalities that have taken place in Victoria.

Kesic delves in greater depth into the Victorian experience with the use of force and reviews the findings from a series of research studies that she and others conducted that examined the use of both fatal and nonfatal force by Victoria Police. These studies included an analysis of all fatalities (48) occurring during the period 1982–2007. The majority of the persons killed during this time were known in some capacity to either the criminal justice or mental health system. More than half had an Axis 1 disorder, and more than a third of these had more than one disorder. Collectively, all of the major mental disorders were significantly overrepresented among the fatalities compared with their estimated prevalence in the general community.

In a separate study of nonfatal use of force by Victoria Police, Kesic and her colleagues found a similar overrepresentation of persons with some form of mental disorder. She concludes that findings like these reinforce, among other things, the need for better and ongoing training for operational police regarding how best to manage their interactions with this group of persons. Many operational police still associate mental illness with aggression and violence, and accordingly themselves act in such interactions in a forceful and assertive manner when it would be preferable to utilise better de-escalation and communication skills.

Clifford reports some of the findings from her own research about the ways in which fatal police shootings of mentally ill persons in crisis are represented and interpreted by and between news media and people traumatised by these events. She suggests that one of the contributing factors to poor relationships between police and mental health consumers and carers can be found in news media coverage of fatal mental health crisis interventions that perpetuate inappropriate stereotypes of both the police and the mentally ill. She also suggests that greater account should be taken of the views of consumers and carers in formulating the boundaries of risk communication as it relates to mental health crises in the community, and in incorporating lived experience in the public discourse surrounding these events. Further, initiatives like the MHIT in NSW and the MHIP in Queensland should not be seen as an alternative to filling service gaps within the health and disability support system.

Frequent Presenters

Chapters 10 and 11 examine a range of complex and difficult issues associated with mental health consumers who are in frequent contact with police and other agencies. In Chapter 10, Gina Andrews and Eileen Baldry emphasise that while there is no universally agreed upon definition of a mental health frequent presenter (MHFP), such persons are mental health consumers with multiple needs who frequently present in a crisis state to a cross section of emergency services (police, ambulance, and hospital emergency departments). They often fail to have their complex mental health, social, and economic needs met, relapsing rapidly and then repeating their presentation to emergency services. Emergency services invest substantial and disproportionate resources to manage this group of MHFPs.

Andrews and Baldry indicate that while a paucity of data exist in Australia about the nature and scope of this aspect of emergency care, the existing local and international research literature has identified a number of common characteristics of the MHFP population. Consistently, these characteristics include requiring intensive health treatment, having an early onset of mental health problems, suffering from treatment-resistant severe mental disorders, exhibiting co-morbidity, and coming into contact with police whether as a result of their mental disorder or as a perpetrator or victim of a crime.

Andrews and Baldry's chapter contains six illustrative MHFP cases drawn from independent research conducted by Andrews utilising the NSWPF's computerised operating policing system (COPS). These unique and highly informative data reveal much about the realities of police and other emergency services interactions with the MHFP population, and the demands these interactions place upon already thinly stretched emergency services resources. The authors go on to identify and discuss a number of interagency programmes that have been put in place in a range of juris-dictions in Australia and overseas to provide suitable case management of MHFPs. Those programmes, which have been properly evaluated, suggest case management can have positive effects for service providers and con-sumers alike, with a reduction in the number of presentations to emergency services and a stabilisation of the mental condition of consumers. But to be effective, programmes have to be flexible, individualised, and comprehensive in addressing the often very complex needs of each consumer.

In Chapter 11, Eileen Baldry and Leanne Dowse explore in greater depth, and utilising a different dataset, a number of case studies involving consum-ers with complex needs who had been in contact with a range of NSW agen-cies, including the NSWPF. Their groundbreaking research obtained data on the lifetime involvement of more than 2,700 individuals in contact with NSW police, health, corrective services, juvenile justice, legal aid, courts, social housing, disability services, and child services. As the various case studies show, the individuals involved, many of them indigenous Australians, were highly disadvantaged people with multiple mental and cognitive impair-ments and problematic alcohol and drug use.

Baldry and Dowse note that the research literature to date has tended to concentrate on police work with people with a single mental impairment, and very little is known about their work with people with multiple impairments. Police often find that such individuals may not be accepted into the mental health system for a number of reasons, including lack of space, because they are deemed not ill enough or need to be dealt with by the criminal justice sys-tem, or because they have other diagnoses that preclude them from admis-sion to a psychiatric service.

As Baldry and Dowse stress, current police training tends to be largely focussed on the recognition of various mental disorders and does not gen-erally extend to the development of a capacity to recognise a cognitive impairment, let alone both a mental and a cognitive impairment. Baldry and Dowse's own research has revealed that many operational police do suspect that a person may have a number of problems, but their capacity to recognise, ascertain, and respond to such a person is limited by a lack of a coherent policing framework to deal with this group, and by a lack of information or assistance from various support services.

Baldry and Dowse's research shows that in NSW, and almost certainly elsewhere in Australia, police currently have great difficulty knowing what to do or how to handle this group of people for whom they have become, by default, the principal care manager. This is clearly a highly unsatisfactory situation that requires both recognition and the development of an integrated multiagency programme in response that is made available in disadvantaged urban and rural areas of NSW.

Examining Decision Making

Simon Bronitt and Jane Gath, in Chapter 12, explore certain aspects of mental health decision making by police and paramedics in Australia. They focus on the use of emergency examination orders (EEOs) in Queensland that are provided for under the provisions of the Queensland Mental Health Act (MHA) 2000. Such an order may be made by a police officer or ambulance officer who reasonably believes:

(a) a person has a mental illness; and
(b) because of the person's illness there is an imminent risk of significant physical harm being sustained by the person or someone else; and
(c) proceeding under division 2 [obtaining an order from a magistrate] would cause dangerous delay and significantly increase the risk of harm to the person or someone else; and
(d) the person should be taken to an authorised mental health service for examination to decide whether a request and recommendation for assessment should be made for the person. (MHA 2000, Section 33)

It should be noted that similar powers, albeit couched in somewhat different terms and not always including ambulance officers, are to be found in mental health legislation in all Australian jurisdictions. So, too, are provisions similar to Section 9 of the Queensland MHA 2000, which states that any power or function under this act relating to a person who has a mental illness must be exercised or performed so that:

(a) the person's liberty and rights are adversely affected only if there is no less restrictive way to protect the person's health and safety or to protect others; and
(b) any adverse effect on the person's liberty and rights is the minimum necessary in the circumstances. (MHA 2000, Section 9)

Bronitt and Gath state that notwithstanding these principles, there has been a systematic failure to adhere to them by frontline decision makers in Queensland. People with mental health issues are routinely denied their rights to autonomy, being made the subject of EEOs even though displaying little or no evidence of impaired capacity or lacking in ability to consent to treatment. They suggest this practise is prevalent in part because of the desire to mitigate the risks of inaction, which might include being the subject of a civil suit for negligence. This fear, say Bronitt and Gath, is unfounded and a clear misunderstanding of Australian law and practise. Decision making by police and paramedics is always likely to be beset by uncertainty. Frontline decision making involves discretionary judgment, and discretion needs to be recognised and valued more explicitly in policy and protocols, rather than being defensively pushed out of existence.

Mental Illness and Suicide Among Police Officers

The final chapter in Section II of the book, with its focus on Australia, Chapter 13, is by Stephen Barron, a former police officer in the NSWPF and an expert on issues associated with the mental well-being of law enforcement personnel. As Barron indicates, mental health is a growing concern in all policing organisations. The costs of sick leave, unplanned leave, and workers' compensation form a significant and expanding impost on policing resources and a major human resources challenge for police leadership. While many police organisations utilise the services of in-house or outsourced mental health professionals, the common myth that the profession of policing is inherently dangerous is challenged by the increasing number of officers who report that the organisation is a significant contributor to police officer stress. The link between mental health and physical health of police officers is not new, but recent research into police officer self-harm and suicide indicates that the organisational factors that contribute to this area are significant. Barron seeks to bring together much of the relevant and recent research into the field of police officer mental health. He concludes that police organisations are obligated to review the growing research into the occupational stress of police officers and develop effective, organisationally based strategies to minimise the impact of the police organisation on its members.

Section III: The Developing World

The three chapters in the concluding part of the book consider the circumstances surrounding police interactions with persons with mental illnesses that occur in less developed nations of the world. There is in general only very limited information available about this topic in the countries of the South, and little significant empirical research. Yet as the World Health Organisation (WHO) has emphasised (see Chapter 14), mental disorders are not the prerogative of the countries of the North, and their prevalence is not confined to any one region or country around the globe. Thus, police are as likely to encounter persons who have a mental disorder as a part of their work in Papua New Guinea (PNG) as they are in Australia, although the way in which they respond to this encounter may vary considerably from place to place as a result of different cultural beliefs and values as well as the types of health and allied resources available.

In Chapter 14, Duncan Chappell considers the challenges that face Australia's near neighbour and former colony, PNG. These challenges are really immense, ranging from overcoming deeply entrenched fear and prejudice regarding those who have a mental illness to preventing such persons being killed as dangerous sorcerers. The PNG police themselves clearly share the values and beliefs of the society in which they live, which adds to the complexity of the situation, as does their lack of understanding of and respect for the basic rights of persons coming into police custody, whether because of criminal behaviour or a mental disorder. As Chappell notes, in a scathing report on a recent mission to PNG, the United Nations special rapporteur on torture condemned the shocking conditions for detainees, including some mentally ill persons, which he witnessed in PNG police lockups.

In earlier chapters, mention has been made of the inadequacy of the resources made available in a number of jurisdictions in countries of the North for the care and treatment of persons with mental illnesses. However, these complaints seem almost trite when matched against the availability of such resources in a country like PNG, which has very few trained mental health professionals and scant ability to provide either community or institutional care and treatment.

Fleur Beaupert, in Chapter 15, describes a situation somewhat similar to that found in PNG in her overview of policing and mental health in the vast continent of Africa. As she emphasises, the unique features of the mental health and policing landscapes in Africa need to be understood, as well as country-specific factors in health and healing systems and urban and rural differences, before seeking to introduce any new policing models relating to persons with mental illnesses. Her analysis leads her to conclude that given the pervasiveness and popularity of traditional healers throughout Africa, these healers should not be ignored but co-opted in various ways to play a useful role in police and mental health interactions. She also points to the need for new legislative initiatives in many countries to replace outdated and outmoded statutes originating from colonial days.

In the final book chapter, Chapter 16, Sharon Ingrid Kwok, T. Wing Lo, and Percy Lee describe the state of interactions between police and persons with mental illnesses in Hong Kong. It must be admitted that it is really a misclassification to include Hong Kong in the developing world since it is rated by the World Bank as a high-income jurisdiction, a rating that is supported, among other things, by Hong Kong's continuing status as one of the world's major financial and trading centres. It remains, however, a special administrative region (SAR) of the People's Republic of China (PRC) and, although having substantial independence from the PRC, is still subject ultimately to its control. Hong Kong, with a population of more than 7 million persons, is one of the most densely settled areas in the world, and has a police force of more than 28,000 officers.

Kwok and her colleagues indicate that during the past two decades, including the entire period since Hong Kong ceased in 1997 to be a British colony, community policing concepts have been practised in the SAR, which has resulted in increased public expectations of police services at large. These expectations have extended to dealing with mental health crises. Like their counterparts elsewhere around the globe, it is usually the police who are the first point of contact in Hong Kong in responding to such crises, and how the police perform this function can have significant consequences for all involved.

The authors describe two highly publicised cases occurring in Hong Kong where mentally ill persons were involved in violent confrontations with police that resulted in injuries (in one circumstance fatal) to both these persons and the police. These cases provoked a review of police practices and procedures that were found to be deficient in a number of ways. In the chapter, these cases are supplemented with interview data obtained from operational police and health workers about their views concerning the management of mental health-related incidents. In the case of the police, these interviews make clear the uncertainties surrounding the exercise of their discretion when handling these incidents, with a preference, where possible, to make an informal disposition of the matter rather than detaining and referring a mentally ill person for assessment and treatment. The police also felt their training about mental health issues was inadequate, as were the guidelines for the management of nonviolent persons involved in a mental health crisis. There were also no effective mechanisms in place to facilitate collaboration among police, mental health professionals, and other agencies in responding to the more complex needs of mentally ill persons.

Although by no means ideal, the overall management of this aspect of policing in Hong Kong would seem to be manifestly of much greater sophistication and substance than the situation described in the preceding chapters on PNG and Africa. It is also unfortunate that time and space constraints precluded an examination in this book of the handling by police of these issues across the SAR border in mainland China. Indeed, such constraints also resulted in the world's largest democracy, India, being left out of consideration. It must be left to future researchers and commentators to fill these admitted gaps in our knowledge, but it is hoped that the material that has been presented offers a fresh, balanced, and informative account of a policing function of still growing import, significance, and debate in contemporary society.

About the Editor

Duncan Chappell, a lawyer and criminologist, is currently an adjunct professor in the Faculty of Law at the University of Sydney, Australia; a conjoint professor in the School of Psychiatry in the Faculty of Medicine at the University of New South Wales, Australia; and an adjunct professor in the School of Criminology at Simon Fraser University in Vancouver, Canada. He is also chair of the International Advisory Board of the Australian Research Council Center of Excellence in Policing and Security. He is a past president of the New South Wales Mental Health Review Tribunal and a past director of the Australian Institute of Criminology.

Contributors

Gina Andrews was the senior policy officer for mental health, NSW Police Force, 2006–2012. She is passionate about the topic of mental health frequent presenters to police, and has represented the NSW Police Force on this topic for several years. In 2011, she represented the NSW Police Force on this topic at the *International Mental Health Law Conference* in Berlin. Gina Andrews started her career in 1998 as a graduate with the Australian Commonwealth's Department of Immigration and Multicultural Affairs, and has since worked at the NSW Cabinet Office, NSW Ministry of Police, and currently works as an advisor in the Commonwealth's Department of Prime Minister and Cabinet. She has a B.A. Hons., a master's in social policy and planning from London School of Economics, and a master's in administrative law and policy.

Gina Andrews
Sydney, New South Wales, Australia
gina.andrews@optusnet.com.au

Eileen Baldry (Ph.D.) is professor of criminology in the School of Social Sciences and deputy dean in the Faculty of Arts and Social Sciences at the University of New South Wales (UNSW), where she has been an academic since 1993 teaching social policy, social development, and criminology. Her research focuses on social justice matters, including mental health and cognitive disability in the criminal justice system, homelessness and transition from prison, indigenous social work, community development and social housing, and disability services, and she has numerous publications in and is chief investigator of a number of large national grants in these areas. She is involved in a voluntary capacity with many development and justice community agencies. She was awarded the 2009 NSW Justice Medal and is currently president of the New South Wales Council of Social Service.

Eileen Baldry
School of Social Sciences
University of New South Wales
New South Wales, Australia
e.baldry@unsw.edu.au

Stephen Barron is a retired police officer with over 27 years of operational, investigative, and command experience with the New South Wales Police Force (Australia). He has master's degrees in criminology and psychology, and a professional doctorate in forensic psychology. He has maintained a private practise in Melbourne since 2007, and many of his clients (and their families) are drawn from policing and emergency services personnel. He currently teaches at Charles Sturt University on psychological aspects of arson and consults with a range of state and federal enforcement agencies. He is the author of a number of peer-reviewed articles on police officer suicide and most recently was featured as a psychological consultant in a TV series on criminal offending. He is a member of many professional organisations, including the International Chiefs of Police Association (Police Psychological Services Section) and the Australian Psychological Society.

Stephen Barron
Mentone, Victoria, Australia
barronpsych@gmail.com

Fleur Beaupert is a lawyer and independent researcher, with a background in the interaction between mental health and the law. She has lectured for the University of Sydney and University of Western Sydney law faculties and worked as a solicitor for NSW Legal Aid's Mental Health Advocacy Service. She was the doctoral candidate on an Australian Research Council funded project comparing the operation of Australian mental health tribunals, graduating with a Ph.D. from the University of Sydney in 2012. She is currently working as a project officer with the NSW ombudsman.

Fleur Beaupert
Newtown, New South Wales, Australia
fbeaupert@gmail.com

Simon Bronitt is a professor at Griffith University and director of the Australian Research Council Centre of Excellence in Policing and Security. Previously, Professor Bronitt held positions at the Australian National University, including professor of law and director of the National Europe Centre. He has published widely in the fields of criminal law, health care law, policing, and human rights.

Simon Bronitt
Griffith University
Mt. Gravatt, Queensland, Australia
s.bronitt@griffith.edu.au

Katrina Cli⊠ord, a former journalist, is now a lecturer in the School of Social Sciences at the University of Tasmania. Her current research examines the ways in which fatal police-involved shootings of mentally ill individuals in crisis are represented and interpreted by and between news media and key stakeholders, who are often traumatised by these critical incidents. She was previously involved as a research assistant on Charles Sturt University's independent evaluation of the NSW Police Force Mental Health Intervention Team programme.

Katrina Clifford
Faculty of Arts
University of Tasmania
Hobart, Tasmania, Australia
Katrina.Clifford@utas.edu.au

Terry G. Coleman was a police officer in Calgary and Moose Jaw for 39 years, including 10½ years as Moose Jaw's chief of police. Subsequently, from 2007 to 2009, he was deputy minister of corrections, public safety and policing, and deputy minister of municipal affairs in Saskatchewan. He is a longtime member of the Canadian Association of Chiefs of Police (CACP), having been a director as well as co-chair of the CACP Police/Mental Health Committee. Coleman has a master of human resource management, a master of arts—police studies, and a Ph.D. from the University of Regina, Canada. His research focus was the measurement of organisational performance in police organisations. He is an adjunct professor at the University of Regina.

Terry Coleman
PMHL Solutions
Moose Jaw, Saskatchewan, Canada
PMHL@nintu.net

Dorothy Cotton is a registered psychologist and a diplomate in police psychology. She has been extensively involved with the Canadian Association of Chiefs of Police (CACP) in developing strategies to develop and improve police interactions with people with mental illness through programme development, research, and training. Dr. Cotton has worked for the Canadian federal correctional system, as well as being chief psychologist and director of the forensic program at a provincial psychiatric hospital. She is an adjunct professor at Queen's University, past president of the College of Psychologists of Ontario, and a fellow and a member of the board of directors of the Canadian Psychological Association. Dr. Cotton received a Diamond Jubilee Medal in 2012 for her extensive work in regard to police interactions with people with mental illnesses. Both she and Terry G. Coleman have also served as members of the Mental Health and the Law Advisory Committee of the Mental Health Commission of Canada (MHCC). Together the authors are the principal consultants of PHML Solutions, whose focus is on police–mental health system issues in Canada.

Dorothy Cotton
PMHL Solutions
Kingston, Ontario, Canada
PMHL@nintu.net

David Donohue has 20 years' experience as a NSW police officer. His current role is commander, St. George Local Area Command, at the rank of superintendent. He holds a master of leadership and management (policing) (Charles Sturt University, 2011), graduate certificate in applied management (Charles Sturt University, 2009), diploma in security (risk management) (Canberra Institute of Technology, 1999), and business management certificate (Australian Institute of Management, 2000). He also has four years' executive-level management in the private sector. Superintendent Donohue has been the NSW Police Force corporate spokesperson, mental health, for over five years, and pioneered its development and trial of the Mental Health Intervention Team (MHIT) in the New South Wales Police Force. He commanded the trial of the MHIT for 2½ years, and has overseen its implementation since.

David Donohue
St. George Local Area Command
Kogarah, NSW
donol dav@police.nsw.gov.au

Leanne Dowse, Ph.D., is a senior lecturer in social research and policy in the School of Social Sciences, Faculty of Arts and Social Sciences, University of New South Wales (UNSW). Her primary research interest is in the application of models of critical inquiry to the study of disability and, in particular, intellectual or cognitive disability. Her work addresses issues for people with complex needs, including mental health disorders, cognitive disabilities, and other dimensions of social disadvantage in the criminal justice system; questions of theory, policy, and practise in relation to people with disabilities (and in particular cognitive disabilities); the dynamics of gender, ageing, race, and ethnicity; and contemporary cultural discourses of disability. She is interested in methodological approaches to the study of disability and in the area of research methods skill development and training for researchers in the social sciences.

Leanne Dowse
School of Social Sciences
University of New South Wales
New South Wales, Australia
l.dowse@unsw.edu.au

Laura Draper served as a policy analyst at the Council of State Governments (CSG) Justice Center, working mainly on law enforcement projects. She helped to coordinate projects relating to the law enforcement response to people with mental illnesses as well as police-involved reentry strategies. She received her B.A. from Case Western Reserve University, her M.Phil. from the University of Cambridge (England), and her M.S. from the University of Pennsylvania. In August 2011, she started law school at the New York University School of Law.

Laura Draper
Brooklyn, New York
laura.e.draper@gmail.com

Jane Gath is a nurse practitioner in the field of mental health with extensive experience within the area of mental health crisis, assessment, and treatment. She obtained her master of nurse practitioner in 2009 from the University of Newcastle, NSW. She is a member of the Australian College of Nurse Practitioners and the Australian College of Mental Health Nurses.

Jane Gath
Redland Hospital
Queensland, Australia
s.bronitt@griffith.edu.au

Dragana Kesic is a registered clinical forensic psychologist working at the Victorian Institute of Forensic Mental Health and a research fellow at the Centre for Forensic Behavioural Science at Monash University in Melbourne, Victoria. Her main research area of interest is examining the issues present at the interface between police and people experiencing mental disorders.

Dragana Kesic
Centre for Forensic Behavioural Science
Victoria, Australia
dragana.kesic@monash.edu

Sharon Ingrid Kwok, M.Sc., was a lecturer in the Division of Social Studies, City University of Hong Kong. She is currently a Ph.D. candidate in the Department of Applied Social Studies at the City University of Hong Kong.

Sharon Ingrid Kwok
City University of Hong Kong
Hong Kong, China
sikwok@cityu.edu.hk

Percy Lee, M.S.Sc., is a police officer and a graduate student of the Department of Applied Social Studies, City University of Hong Kong, China.

Percy Lee
Department of Applied Social Studies
City University of Hong Kong
Hong Kong, China
sstwl@cityu.edu.hk

T. Wing Lo is professor of criminology and social work at City University of Hong Kong. He graduated with a Ph.D. in criminology from the University of Cambridge, UK, in 1991.

T. Wing Lo
Department of Applied Social Studies
City University of Hong Kong
Hong Kong, China
sstwl@cityu.edu.hk

Rhonda Moore has a background as a research librarian, with a B.A. from the University of Sydney, Australia, and a postgraduate diploma of librarianship from the University of New South Wales, Australia. Her research and writing since the 1980s have focussed on policing and allied criminological issues, notably drug use. Her publications include numerous journal articles and co-authored books, including *Drugs in Australian Society: Patterns, Attitudes and Policies.*

Rhonda Moore
Balmain East, NSW, Australia
chappell@bigpond.net.au

Blake Norton serves as an advisor and technical assistance provider on Justice Center projects that focus on law enforcement issues and community partnerships. Before joining the centre, Blake spent more than 18 years with the Boston Police Department, where she helped shape the agency's prisoner reentry efforts and successfully worked with citizens and faith-based organisations to advance consensus-based strategies for improving public safety.

She designed and managed the police department's community affairs activities, including programmes for court-involved and at-risk youth. She received her B.A. from the University of Massachusetts and her M.Ed. from Boston University.

Blake Norton
Council of State Governments
Bethesda, Maryland
bnorton@csg.org

Queensland Police Service (QPS) is the law enforcement agency responsible for the policing of the Australian state of Queensland. With a sworn personnel of about 10,600 officers, it operates across an area of approximately 1.7 million square kilometres. Queensland, Australia's second largest state, with a population of about 4.5 million, stretches from the border with Papua New Guinea in the north to the state of New South Wales in the south. The QPS Mental Health Intervention Program (MHIP) administrative headquarters is located in the state's capital city of Brisbane in Queensland's most populous southeast region.

MHIP/QPS
Michael Mitchell, Senior Sergeant
Operations Support Command
Brisbane, Queensland, Australia
mitchell.michaelg@police.qld.gov.au

Melissa Reuland consults on projects related to the police response to people with mental illness. Reuland currently is working with the Council of State Governments (CSG) Justice Center and the Police Executive Research Forum (PERF) developing products that support expansion of specialised responses to people with mental illnesses. Reuland and colleagues prepared several documents, including *Tailoring Law Enforcement Initiatives to Individual Jurisdictions, A Guide to Research-Informed Policy and Practice, Strategies for Effective Law Enforcement Training,* and *The Essential Elements of a Specialized Law Enforcement-Based Program.* Reuland worked at PERF from 1994 through 2004, where she was a senior research associate. She directed two GAINS/TAPA Center projects on models for law enforcement diversion of people with mental illness, the law enforcement track of CSG's Criminal Justice/Mental Health Consensus Project and PERF's *The Police Response to People With Mental Illnesses* publication.

Melissa Reuland
Baltimore, Maryland
melissareuland86@gmail.com

Tamsin Short is a clinical and forensic psychologist who currently works full-time in clinical practise in Melbourne, Australia. Dr. Short completed her research studies at Monash University in 2011 and went on to conduct further research into the interface between policing and mental illness. Her chapter is based on her doctoral thesis, which examined the relationship between severe mental illness and violent offending. Dr. Short has presented her research at several national and international conferences, and has published in the area of psychosis and violence while working at the Centre for Forensic Behavioural Science in Melbourne. Today, Dr. Short divides her time between working at the Victorian Institute of Forensic Mental Health and practising at community drug and alcohol services in Melbourne, Australia.

Tamsin Short
Victoria, Australia
tamsin.short@forensicare.vic.gov.au

Stuart Thomas is an associate professor in the School of Psychology and Psychiatry at Monash University in Melbourne, Australia. He is also deputy director of the Centre for Forensic Behavioural Science, a collaboration between Monash University and the Victorian Institute of Forensic Mental Health.

Stuart Thomas
Centre for Forensic Behavioural Science
Melbourne, Victoria, Australia
stuart.thomas@monash.edu

Developments in
North America
and Europe

I

Developing a Statewide Approach to Specialised Policing Response (SPR) Programme Implementation

1

MELISSA REULAND
LAURA DRAPER
BLAKE NORTON

Contents

While mental health-related calls for service may be a relatively small proportion of total calls for service—approximately 7% of all calls[*]—they are among the most complex and time-consuming. Police encounters with people who have a mental illness who are in crisis can prove to be pivotal events where enhanced linkages to treatment can potentially prevent future serious incidents. Ultimately, focussed attention on improving the police response in

---

[*] Teller, J.L.S., Munetz, M.R., Gil, K.M., & Ritter, C. (2006). Crisis intervention team training for police officers responding to mental disturbance calls. *Psychiatric Services*, 57, 232–237; Deane, M.W., Steadman, H.J., Borum, R., Veysey, B.M., & Morrissey, J.P. (1999). Emerging partnerships between mental health and law enforcement. *Psychiatric Services*, 50, 99–101.

these encounters can reduce victimisations and repeat calls for service, thus improving the lives of people with mental illnesses.

Failure to address these calls correctly can have tragic consequences for the individual, the officer, and the public. Officers have limited options—either informally resolve the incident at the scene, transport the person to mental health services, or make an arrest. Officers who try to connect the individual to services can spend hours in hospitals or other facilities waiting to admit the individual for an emergency mental health evaluation, during which time they cannot respond to other calls.*

In response, some law enforcement agencies are partnering with community service providers to develop programmes that prioritise safety and treatment over incarceration, when appropriate. The two most prevalent specialised policing response (SPR) approaches are crisis intervention teams (CITs) and co-responder teams. The CIT programme was developed in Memphis, Tennessee, in 1988, when the Memphis Police Department confronted a terrible tragedy—a person with mental illness had been killed by police. Through partnership with the National Alliance on Mental Illness (NAMI)† the police department developed a specialised police response that improves safety during police encounters with people with mental illness through enhanced, immediate crisis de-escalation. This approach hinges on a self-selected cadre of officers trained to identify signs and symptoms of mental illness, de-escalate the situation, and connect the person to treatment.

In the late 1980s, law enforcement and mental health communities in Los Angeles City and County in California were confronting another dimension of this problem. These communities were concerned with the frequency with which people in crisis who interact with police did not become engaged in treatments and services. Because police are limited by time and inefficient access to resources and knowledge about crisis, they left scenes with only a short-term resolution in place. For these agencies, the critical part of their approach is the linkage to community-based mental health services—a linkage mental health practitioners provide. Consequently, these agencies developed co-responder teams that pair law enforcement officers with mental health professionals to respond to scenes involving a person in mental health crisis.

---

* Green, T.M. (1997). Police as frontline mental health workers: The decision to arrest or refer to mental health agencies. *International Journal of Law and Psychiatry*, 20, 469–486.
† The National Alliance on Mental Illness (NAMI) is the United States' largest grassroots advocacy organisation devoted to improving access to mental health services, treatments, and supports. More information about NAMI can be obtained from its website: www.NAMI.org.

Evidence suggests that when appropriately implemented, these specialised police response (SPR)[*] programmes can be quite successful, including decreasing numbers of injuries to officers and improved linkages to mental health treatment.[†]

SPR Programme Replication Strategies

Following the groundbreaking efforts in Memphis and Los Angeles, these programmes have spread to new communities by word of mouth, or in response to a tragedy.[‡] Practitioners and advocates traditionally have travelled to visit known programmes, and then adapted approaches to their jurisdiction's needs.[§] But as the demand has increased, it is no longer feasible for interested communities to learn from the programme originators. Another barrier to widespread programme implementation is the sheer volume of police departments in the United States. Recent census research indicates there are approximately 18,000 state and local law enforcement agencies in the United States, about half of which have fewer than 10 sworn personnel.[¶] Understandably, most agencies lack the capacity and expertise to send a team to another agency for a week, and then tailor the programme to their own jurisdiction's unique needs.

In the United States, a branch of each state's government oversees the administration of mental health services for those in that state. Typically, states have a Department of Mental Health, which may stand alone, or be part of a larger Department of Health or Human Services.[**] These state agencies receive funding from a variety of sources—the federal government as well

---

[*] The term specialised policing response is used as an umbrella term to include the two main variations described (CITs and co-responder models).

[†] Reuland, M., Schwarzfeld, M., & Draper, L. (2009). *Law enforcement responses to people with mental illnesses: A guide to research-informed policy and practice.* New York, NY: Council of State Governments Justice Center; Reuland, M. (2004). *A guide to implementing police-based diversion programs for people with mental illness.* Delmar, NY: Technical Assistance and Policy Analysis Center for Jail Diversion; Dupont, R., & Cochran, S. (2000). Police response to mental health emergencies—Barriers to change. *Journal of the American Academy of Psychiatry and Law,* 28(3), 228–244.

[‡] Reuland, 2004.

[§] Ibid.

[¶] Information on the numbers and types of law enforcement agencies in the United States can be obtained from the Bureau of Justice Statistics at http://bjs.ojp.usdoj.gov/index. cfm?ty=tp&tid=71.

[**] Massaro, J. (2007). *Overview of the mental health service system for criminal justice professionals.* Delmar, NY: National GAINS Technical Assistance and Policy Analysis Center for Jail Diversion.

as state and local revenues—and allocate those funds to individual counties. These county agencies then either directly offer mental health services or contract with private entities to offer them.

Important for the purposes of specialised policing response programmes is that each state government has the authority to create the laws that authorise police powers to take someone into custody for an emergency mental health evaluation.* These laws vary considerably across the United States— some states permit police to make this determination alone, and others require the involvement of mental health personnel in addition to or instead of the officer.

As such, state-level policy makers and legislators are uniquely positioned to provide support to communities within their state in their efforts to improve police responses. For example, state legislatures can offer incentives for partnerships among law enforcement, the community, and the mental health system. In 2009, the Virginia legislature authorised the state's Department of Criminal Justice Services to support CIT programmes throughout the state by convening stakeholders and providing information about CIT programmes and how to implement them.† Statewide coordination can also facilitate regional pooling of resources, which could particularly benefit rural areas where sparse populations and small police departments must rely on distant mental health resources. A statewide structure could also help ensure that more than a smattering of jurisdictions nationwide will implement programmes to improve responses to people with mental illnesses.

The U.S. Department of Justice, Bureau of Justice Assistance provided funding to the Council of State Governments Justice Center‡ to explore statewide efforts to implement SPR programmes in 2009. This study identified states with a statewide coordination effort that promotes local law enforcement specialised policing response (SPR) programmes and determined how these statewide coordination programmes are structured, which elements of these statewide strategies are promising, and what challenges exist. This chapter reviews the findings from this work.§

* Massaro, 2007.
† Department of Criminal Justice Services. (2011). Assessing the impact and effectiveness of Virginia's crisis intervention team programs FY2011 (§ 9.1-190). Retrieved March 1, 2012, from http://leg2.state.va.us/dls/h&sdocs.nsf/By+Year/RD3062011/$file/RD306.pdf.
‡ The Council of State Governments Justice Center is a national nonprofit organisation that serves state-level policy makers in the United States. For more information about the Justice Center, visit their website at http://justicecenter.csg.org.
§ Reuland, M., Draper, L., & Norton, B. (2012). *Statewide law enforcement/mental health efforts: Strategies to support and sustain local initiatives.* New York, NY: Council of State Governments Justice Center.

Statewide Coordination Efforts Defined

A statewide coordination effort is one where a state-level organisation leads an effort to promote SPR programme development by coordinating collaboration among other state-level law enforcement, mental health, and advocacy organisations. State-level organisations can include state mental health organisations or state-level advocacy organisations, such as the National Alliance on Mental Illness and mental health associations.* Further, a statewide collaborative group must support community collaboration at the local level, develop and implement training for communities statewide, collect data on the statewide efforts, and establish mechanisms to facilitate ongoing success.

This definition encompasses the three prongs of an effective statewide effort: (1) a state-level structure designed to promulgate the spread of SPR throughout the state, (2) strategies to maintain the quality of these programmes such that they adhere to the essential elements of SPR programmes, and (3) mechanisms to ensure sustainability of programmes over time (Table 1.1).

The Justice Center staff identified eight states with sustained statewide coordination efforts. Project staff selected three states for site visits based on the depth of their experience and a range of approaches taken. Project staff visited communities, both large and small, in each state to inventory the states' structure, approaches, and rationale for their decisions.

The Importance of Tailoring SPRs to Communities

When a state embarks on a statewide SPR implementation effort, planners typically have a particular model in mind—often a crisis intervention team (CIT) approach. However, not all communities will be willing or able to implement all elements of a CIT programme. This is partly because research has demonstrated that selection of SPR programme elements depends on two distinct community features: its problems and its characteristics.† For statewide approaches to succeed, therefore, planners must allow the jurisdictions they recruit some flexibility to tailor their SPR programmes to their own needs.

---

* Mental health associations exist in many states to provide education and advocacy on behalf of individuals with mental illnesses.
† Reuland, M., Draper, L., & Norton, B. (2010). *Improving responses to people with mental illnesses: Tailoring law enforcement initiatives to individual jurisdictions.* New York, NY: Council of State Governments Justice Center.

Table 1.1   Essential Elements of SPR Programmes

Element	CIT	Co-responder
Collaborative planning and implementation	Organisations and individuals affected by police encounters with people with mental illnesses work together in one or more multidisciplinary groups; the purpose of these groups is to determine the response programme's characteristics and guide implementation efforts.	
Specialised training	Intense training is provided to a group of officers to improve their ability to de-escalate crisis.	All officers receive some training on crisis de-escalation, and a small group receives intense training on these skills.
Call taker and dispatcher protocols	Call takers and dispatchers identify critical information to direct calls to the appropriate responders, inform the law enforcement response, and record this information for analysis and as a reference for future calls for service.	
On-scene stabilisation and de-escalation	The group of officers who are trained to handle calls involving mental illness are dispatched to those scenes.	The small group of officers who are trained to handle calls involving mental illness ride with mental health professionals. This team is dispatched to those scenes.
On-scene assessment of the signs and symptoms of mental illnesses, and the subsequent disposition	Trained officers make the assessment of mental illness involvement and select the appropriate disposition.	Trained officers working in teams with mental health professionals make this assessment and select appropriate disposition together.
Confidentiality and information exchange	Law enforcement and mental health personnel have a well-designed procedure governing the release and exchange of information to facilitate appropriate communication while protecting the confidentiality of community members.	
Transportation and custodial transfer	Officers take into custody and transport those individuals who meet the criteria for emergency evaluation or who are being arrested.	Officers can take into custody these individuals also. Mental health professionals can assist in transporting those who are not a danger.
Specialised crisis response sites and treatment supports and services	Specialised police-based response programmes connect individuals with mental illnesses to comprehensive and effective community-based treatment supports and services.	
Organisational support	The law enforcement agency's policies, practises, and culture support the specialised response programme and the personnel who further its goals.	
Programme evaluation and sustainability	Data are collected and analysed to help demonstrate programme impact and to inform modifications to the programme. Support for the programme is continuously cultivated in the community and police department.	

Table 1.2   Community Problems and Related SPR Options

Problem	Problem Causes	SPR Options
Unsafe encounters	Lack of information about signs and symptoms of mental illness Lack of tools to de-escalate crisis behaviour	Education about mental illness Call taker protocols that gather relevant information related to safety De-escalation skills training
Frequent arrests/strains on police resources	Inefficient access to limited mental health resources	Streamlined intake procedures for police at mental health facilities Involve mental health professional in on-scene response to access information to assist in appropriate placement Partner with other emergency medical providers (e.g., ambulance services)
High utilisation of emergency services	Difficult to treat populations, who are often homeless or have co-morbid substance use problems	Law enforcement partners with mental health professionals to craft individualised solutions Draw on partnerships with wide range of service providers (e.g., housing, social services)

Table 1.2 offers examples to illustrate how various problems, and their causes, typically compel a community to develop a SPR, and how that information drives the selection of specific SPR programme elements. It is important to note that any separation of problems into distinct categories is somewhat artificial, as they often overlap and relate to one another. Three main problem areas are addressed below: unsafe encounters, frequent arrests and strains on law enforcement resources, and high utilisation of emergency services.

The solutions to these problems—including changes to law enforcement training, policies, and procedures—must also fit within the community's characteristics. As distinct from the previous discussion about problems and their impact on the specialised response programme, jurisdictional characteristics are largely static features in a community, which policy makers must work around in the short term. For example, while it is certainly possible to change the laws that govern police custodial arrangements for people in need of emergency mental health evaluation, changing these laws would likely take many years. These characteristics will significantly impact the ways in which programme responses are designed and implemented. Training officers on diversion and other strategies, for example, will be ineffective if mental health resources in the community are unavailable or lack the capacity to support this shift.

Table 1.3 examines four jurisdictional characteristics that shape programme responses: law enforcement agency leadership style, mental health

Table 1.3   Community Characteristics and Related SPR Options

Characteristic	Dimensions of the Characteristic	SPR Options
Law enforcement agency leadership style	Leaders who believe specialised units are needed to address particular crime areas Leaders who are generalists and expect all officers to be able to respond to all incidents	Specialists train a cadre of officers who volunteer for the team and meet certain selection criteria. Generalists are more likely to train the entire department. In these cases, a select group of officers may still get more advanced training.
Mental health system resources	Limited mental health resources	Law enforcement develop better screening to assess those people who meet the criteria for emergency evaluation, and divert those who do not to another resource. Mental health partners facilitate enrolment in benefits for clients who have no insurance.
State law on police role in emergency mental health evaluation	Many states require law enforcement to maintain custody of a person who meets the criteria for emergency evaluation until a mental health professional conducts a more thorough assessment and finds an inpatient bed.	Detail law enforcement or hospital security staff to the emergency department or other mental health facility to manage custody during the assessment process.
Jurisdiction size	Population size and density Geographic size and type	Limit specialised patrol responses to those areas in large cities that generate the largest number of calls for service. Partner with ambulance service providers as a "force multiplier" in large, rural areas. Develop regional partnerships to capitalise on shared resources.

system resources, state law regarding police role in emergency mental health evaluation, and demographics and geography.

The next two sections review (1) how states structure the statewide coordination effort (e.g., which agency takes the lead, what other agencies partner in the effort, how the organisation recruits new jurisdictions) and (2) how states maintain adherence to the essential elements of SPRs (e.g., curriculum development, training, or data collection) while still allowing for flexibility. Variations among the states illustrate that there is no single path to success, but rather, implementation strategies must be tailored to individual states' strengths and weaknesses.

Statewide Coordination Efforts Structure

Each statewide effort begins with an organisation working at the state level that determines there is an interest in spreading SPRs throughout the state. This lead organisation gathers support of partner state-level organisations, determines its mission and goals, and identifies needs and avenues for funding. Once the state-level collaborative is in place, partners decide how to proliferate the SPR programme, which entails recruiting and persuading jurisdictions to join the effort. This section describes these two aspects of the statewide structures in the states' Justice Center staff studied for this project.

Lead State-Level Organisations

Of the eight states actively engaged in statewide programmes, the lead state-level agency fell into one of three categories: advocacy, mental health, or law enforcement. The three states chosen for site visits were selected partly because their lead organisations were different—one is led by an advocacy-based organisation, one is coordinated through a mental health agency, and a local police department manages the last. Although all of the lead agencies work closely with their partners in the other two domains, there are distinct advantages and challenges to being in the lead role positions.

The advantage of having the effort led by an advocacy group is that it places the coordination within a group most familiar with the needs of mental health consumers. In fact, in most communities around the nation that have begun specialised policing responses, the local advocacy group has been instrumental in instituting the change. A challenge for advocacy groups is that they are outside of the government entities charged with providing service to this population, and therefore have little leverage over them.

The advantage of having the effort coordinated through the mental health agency is that it brings in-depth knowledge of the mental health system and its available resources. The mental health authority in each state also has direct control over how funds are dispersed through the state and for what purposes, and can influence local mental health providers to collaborate with police. The availability of funding streams and a wide range of mental health treatment options is critical to the success of these specialised programmes. State-level mental health lead agencies have leverage over how and what kind of mental health services are delivered. Although their sphere of influence is limited to publicly funded mental health services, they can also influence private providers and marshal their support.

The advantage of having the effort coordinated through law enforcement is that law enforcement agencies now represent the frontline responders for many people with mental illnesses and are arguably the least prepared for that role. These agencies have the most to gain from implementing specialised policing programmes, but may not recognise the benefits of the programmes. Law enforcement agencies that have experienced positive outcomes are in the best position to persuade other agencies.

Housing a statewide effort in a law enforcement agency also has a unique set of challenges. First, there is no recognised state-based organisation in law enforcement in the United States (as there are in advocacy and mental health). When individual police departments do take the lead, they must garner the respect of the agencies in their state to act in this role. Another challenge is that the director and coordinator of these programmes serve at the discretion of their supervisors. If the chief executive officer of the law enforcement agency does not support the statewide effort, the programme would suffer.

Recruitment Structures

Most statewide efforts pay programme coordinators to do the work of recruiting and maintaining the individual programmes across the state. Some states have two coordinators—one each from mental health and law enforcement—who work together to recruit agencies to the statewide effort. These coordinators use two general strategies to recruit new jurisdictions to participate in the statewide effort—a regionalised approach or a centralised one.

In the first, a regionalised coordination approach, state organisers recruit a primary law enforcement agency in a catchment area* or county, work closely with community partners from law enforcement, mental health, and advocacy to get a SPR programme up and running, and then identify a regional CIT coordinator who is responsible for recruiting other communities within their area. Programme coordinators at the state level typically respond to a request from an advocate at the local or county level by meeting with stakeholders in the region and presenting information on the SPR programme elements. They then support building the training capacity in that catchment area. This approach is useful because the single mental health service provider that serves the single area provides consistency in the rules and protocols throughout that area.

In the second approach, a centralised coordination approach, staff at the state-level organisation coordinate recruitment of all communities across the state. Although training may be regionalised, the state-level organisation

* Most state mental health departments in the United States divide the state into catchment areas. Typically, a single mental health provider then serves residents in need in that area. Catchment areas typically include more than one police jurisdiction.

remains the main point of recruitment or access to the training. In this strategy, statewide programme coordinators begin by recruiting agencies they know to be willing or that are already involved in a SPR programme and snowball from there.

Outreach Strategies

Whether the recruitment structure is regionalised or centralised, state coordinators and their emissaries engage in several strategies to recruit communities to the statewide programme. Included are making presentations (e.g., to regional chiefs of police meetings, university security leaders, executive summits), debriefing a department after a tragic incident (e.g., educate the department when there is an officer-involved shooting with someone with a mental illness in a community about ways CIT can reduce injuries, or connect the agency with a CIT coordinator in another community), and enlisting the assistance of the State Attorney's Office, which carries a lot of weight with police departments.

Maintaining Adherence to SPR Elements

The spread of SPR programmes in the United States was initially accomplished through informal channels; typically, one department reached out to another with expertise in SPRs, either in anticipation of a tragic incident or in response to one. Because this pattern of programme replication was managed through lengthy one-to-one communication, programmes often closely resembled the original department's efforts. Programme originators strongly advised agencies to maintain all components of their own SPR programmes, and precise replication was often achieved.

With the advent of statewide implementation efforts, oversight of how comprehensively programmes are actually implemented in recruited localities becomes a major focus of the coordination efforts. This section describes mechanisms state coordinators use to ensure programmes substantially address 3 of the 10 essential elements described earlier: collaboration, training, and law enforcement and mental health agency policies.

The unique jurisdictional needs are sometimes at odds with the statewide planners' focus, however.* For example, states often wish solely to proliferate crisis intervention team (CIT) programmes. However, as discussed in previous sections, the CIT model does not address a full range of community problems. The CIT model is designed to improve safety during police

* Reuland, Draper, & Norton, 2010.

encounters. If a community is not having a problem with safety, elements of the CIT model will not be seen as necessary. Therefore, the state-level oversight and approach must also allow for flexibility to accommodate the individual community's problems and characteristics.

Collaboration

The first step in developing a SPR programme is to establish collaboration at the local level, including all relevant stakeholders. Some states convene a community stakeholder planning meeting to develop and define the programme model, and provide suggestions and examples from other departments to help influence the community to develop a programme. Subsequent to these initial efforts, programme coordinators initiate a dialogue between the local law enforcement department and their mental health authority to demonstrate what procedures the mental health providers can develop to assist the agencies.

Another state has a mentor system, in which the state programme coordinator pairs a seasoned SPR coordinator from another area with a community interested in developing SPR. The primary role of this coordinator, who is paid, is to help the community customise the training curriculum. The coordinator helps the community to identify trainers, provides funding for training, and fosters the creation of an advisory group at the local level.

Because each community in the state will have different issues and problems to address, local-level collaborations often go well beyond a core stakeholder group composed of local law enforcement, the mental health authority, and advocacy groups.

For example, some communities now partner with fire departments and emergency medical services (EMS) personnel to respond to mental health crises in addition to law enforcement. These communities consider these events within the realm of medical professionals' responsibility. Because these responders may lack training in this area, these communities have shifted their training focus to include fire department and EMS personnel to enhance their responses to people in mental health crisis. Partnering with fire departments and EMS can be difficult to achieve, however, when resources are scarce or when these professionals view incidents involving people with mental illnesses as unsafe.

Several components of the existing mental health services delivery system will also need to be included in these local collaborations. For example, most communities must coordinate with hospital emergency departments and build relationships with emergency medicine physicians to facilitate medical clearance before individuals in crisis can be evaluated for mental health services. In addition, those communities with mobile crisis teams must integrate them into other SPR response protocols.

Training

Statewide coordinators use two strategies to control fidelity to the core elements of training. In the first strategy, the statewide group creates the curriculum and requires officers throughout the state to attend an academy they run. In these cases, the curriculum includes core content (e.g., de-escalation, psychiatric diseases, suicide assessment/intervention) and adds new blocks of instruction when appropriate (e.g., autism spectrum, veterans, post-shooting trauma). The advantage of this approach is that it connects agencies to training and does not "recreate the wheel." Further, the consistency of the training has allowed some states to obtain Police Officer Standards and Training (POST) Council certification for parts of the curriculum. The POST certification makes the training desirable for law enforcement agencies that are often required by law to provide 40 hours of annual in-service training to officers.

This approach can also be regionalised such that the statewide group sets up separate training centres within a defined state region (e.g., catchment areas). These regional training centres only train officers from within that region. In this approach, statewide planners develop a set of requirements for each regional academy, including which topics to include and what site visits to conduct. They are essentially replicas of state-developed training. However, these regional academies are allowed autonomy to make changes to suit their jurisdiction. To ensure consistency across the academies, each uses the same end-of-training examination, and all officers who have successfully completed the training are certified by a state agency.

In the second strategy, the statewide effort requires jurisdictions to develop their own curricula based on a set of core elements. The resulting curriculum is then reviewed by state coordinators to ensure it is comprehensive. In these states, individual jurisdictions often reach out to their colleagues in other areas to review existing curricula as part of their own training development process. State coordinators often have chosen this approach because they believe the curriculum development process is an essential component of partnership development in the locality, and it allows for the locality to include important area-specific information where needed.

Law Enforcement and Mental Health Agency Policies

In all of the states visited for this project, state planners arrange for someone from the individual law enforcement agencies involved in the SPR programmes to act as the CIT coordinator. The specific responsibilities of this individual may vary in each state, but the intention is the same—this individual will be the liaison between the statewide planners and the jurisdiction, and will be responsible for ensuring that the law enforcement agency makes necessary policy changes. One state encourages each community to have three coordinators—one from law enforcement, one from mental health, and one from advocacy—although this is not required. Many agencies have trained officers but do not have a CIT coordinator.

In another state, individual communities recruit a mental health clinician to act as the liaison between the law enforcement officer and the mental health system. These CIT clinicians are paid by the state, which is very unusual. This state uses an additional strategy to ensure that local law enforcement agencies make necessary policy changes: They require each agency to develop a SPR policy before they can receive reimbursement for their officers' overtime spent in training. The state-level lead agency specifies the core elements that all agencies must include in their policies, and provides sample policies from a variety of departments to illustrate acceptable options. The agency does grant latitude in the policy's specifics. In general, the policy must state that when there is a mental health-related incident, a specially trained officer should be directed to the call, and when that officer is on the scene, they are able to use all the tools available to them, including all partner agencies.

Sustaining Statewide Coordination Approaches

Although many states are in the process of collecting and analysing data on the effectiveness of their programmes, the majority of findings at present are anecdotal. Site visit participants note that officers have increased awareness of the problems experienced by people with mental illness, and that programmes have led to other collaborations and referrals. Across the board, these programmes appear to be successful in directing people with mental illness away from jails and to mental health services, particularly when they focus on follow-up.

Each state maintains contact with and provides assistance to localities within the state to share information about the state's efforts and discuss roadblocks or problems. State representatives provide these contacts in a variety of ways, including hosting quarterly meetings or annual meetings, sending newsletters, and setting up listservs and Google groups. Annual symposia arranged in each state serve as refresher training and as networking opportunities among officers from different agencies, as does the International Crisis Intervention Team annual conference.*

Some of the contact between the statewide planners and the localities is more informal; programme coordinators often regularly respond to telephone

---

* The International CIT organisation has organised an annual conference on crisis intervention teams since 2002. Each year a different law enforcement agency hosts the conference and works with the International CIT organisation on planning. For more information about this conference, visit http://www.citinternational.org/.

calls and emails from localities to address issues, challenges, or share new ideas about how to expand specialised programmes. Ongoing training is another way to maintain programme interest and success and refresh skills.

The statewide efforts rely on the individuals who are committed to improving the police response to people with mental illness. To enhance the ability of programmes to continue beyond the careers of these individuals, statewide planners recommend engaging police chiefs, elected officials, the Attorney General's Office, and the advocacy community. Community demand draws more attention to the programmes and their successes, and can increase the likelihood of their continuance.

Next Steps for Statewide Efforts

This project identified 13 states that were either well into the statewide implementation process or at the early planning stages for such an initiative. The statewide SPR implementation strategies project staff identified have the potential to transform the way in which SPR programmes are implemented in the United States. What was once a seemingly haphazard, case-by-case spread of SPR programmes across the United States now has the potential to dramatically increase not simply the number of programmes in the country, but the quality of those programmes and the likelihood they will succeed.

The potential for more statewide SPR implementation efforts may depend on the size of the state, or other important characteristics, such as funding availability and the features and capacity of the mental health system. The federal government has taken an interest in spreading these kinds of programmes. In 2004, the U.S. Department of Justice, Bureau of Justice Assistance funded the Justice Mental Health Collaboration Project (JMHCP), which provides grants to communities wishing to plan and implement a jail diversion programme. These grants fund police-based programmes, as well as court and corrections initiatives, and the number of grantees and funding varies every year.

Although this research demonstrates that a statewide structure can have important consequences for SPR programme replications, one of the states identified at the onset of the project reported that it had actually completed its statewide initiative. In this state, planners had set up regional centres to assume the responsibilities of the state-level coordinators in managing training, collaboration, and programme sustainability. Once the transition was complete, the state-level structure was disbanded.

Whether future increases in programme implementation lie in a regionalised or statewide model, SPR programme replications are desirable given the potential these programmes have to improve the circumstances of individuals whose mental illnesses put them at risk for criminal justice involvement.

Improving Relationships Between Police and People With Mental Illnesses
Canadian Developments

2

DOROTHY COTTON
TERRY COLEMAN

Contents

Like their counterparts in many other countries, Canada's twenty-first-century police service employs a contemporary policing model that reflects a systems and community-based approach to service delivery. Thus, police services have emerged to be an integral part of the extended mental health system, devoting significant resources to interactions with people with mental illnesses (PMI).* Most Canadian police services have developed some form of specialised service for PMI, including dedicated staff for this purpose, in-service education and training for police personnel including police officers, and interagency agreements with their mental health system counterparts. While the nature and quality of services provided by Canadian police services to PMI has improved significantly in the last decade, and generally PMI are more positive than negative about their interactions with police services,

---

* There is little agreement in Canada about what term is most appropriate to use to refer to people with mental illnesses. With apologies to those who might disagree, this chapter will use the acronym PMI (person with a mental illness) as well as the term *consumer*.

the relationship remains, at times, ambiguous and ambivalent. To quote one participant in a study of the experiences of people who have a mental illness and who have also had contact with police:

> I've got some really negative ones [experiences with the police], and I've got some quite positive ones, so, you, know, averaging out, it's right in the middle.... Because I've met a lot of good police people, who have been kind and knowledgeable, and they really helped me when I was really low or high as the case may be. And there are some good ones out there. And I think they really want to do a good job, and sometimes they want to do a good job and they just don't know how. They're just good people, with not the right skills ... and sometimes they're jerks. (Brink et al., 2011, p. 69)

A similar ambivalence has been evident among police services and police officers. For many years, there was a sense by police that they should not be playing a primary role in the management of people in the community with mental illnesses. For example, as recently as the late 1990s, a police chief in Ontario picketed a conference on mental illness, carrying a sign that read, "We are not mental health workers." However, there is no doubt that there have been significant developments in the area of police–mental health liaison in the past decade. In this chapter, we will examine the trends as well as the relationship between police and PMI in the Canadian context, with particular attention to the questions:

- What is the nature of interactions between police and PMI?
- What is the social context within which interactions between police and PMI occur in Canada?
- How do police and PMI view each other?
- What kinds of formal mechanisms and programmes exist within policing to support their work with PMI?
- Where are things headed—and where do they need to head?

What Is the Nature of Interactions Between Police and PMI?

Interactions between police and PMI in Canada take a variety of forms. Generally, they include:

- Apprehensions under the respective provincial/territorial mental health act (MHA)
- Arrests for a criminal offence in which the accused person appears to have a mental illness

- Minor and noncriminal disturbances in which a person appears to be mentally ill
- Situations in which a PMI is the victim of an offence
- Situations in which family and support persons of PMI call police for assistance
- Social support and informal contacts by police

All provincial/territorial mental health acts in Canada authorise police to apprehend a person who appears to be mentally disordered and has displayed indications of actual or potential harm or disorderly conduct, in circumstances in which it is not practical to use a physician or judge to obtain a psychiatric examination (Gray, Shone, & Liddle, 2008). This is the most commonly used authority that police have available to deal with people who are apparently mentally ill yet have not committed an offence. Indeed, it is generally the only specific power police have in regard to PMI.

When an offence has been committed, police commonly employ discretion about whether or not to arrest. When exercising such discretion, police arguably do so for one of two reasons: (1) the primary purpose of protecting the public and (2) the purpose of acting in a paternalistic role to safeguard disabled individuals (Bloom & Schneider, 2006). Thus, police may decide to take no further action, issue a warning, divert a person to the mental health system, or proceed with criminal charges. The discretion afforded police can also have the unfortunate side effect of enabling police to use the criminal justice system as an access point to mental health services through diversion programmes or mental health courts, or by allowing access to provisions under the Criminal Code for various types of mental health intervention.

As will be discussed later in this chapter, mental health services are not always readily available in Canada—and in any case, individual rights and freedoms generally preclude forcing treatment upon someone who does not want it. However, a formal criminal charge can result in a court order for an assessment for fitness to stand trial, an assessment to determine if the PMI was "not criminally responsible" for the offence,* or an order for treatment (in very limited circumstances). Not surprisingly, as the number of general mental health beds has decreased in Canada, the number of forensic beds has increased (Schneider, Bloom, & Heerema, 2007).

While crisis calls and mental health apprehensions may be the most notable types of interactions between police and PMI, they are far from being the most numerous forms of contact. A study conducted in a typical small

---

* Part XX.I of the Criminal Code of Canada addresses issues related to mental disorder, including fitness to stand trial and verdicts of not criminally responsible on account of mental disorder.

Canadian city (Belleville, Ontario, population 45,000) suggested MHA apprehensions accounted for only 8% of police interactions with PMI (Belleville Police Service, 2007). This study revealed that people who appeared to be mentally ill made up about 6% of suspects with regard to an offence and 4% of those charged by police.

However, the nature and extent of police interaction with PMI varies significantly depending on location. In Vancouver a different picture emerges. A study in Vancouver (permanent population of approximately 611,000, with a metropolitan population of approximately 2.2 million) suggested between 23% and 49% of police calls for service involved a PMI (Wilson-Bates, 2008). The most rigorous Canadian investigation concerning police interactions with PMI (Hartford, Heslop, Stitt, & Hoch, 2005) was conducted in London, Ontario (population of approximately 352,000). Key findings included:

- PMI had 3.1 times more interactions with police than the general population.
- PMI were twice as likely to be reinvolved with police as the general population (79.9% vs. 38.3%). This reinvolvement happened sooner for PMI. Fifty percent of those with mental illness were reinvolved with police within 59 days (vs. 681 days for those in the general population).
- Almost twice as many PMI were charged or arrested during the study period compared to the general population.
- Forty percent of offences for which PMI were charged were for minor, nuisance type offences.
- Once charged, PMI were more likely to spend time in custody both prior to conviction and as part of their disposition (37% and 57%, respectively). PMI were more likely to be convicted.
- PMI were offenders in violent crimes as often as the general population.
- Events involving PMI represented a considerable cost to the London Police, estimated to be between 3% and 9% of the annual operating budget.

Although studies from these three different jurisdictions all arrive at different conclusions, they illustrate the issue of frequent and resource-intensive encounters between police and PMI. When one considers that these studies do not include informal supportive contacts or more positive interactions that occur between police and PMI, it seems likely that the frequency is much higher than reported. Nandlal, Cotton, and Coleman (2006) examined the phenomenon of police providing social support to PMI and found that police were often engaged in a variety of psychological, emotional, and instrumental social supports. Indeed, these types of interactions are consistent with the contemporary policing models espoused by the majority of Canadian police services.

It is worth noting that most police–mental health joint response programmes in Canada do not focus solely on crisis situations, but rather include the broader range of interactions that might occur between police and PMI. This is appropriate given the relative rarity of extremely negative outcomes between police and PMI. For example, deaths from interactions between PMI and police are, fortunately, rare. Between 1992 and 2002, for example, there were 11 such occasions across Canada (Coleman & Cotton, 2005). Needless to say, even one such death is too many. But it remains the case that the preponderance of interactions between police and PMI in Canada involve neither crisis situations nor violence.

The Social Context

There are a number of social, legal, and demographic factors that affect interactions between police and PMI in Canada. Factors such as climate, population density, geography, and ethnic diversity have indirect but considerable effects. In brief, much of the country is in the northern half of the northern temperate zone. This is relevant because PMI who might lack the judgement to dress appropriately or seek shelter in the winter may be at risk of harm in these circumstances. An apprehension under the MHA is therefore sometimes used as a protective measure by police.

There is also considerable variation in population density across Canada. While Canada has the second largest land mass in the world (just under 10 million square kilometres), its population is only slightly over 33 million. Almost 80% of the population lives in urban areas of 10,000 people or more (Population density of the provinces and territories, 2008); however, there are remote areas where the nearest mental health service might be a one-day drive away—or not accessible by road at all. It is a challenge to provide services to isolated low-density areas and for mental health and police services to work together in these situations.

In addition, Canada is a country of many cultures, with one of the highest national immigration rates in the world (Census shows Canada truly multicultural, 2003). Canada has a national policy in support of multiculturalism (Burnet, 2008) and endeavors to provide all services in a culturally appropriate manner. The wide variety of ethnic and cultural groups poses challenges for both police and mental health agencies. Many cultural and immigrant groups hesitate to make use of mental health services because of the stigma as well as the limited availability of culturally appropriate services. Similarly, some immigrants actively avoid interactions with police based on experiences in their home countries—as well as perceptions of possible racial bias.

These static factors interact with social changes and dynamics. The most obvious of these has been the reduction in the number of psychiatric hospital beds. Deinstitutionalisation in Canada began in the 1970s and continues. Between 1985 and 1999, for example, the average number of days of care in psychiatric hospitals in Canada decreased by 41.6% (Sealey & Whitehead, 2004). While some community services have been developed, they do not adequately replace the care that was provided in psychiatric hospitals (cf. Sealey & Whitehead, 2004). In addition, government planning for community services post-deinstitutionalisation was generally inadequate. A review of government documents related to deinstitutionalisation reveals little mention of potential effects on police services, or indeed the criminal justice system as a whole.

Simultaneous to the deinstitutionalisation movement, there were also considerable changes in mental health legislation. As Gray et al. (2008) pointed out, since the 1970s the trend in Canadian mental health law reform has been to increase rights protection to people involuntarily detained in the hospital and decrease the number of people subjected to compulsory admission and treatment. Today, most legislation allows only for dangerous persons to be detained, and there are extremely limited provisions for involuntary treatment. These changes emerged during an era characterised by an increased emphasis on the human rights and freedoms of people with mental illnesses, and when the voice of the mental health consumer finally began to be heard within Canadian society. While the desirability of these changes continues to be subject of debate, their effect is nevertheless evident in the increase in interactions between police and PMI.

A phenomenon simultaneous to deinstitutionalisation and mental health law reform has been the increased numbers of homeless people in Canada, many with a history of mental illness often in conjunction with substance abuse and addiction. Laird (2007) observed that while reliable data are difficult to obtain, the number of homeless people in Canada increased dramatically between the mid-1990s and the mid-2000s, sometimes at triple digit rates. Riordan (2004) noted 66% of homeless people have a history of mental illness. Not surprisingly, homeless people have a higher rate of interaction with police than other people. For instance, Riordan (2004) noted that 30% of homeless people spent time in police custody in the year prior to becoming homeless. Zakrison, Hamel, and Hwang (2004) reported that 61% of homeless people in a Toronto shelter interacted with police in the previous year.

Social factors affecting mental health care have implications for police services and the population as a whole. While Canadians enjoy an accessible government- funded and -operated health care system, mental health care lags behind other aspects of health care in terms of availability. Indeed, Canada only adopted its first mental health society in 2012. Integral to this strategy is the investigation of issues related to mental health and the law, including interactions between PMI and the criminal justice system in general and police in particular. As a result, the MHCC has pursued a series of police projects, including reviews of police education and training curricula. Development of learning programmes and partnerships is considered integral to the proposed mental health strategy, as is a concern about the broader issue of overinvolvement of PMI in the criminal justice system at all levels.

How Do Police and People With Mental Illnesses View Each Other?

Of particular interest is a unique study funded by the MHCC that examined police interactions with PMI from the standpoint of the consumer rather from that of the police (Brink et al., 2011). The results indicate that while PMI are somewhat less positive about police than is the general public, they are nevertheless more positive than negative. Not surprisingly, participants in this study expressed concerns about police use of force, about the relative insensitivity of some police officers, and about the need for police officers to be educated about mental illness. Many described their interactions with police personnel as positive and were appreciative of the assistance that police had provided, particularly in times of crisis. Conversely, some felt they had been treated disrespectfully and with more force than necessary. There was general interest by participants in establishing not only closer working relationships between police and the mental health community, but also for increased civilian oversight of police in this area. While this unique study has been used to inform the development of a Canadian model of police education and training, at the same time it points to the strength of the existing programmes and the value of education and training. It also clearly emphasises the complexity of services that police are called upon to play a role in in the lives of PMI.

Police attitudes toward PMI are similarly mixed. A sense of ambivalence toward PMI was evident in the study of police attitudes by Cotton (2004). While most officers (80%) agreed that dealing with PMI is part of a police officer's role, and that police need special training to carry out this role, about 50% felt that PMI take up more than their fair share of police resources. A considerable minority (38%) felt if mental health services were adequate, the police would not be put in the position of having to deal with mental illness-related issues. Members of the three police services surveyed in this study did not display high levels of authoritarianism or significantly socially restrictive attitudes toward PMI. In fact, they were at least as benevolent as the general public, based on a comparison with a community sample (Taylor & Dear, 1981).

These findings do, however, reflect a basic dilemma. When a person appears to be mentally ill and is acting in an unusual manner, it is the police who are expected to address and resolve the situation. Yet the police find themselves in the untenable position of having a social expectation to "do something," while at the same time having no clear reason to arrest, and knowing that there is little in the way of specific provisions under the MHA to address the situation unless the individual in question is acutely homicidal or suicidal.

Research conducted by Inspector Frank Trovato, then a member of the Toronto Police, similarly noted: "On the one hand, officers feel a profound obligation toward EDPs [emotionally disturbed persons] ... while, on the other hand, they feel the public needs protection from them" (Trovato, 2000, p. 81). Trovato (2000) assessed police attitudes toward PMI in a sample of 374 Toronto police officers. Their responses indicated a high degree of benevolence, which is described as representing a view of care for PMI that is a societal obligation and reflecting a belief in advocacy for these individuals. Trovato's results indicated that police displayed a generally positive orientation toward PMI, but at the same time, a relatively socially restricted view. In addition, he found that while officers ascribed in theory to principles of benevolence and a "mental hygiene ideology," their behaviour was more consistent with authoritarian and socially restrictive views. One particularly intriguing aspect of Trovato's work was the inclusion of qualitative information in the form of comments and observations by the police about other aspects of their attitudes toward working with PMI, especially in reference to how they viewed their role as police officers, and to what they attributed the increasing amount of contact. There were some general themes that emerged. Some officers clearly thought that there were serious flaws in the mental health system. Others made observations about the appropriateness of the role of police in this type of work.

Taken together, these studies suggest that there is significant goodwill and cooperation between PMI and police in many instances—but again, that there is room for improvement, and that role issues and a sense of ambivalence remain.

What Kinds of Formal Mechanisms and Programmes Exist Within Policing to Support Their Work With People With Mental Illnesses?

In Canada, because health care and policing are constitutionally delegated to each province, systems and some laws vary across the country. The approximately 230 Canadian police organisations include municipal, provincial, and federal services. They vary in size from approximately 100 municipal police services with fewer than 25 officers, to 12 provincial and municipal police services with more than 1,000 officers. The largest is the Royal Canadian Mounted Police (RCMP), with more than 17,000 officers* (Police Sector Council, 2006). Similarly, mental health services vary significantly. Thus, the nature and extent of the police role with PMI varies depending upon the nature and extent of the local mental health services and programming. As recently as 2001, dedicated programmes within police services to address issues related to PMI were still rare (Cotton, 2001) in that only about 10% of Canadian police services had any kind of formal mechanism in place to work with PMI. However, arguably the first formal dedicated programme appears to have been developed in London, Ontario, in the late 1960s. Little information is available about the origins and impetus for this programme. However, not long after the London programme was established, another joint response model was developed in Vancouver, British Columbia. The origins of Vancouver's programme provide some insight into the nature of police interactions with PMI in Canada.

According to Levine (1979), Vancouver's "Car 86 and Car 87" programmes arose in the context of a justice reform movement whose aim was "to explore new avenues to solve old problems" (p. II-2), and to explore ways to use police and community resources to develop diversionary and preventative programmes, including methods of informal dispute resolution. The programme that arose was essentially a joint police–mental health mobile response programme, in which a police officer and a mental health worker would respond jointly to calls that involved a person who appeared to be mentally ill. What is significant about the origin of this programme (and its subsequent impact in Canada) is that the impetus did not arise from a violent incident, a shooting or other death—as has been the case in many jurisdictions outside Canada. Canada's first formal police response developed in the context of community policing and philosophical shifts in the application of law. As will be noted later in this chapter, this may well account for an essential difference in the model of police response that is predominant in Canada as opposed to some other Western countries (notably, the United States).

The shift toward community policing has continued since the Levine report was written in the 1970s. Most police organisations in Canada now consider themselves to be community (contemporary) policing organisations (Coleman, 2006). Several of the fundamental principles of contemporary policing (Coleman, 2005) apply directly to police interactions with PMI:

---

* In addition to their role as federal police, the RCMP also contracts to some provinces and municipalities for their policing. This is in addition to the aforementioned jurisdictions policed by their own police services.

- A conscious focus on delivering quality and valued customer/client service
- Consultation and collaboration internally and with the community
- Procedural justice
- Ethical conduct
- Decentralisation of authority and decision making
- Increased communication by actively sharing information internally and externally with the community
- An outcome focus

Thus, the contemporary policing model includes a focus on a preemptive operation where vulnerable PMI are identified and provided with instrumental assistance and interventions to avert more serious problems, such as arrest, involuntary hospitalisation, or even serious physical harm to the PMI (or to police). In concert with the philosophy of contemporary policing, such assistance and intervention is achieved through communication, cooperation, and collaboration with other agencies, such as mental health care providers. In relation to police interactions with PMI in particular, these principles have led to three major developments:

- The establishment of guidelines for police services about how to develop relationships with the mental health system
- Specialised education and training for police personnel about mental health, mental illness, and mental health resources
- A variety of formal joint response initiatives between police services and mental health agencies

Guidelines for Police Working With the Mental Health System

The Canadian Association of Chiefs of Police (CACP) has played a significant leadership role in facilitating the development of a knowledge base, encouraging communication and exchange of ideas, and developing guidelines for police services to assist in programme development.[*] During the years when formal mechanisms to enable police to work with PMI and the mental health system were evolving, it became clear that while there was no single model or approach that meets the needs of all Canadian jurisdictions, some common elements were evident in successful approaches. These form the basis of guidelines that were developed by CACP (Cotton & Coleman, 2006) to

---

[*] These guidelines and other information about the CACP's activities in this area are available at www.pmhl.ca.

encourage police services to establish an organised and coherent approach to issues related to PMI. At the same time, the guidelines allow flexibility for each police organisation to develop services that reflect local needs. The principles of these guidelines include:

- Designating specific police personnel responsible for mental health-related issues
- Establishing formal liaisons with the mental health system through both local or regional liaison committee participation and development of individual contacts
- Providing appropriate and ongoing education as well as training for all officers as well as dispatch, communications, and victim services personnel, and ongoing access to information about mental illness
- Having a method for accessing mental health expertise on a case-by-case basis
- Making information available for police personnel and for families/consumers about local mental health resources
- Creating a data collection system to enable analyses, and thus inform improvement, development, and monitoring of interactions with PMI

The guidelines also speak to the need for a proactive police leadership, and a stigma-free, ethical, and respectful police environment.

Education and Training

Education and training has been identified as a concern by a number of findings from fatality inquiries/inquests after a PMI has died as a result of an interaction with police (Coleman & Cotton, 2005). As noted earlier, police officers themselves have requested such learning—and PMI have indicated that police should receive such training. Cotton and Zanibbi (2003) found that 76% of Canadian police officers in three police services surveyed already had some basic training, but that levels of knowledge were variable. Most police officers were well aware of the obvious signs and symptoms of mental illness, as well as being aware of some practical strategies and skills that would be useful in interactions with PMI.

A survey of Canadian police academies/colleges (Cotton & Coleman, 2008) indicated that all institutions responsible for basic police training and education include some instruction during basic training about working with PMI. However, the extent of this varies significantly (from 1 to about 30 hours). Similarly, a study with regard to Canadian in-service police education and training found it to be highly variable (Coleman & Cotton, 2010).

A recent review of existing programmes, both within Canada and internationally, has led to the development of the comprehensive aspiration model of police education and training, the TEMPO model (where TEMPO refers to Training and Education about Mental Illness for Police Organizations)* (Coleman & Cotton, 2010). This model, developed in conjunction with the Mental Health Commission of Canada, draws heavily on existing Canadian programmes. While it also reflects the trends in other countries (such as crisis intervention training in the United States, for example), it is adapted to reflect the unique Canadian context within which police–PMI interactions occur. It is a multitiered model intended to provide education for all members of a police organisation (not only officers but also support staff). It includes significant emphasis on a human rights perspective and the need to address stigma. It also emphasises the role of PMI themselves in educating police.

Police Response Models

Given the variety of police organisations, mental heath systems, and geographical and demographic considerations in Canada, it is not surprising that there are many different Canadian response strategies and models. That is, there are various ways police work with the mental health system to minimise criminalisation of PMI, divert them from the criminal justice system, and connect them with appropriate supports. Informal diversion of PMI from the criminal justice system is an inherent part of police work facilitated through police discretion.

In some jurisdictions, however, informal mechanisms have been developed into formal joint response initiatives, and police-based precharge diversion programmes. The latter are typically directed toward PMI who have committed minor nonviolent offences. Best police diversion practices identified by Livingston (2008) and Hall and Weaver (2008) include:

- Appropriate education and training and tools for officers and dispatch/communications personnel
- Appropriate mechanisms for officers for on-site assessment and disposition
- A specialised crisis response location where police can take PMI, rather than to the hospital or jail

A common feature of most response initiatives is community-based liaison committees with representation from numerous stakeholders, including

---

* While the acronym TEMPO was originally construed to refer to education and training for police *officers*, subsequent development of the model has resulted in a change to the word "organizations" in order to emphasise the need for training for all employees.

police, others in the criminal justice system, key members of the mental health system, consumer and family groups, other first responders, and housing agencies. The liaison committee is a primary component in joint police–mental health initiatives to ensure that communications between partners takes place and programme design meets the needs of PMI. Notwithstanding this, the way in which individual police services operationalise working relationships with the mental health system, by necessity, varies significantly across the country. Current models used in Canada include:

- **A designated mental health officer:** Most Canadian police services with more than 50 police officers have designated at least one officer as the mental health officer. Their primary task is to be the contact between the mental health and police/criminal justice agencies. In some organisations, this officer may also provide direct response to situations involving a PMI.
- **Mobile crisis teams:** This is arguably the predominant Canadian model employed by many large urban centres. While the specifics of such programmes vary, their essential characteristic is that police and mental health workers co-respond to calls for service involving a PMI. Calls may come directly to the mobile response team from the police dispatcher, or the mobile team may be dispatched after initial response by other first responders. The presence of a mental health worker on the scene provides immediate and more accurate assessment of the scope of the mental health problem, and more efficient referral to appropriate mental health services. In some instances, mobile teams also provide both proactive and follow-up services. The presence of a police officer provides for immediate safety and stability in the event of violence or danger, and affords the use of police powers pursuant to the mental health act when apprehension is appropriate. Adaptations of this model exist in rural areas, sometimes via telephone consultations rather than face-to-face assessment by a mental health worker.
- **Crisis intervention team (CIT):** This model, which arose in the United States from concerns about safety for officers and PMI, dominates the field in the United States but is less common in Canada. This is a police-based response as opposed to a joint response. Specially selected and trained police officers are designated to respond to problematic situations, usually at the request of other first responders already in attendance or en route. An enhanced "value-added CIT" has been developed in British Columbia (Hall & Weaver, 2008) and offers community-based cross-training to a core group of first responders (police, ambulance paramedics, emergency room

psychiatric nurses, dispatchers, corrections officers) with appoint-ment of post-training CIT liaisons in each agency in order to main-tain relationships and collaboration in the community. This model is also used in a few smaller jurisdictions where the number of calls for service is insufficient to warrant a dedicated mobile response team or where geography makes reliance on prompt response by mental health personnel impractical.

- **Comprehensive advanced police response:** Some jurisdictions have developed strategies whereby all police first responders receive advanced mental illness education and training. While such advanced training for all officers is an admirable goal, and consistent with the principles outlined in the TEMPO model, it presents logistical and financial challenges, particularly for large police services. However, it might be the only option for small or rural police services in areas where mental health services are scarce or remote for a timely cri-sis response.

- **Sequential response model:** In jurisdictions where mental health services are available locally but the number of calls for service to police does not warrant a full-time dedicated response model, police have developed agreements with mental health agencies so that once a situation is stabilised and a police presence no longer necessary, a PMI can be taken to an agency that will immediately assume respon-sibility and ensure that he or she is connected to services (if appropri-ate or desired). This model has been used, for example, in conjunction with court diversion services in Ontario, and in smaller communities where memoranda of agreement exist between police and the mental health services. In Montreal, mental health workers meet the police at the scene of an event and might take over responsibility at that time, or function essentially as an ad hoc mobile response team and work in conjunction with police to resolve the incident.

- **Community development model:** Some of the most successful coop-erative police–mental health ventures have occurred in areas where there is not a readily apparent programme per se. The Belleville, Ontario, area is one of these areas. In these smaller communities, all police and all mental health agencies are de facto parts of compre-hensive joint response schemes. Such a strategy requires committed leadership by police and mental health organisations, as well as fre-quent education and training of all first responder officers, mental health workers, and active interagency liaison committee members.

---

* This model is often called the reception centre model in the United States.

Where Are Things Headed—and Where Do They Need to Head?

Currently, most major police services in Canada have joint liaison ventures in place; all police academies/colleges provide training related to mental illness. CACP has been a leader in facilitating enhanced services for PMI, and the MHCC has recognised and supported the work initiated by CACP. However, obstacles remain—at the practical, operational level, at the programme development level, at the level of knowledge, and at the philosophical level.

While the number of dedicated police–mental health initiatives in Canada has increased, it is difficult to document their outcomes because of a paucity of outcome data. Some of the best data have been generated by the London (Ontario) Police study (Hartford et al., 2005). In 2003, London Police entered a service agreement with the London Mental Health Crisis Service stipulating that the mental health service would respond on scene to police occurrences involving PMI. They also implemented police–mental health training developed by the Ontario Police College. Within one year, the London Police documented involvement with 26% fewer PMI, the median time to reinvolvement was extended by nine days, and there were 25% fewer occurrences involving PMI. Similarly, Baess (2005) reported that although the pairing of police with mental health outreach services in Victoria, British Columbia, almost doubled the calls for service they were able to attend, hospital wait times decreased appreciably, hospital-based resources were required in fewer cases, communication and exchange of information improved, and generally, case disposition better reflected the unique needs of each PMI.

Other joint police and mental health services also report considerable decreases in hospital wait times, increased joint police–mental health response to calls for service, reduction in mental health act apprehensions by police, and generally improved communication and problem solving (D. Dupuis, personal communication, December 15, 2008). More recently, in what is probably the only controlled before-and-after evaluation of an integrated mental health crisis service, researchers in Nova Scotia were able to document some of the anticipated, but to date largely unproven, expectations of joint response initiatives. Kisely et al. (2010) demonstrated that the implementation of such a service can result in increased service utilisation by consumers and families, decreased time expenditures per call for service on the part of police, and greater engagement in mental health services by consumers.

However, some outcomes are difficult to quantify and have yet to be thoroughly researched. The general consensus in the field (cf. No data?) is that joint police–mental health initiatives lead to improved communication, better disposition of cases, more client-centred solutions, better appreciation of the roles of each of the professional groups, more selective and efficient use of emergency room resources, an overall reduced tendency to criminalise and stigmatise mental illness, and greater awareness of mental illness in communities. However, it remains the case that data are sparse and there is need for a more comprehensive understanding of the role of police, as well as both the immediate and longer-term consequences of interactions between police and PMI.

Outcomes also need to be linked more directly to inputs—in terms of financial and human resources. Operationally, programmes are expensive to develop and implement. At least one joint response model in Canada has been disbanded for budgetary reasons. The successful delivery of comprehensive education and training is potentially expensive. Problems also persist in regard to the logistics of police and mental health agencies working jointly—issues related to decision making, budgets, as well as the transfer of mental health and police-related information, for example. Interagency service agreements have addressed these matters in some jurisdictions, but it is difficult to achieve the balance between protection of privacy, community safety, and well-being for the PMI.

At the programmatic level, the (unspoken) focus to date has been on people with psychotic disorders as well as people who might be suicidal. But there are increasingly concerns about a variety of other populations, such as elderly persons with mental health problems, youth with mental health problems, people with developmental delays as well as a mental illness, and the subgroup of PMI who are very frequent users of police–mental health services. These groups present special challenges—and often do not fall under the provisions of mental health acts, further limiting the resources that police have available.

There are gaps in knowledge. There are no national standards for collecting data in regard to police interactions with PMI; this significantly impedes research. Data are strikingly absent in regard to victimisation of PMI as well as positive or social support interactions between police and PMI. The scarcity of data makes it difficult to systematically assess and compare the efficiency or effectiveness of programmes. There is also little known about the experiences and opinions of PMI regarding their interactions with police. The recent landmark study in this area (Brink et al., 2011) has provided some important insights into the consumer experience—but there is clearly more work to be done.

Finally, at a philosophical level, perplexing questions remain about the goal of improving police interactions with PMI. While much of the impetus to date has come from concern about the appropriate use of police resources, there are other fundamental questions. To what extent should the presence of a mental illness mitigate one's responsibility for criminal behaviour? To what extent should police/criminal justice systems continue to be expected to address deficiencies in the mental health subsystem? At what point does public safety override an individual's right to refuse treatment or maintain privacy? What are the long-term desired outcomes of joint ventures? More police involvement? Less? What would people with mental illnesses like police to know—and what do they expect from their police services?

As is always the case, interactions between police and members of the community reflect the values and predominant issues of the society. So it is with interactions between police and people with mental illnesses in Canada. Are police–mental health liaison initiatives an indication of a failure on the part of the health care system—or a legitimate and appropriate police activity? Are these initiatives addressing a fundamental problem or merely serving as a stopgap measure to address a symptom? Answers to these questions require a comprehensive review of Canadian public policy and mental health law at their most basic levels, activities that are far outside the domain of police service provision. In the meantime, there is no doubt that police will continue to be involved in the lives of many people with mental illnesses in Canada.

References

Baess, E.E. (2005). *Integrated mobile crisis response team: A review of pairing police with mental health outreach services.* Victoria, British Columbia: Victoria Police Service and Adult Mental Health and Addictions Services, Vancouver Island Health Authority—South Region.

Belleville Police Service. (2007). *Police interactions with emotionally disturbed/ mentally ill people: A comprehensive analysis and review.* Belleville, Ontario.

Bloom, H., & Schneider R.D. (2006). *Mental disorder and the law: A primer for legal and mental health professionals.* Toronto: Irwin Law.

Brink, J., Livingston, J.D., Desmarais, S., Greaves, C., Maxwell, V., Michalak, E., et al. (2011). A study of how people with mental illness perceive and interact with the police. Retrieved from Mental Health Commission of Canada website: http://www.mentalhealthcommission.ca

Burnet, J. (2008). Multiculturalism. *The Canadian Encyclopedia.* Retrieved December 2, 2008, from http://www.thecanadianencyclopedia.com/index.cfm?PgNm=TCE&Params=A1ARTA0005511

Census shows Canada truly multicultural. (2003). Retrieved December 2, 2008, from http://www.cbc.ca/canada/story/2003/01/21/census030121.html

Closed listserv. Discussion retrieved December 2008 from the electronic mailing list policemhl-l: http://lists.queensu.ca/cgibin/listserv/wa?A1=ind0812&L=POLICEMHL-L&X=6D36DC6AAF450F730E&Y=dhgc%40post.queensu.ca

Coleman, T.G. (2005, November). Policing with a purpose. Paper presented at the 4th Annual Conference of the Canadian National Committee for Police/Mental Health Liaison, Vancouver, British Columbia.

Coleman, T.G. (2006). A study of strategic management and performance measurement in Canadian police organizations. Unpublished master's thesis, University of Regina, Saskatchewan, Canada.

Coleman, T., & Cotton, D. (2005, July). A study of fatal interactions between Canadian police and the mentally ill. Presented at annual conference of the International Association of Law and Mental Health, Paris, France.

Coleman, T.G., & Cotton, D. (2010). *Police interactions with persons with a mental illness: Police learning in the environment of contemporary policing.* Report prepared for the Mental Health Commission of Canada, Calgary.

Cotton, D. (2001). A survey of police/mental health agency liaison models. Unpublished survey.

Cotton, D. (2004). The attitudes of Canadian police officers toward the mentally ill. *International Journal of Law and Mental Health, 27,* 135–146.

Cotton, D., & Coleman, T. (2006). *Contemporary policing guidelines for working with the mental health system.* Ottawa, Canada: Canadian Association of Chiefs of Police.

Cotton, D., & Coleman, T. (2008). *A survey of police academy training at the basic training level related to working with people with mental illness.* Report prepared on behalf of the Human Resources Committee of the Canadian Association of Chiefs of Police and the Mental Health and the Law Advisory Committee of the Mental Health Commission of Canada.

Cotton, D., & Zanibbi, K. (2003). Police officers' knowledge about mental illness. *Canadian Journal of Police and Security Studies, 1*(2), 135–146.

Gray, J.E., Shone, M.A., & Liddle, P.F. (2008). *Canadian mental health law and policy* (2nd ed.). Markham, Ontario: LexisNexis.

Hall, N., & Weaver, C. (2008, March). *A framework for diversion of persons with a mental disorder in BC.* Vancouver, British Columbia: Canadian Mental Health Association—British Columbia Diversion Project.

Hartford, K., Heslop, L., Stitt, L., & Hoch, J.S. (2005). Design of an algorithm to identify persons with mental illness in a police administrative database. *International Journal of Law and Psychiatry, 28,* 1–11.

Kisely, S., Campbell, L.A., Peddle, S., Hare, S., Psyche, M., Spicer, D., & Moore, B. (2010). A controlled before-and-after evaluation of a mobile crisis partnership between mental health and police services in NovaScotia. *Canadian Journal of Psychiatry/La revue canadienne de psychiatrie, 55*(10), 662–668.

Laird, G. (2007). *Homelessness in a growth economy: Canada's 21st century paradox.* Calgary, Alberta: Sheldon Chumir Foundation for Ethics in Leadership.

Levine, P. (1979, April). *Cars 86 and 76: A review.* Report prepared for the Emergency Services Implementation Committee, Vancouver, British Columbia.

Livingston, J. (2008, March). *Criminal justice diversion for persons with mental disorders: A review of best practices.* Vancouver, British Columbia: Canadian Mental Health Association—British Columbia Diversion Project.

Nandlal, J., Cotton, D., & Coleman, T. (2006). Community supports for persons with a mental illness: Social support in interactions with police officers. Poster presented at the Canadian Psychological Association Annual Conference, Calgary, Canada.

Police Sector Council. (2006). Policing. Retrieved November 12, 2008, from www.policecouncil.ca/pages/police.html.

Population density of the provinces and territories. Retrieved December 19, 2008, from http://www.canadainfolink.ca/chartten.htm.

Riordan, T. (2004). *Exploring the cycle: Mental illness, homelessness and the criminal justice system in Canada* (Report PRB 04-02E). Ottawa, Canada: Parliamentary Information and Research Service, Political and Social Affairs Division.

Schneider, R., Bloom, H., & Heerema, M. (2007). *Mental health courts: Decriminalizing the mentally ill.* Toronto: Irwin Law.

Sealey, P., & Whitehead, P.C. (2004). Forty years of deinstitutionalization in Canada: An empirical assessment. *Canadian Journal of Psychiatry, 49,* 249–257.

Taylor, S.M., & Dear, M.J. (1981). Scaling community attitudes toward the mentally ill. *Schizophrenia Bulletin, 7,* 225–240.

Trovato, F. (2000). Community policing and the emotional disturbed persons: Are we meeting their needs? Unpublished master's thesis, Niagara University, Niagara Falls, NY.

Wilson-Bates, F. (2008). *Lost in transition: How a lack of capacity in the mental health system is failing Vancouver's mentally ill and draining police resources.* Vancouver, British Columbia: Vancouver Police Board.

Zakrison, T., Hamel, P.A., & Hwang, S.W. (2004). Homeless people's trust and interactions with police and paramedics. *Journal of Urban Health, Bulletin of the New York Academy of Medicine, 81*(4), 596–605.

European Police and Persons With Mental Illnesses

A Review of the Contemporary Literature

3

RHONDA MOORE

Contents

Introduction

A great deal of research has been done in the United States and progress made in assisting police to deal with encounters with mentally ill offenders. Much has been written about crisis intervention teams and their varying degrees of success in the United States, depending on the particular jurisdiction. While the situation there has been well documented in the literature

(Compton et al., 2008), and to a lesser extent the situation in the UK, Canada, and Australia, outside of these areas there is a lack of research literature specifically on this issue. The purpose of this chapter is to provide some coverage of the situation in Europe (including the UK) from such documentation, as is available.

A review of the literature reveals much about the different legal systems in the UK, Western Europe, the countries of the European Union (EU), and Central and Eastern Europe, and about the treatment and rights of the mentally ill. Although there is considerable information about the nature of mental illness and the laws relating to the detention and incarceration of mentally ill offenders in Europe, very little can be found that specifically relates to policing procedures during interactions with the mentally ill. With the exception of the UK, very few articles came to light that dealt with the issues facing the police and the progress that has been made in overcoming the problems confronting them. Where a particular country has a sufficiently robust economy to support any research into the issue of mentally ill offenders, the research has mainly been done by psychiatrists and other health professionals, government agencies, or human rights advocates, and focusses on the handling and treatment of the offender as patient.

Worldwide there is a need for secure mental health facilities in which to place offenders where they will have access to treatment, and for the resources and programmes for specialised training of police who encounter mentally ill people on a daily basis. Two factors that exacerbate the problem for mentally ill persons and increase the frequency of their encounters with law enforcement officers are homelessness—a common situation, especially for those with a severe mental illness—and stigmatisation, that is, the widespread belief that these people are a danger to the community. These are issues that every country has to deal with.

Methodology

This chapter initially appeared as an article published in *Police Practice and Research: An International Journal* (*11*(4), 2010), but it has been updated to include some recent developments, most notably in the Netherlands, Denmark, and France. Knowledge of these developments was mainly obtained through personal contact with colleagues in the field and through attendance at relevant national and international conferences. However, a further review of electronic databases was also conducted, but without being very productive.

The original article is based on a review of literature found in the following electronic databases covering the areas of health, mental illness, the law, criminology, psychiatry, and policing: ISI Web of Knowledge, Social Science Citation Index, Scopus, National Criminal Justice Reference Service, and

Google Advanced Scholar. Any literature reviews and bibliographies produced from these searches were also followed up. This included only articles in English or with English abstracts. Although the search included the period prior to 2000, with a few notable exceptions, priority was given to the most current articles, mainly those published since that date. Whereas there was a substantial amount of relevant information emanating from the UK, very little was found from other countries that specifically discussed developments in the policing area. Most of the literature dealt with legislation relating to the rights of the mentally ill. Within those limitations what follows is an appraisal of the present situation in Europe for people with mental illness in their interactions with the criminal justice system.

The chapter deals first with the situation in Western Europe generally, then focusses on the UK, since this is where the literature search proved most productive. The effectiveness of antistigma programmes is discussed, followed by a description of a number of successful police station diversion schemes. Mention is made of some of the problems inherent in the role of the "appropriate adult" provided for by the UK Police and Criminal Evidence Act (PACE) legislation. The findings are then outlined of several European studies in the Netherlands, Denmark, France, and Greece. The chapter concludes with a description of the situation in Central and Eastern Europe.

The Situation in Western Europe

"The handling of mentally ill offenders by a criminal justice system is an indicator of the ability of a society to balance public safety interests with the achievements of modern psychiatry and of its ability to incorporate basic human rights principles into penal and mental health practice" (European Commission, 2005, p. 6).

This statement by the European Commission sums up the objectives not just of European countries, but of any contemporary civilised society. Achieving these aims is by no means easy, and those confronted with one of the most difficult aspects of the problem are the frontline police officers. The balance between safety of the public and protecting the human rights of the mentally ill offender is a sensitive matter that varies somewhat according to the culture of the particular country. For example, in English-speaking, German and Scandinavian countries, it is a more formal process requiring a detailed legal framework supervised by judicial authority, compared with Latin countries, where there is a tendency to give health care professionals more discretionary powers (according to the *parens patriae* principle) (see European Commission, 2005, for a detailed account of the legislation of each country).

The Perception of Risk

The issue of perceived risk from people with mental illness (PMI) is one that receives constant attention in every country, as without some awareness and education of the public and police the level of risk tends to be overestimated. This widespread misperception largely contributes to the stigmatisation of PMI and also leads to their high level of incarceration. Their contribution to overall levels of criminality is quite small however—in fact much lower than other social groups (European Commission, 2005).

An exploration of risk carried out by the European Commission (2005) found that people suffering from "organic mental disorders" posed no more risk of criminality than the general population, although aggressive and impulsive behaviour may accompany certain types of brain damage. Substance abuse seems to be a very significant risk factor for offending behaviour. Persons with paranoid schizophrenia or some types of personality disorders are at greater risk of offending, as are those with certain types of affective disorders (see, for example, studies on schizophrenia and homicide rates in Norway by Hartvig & Kjelsberg, 2009, and Sweden by Fazel & Grann, 2004, 2006). There is no increased risk of violence or rate of offending found among those with most other mental illnesses or disorders; however, what does occur is an alarming rate of self-destructive and suicidal behaviour, associated with most depressive disorders.

A review of mental health legislation and detention rates in different European countries by Zinkler and Priebe (2002) found that while there are huge (nearly 20-fold) variations in detention rates, the criteria for detention are fairly consistent when it comes to PMI who are a danger to themselves or others. Different rules that were applied for involuntary treatment were based very largely on the particular patient's health. These variations seem to be influenced by the various professionals' ethics and attitudes, socio-demographic variables, the public's preoccupation about risk associated with mental illness, and the particular legal framework. Detention rates are rising in England, Austria, and the Netherlands—in England this may be due to a growing emphasis on public safety and responsibility for PMI's behaviour in the community being seen as belonging to the courts and statutory authorities rather than to psychiatrists (Zinkler & Priebe, 2002). Changes in mental health legislation are likely to focus on compulsory treatment in the community and detention of those considered dangerous. In Austria and the Netherlands, although there were legislative changes emphasising patients' rights, and that they be adequately informed and legally represented, detention rates have increased sharply. Reliable data from Germany were not available, and in some parts of Italy the low detention rates may be because of a de-medicalised model of mental illness and the abolition of asylums by law in 1978. High detention rates in urban areas probably reflect the degree of homelessness among the mentally ill (Zinkler & Priebe, 2002). Zinkler and Priebe's research, while limited by a lack of comparable data on detention rates collected and published in EU member states and other European countries, as well as the complications of varying translations of key definitions, nevertheless provides useful comparative material.

A Return to Reinstitutionalisation?

A study of England, Germany, Italy, the Netherlands, Spain, and Sweden (Priebe et al., 2005) that sought to establish whether reinstitutionalisation is taking place in mental health care found that what had in fact occurred since 1990 were newly established forms of institutionalised mental health care, and that in all countries the general prison population had increased. There are a number of hypotheses as regards this situation: greater frequency of illness, severity of illness, or both, possibly influenced by increasing use of illegal drugs; loss of social support in traditional families (more women in the workforce); and the definition of mental illness having expanded to include personality disorders. However, Priebe and colleagues suggest that a trend toward reinstitutionalisation may be "driven by a 'zeitgeist' towards risk containment in 21st century European society" (2005, p. 125).

A follow-up study covering the period from 2002 to 2006 of nine European countries—this time including Austria, Denmark, Ireland, and Switzerland—also found a continuing, though not consistent, trend toward increasing provision of institutionalised mental health care throughout Europe (Priebe et al., 2008). A relationship between a lack of psychiatric hospital beds and an increase in prison beds was noted by Penrose in an article as long ago as 1939; then in a 2009 study Hartvig and Kjelsberg, seeking to test Penrose's theories in Norway during the years 1930–2004, found the same relationship. They concluded that Penrose's "law" held up well from the longitudinal perspective in that country.

The United Kingdom

Although mainly independent, police forces in the UK are to a certain extent overseen by the Home Office and also aligned to other organisations, the primary ones being the Association of Chief Police Officers (ACPO), Her Majesty's Inspectorate of Constabulary (HMIC), the Independent Police Complaints Commission (IPCC), the National Police Improvement Agency (NPIA), and the Crown Prosecution Service (CPS). The ACPO, in association with the government and the Association of Police Authorities, is primarily responsible for the direction and development of the police service in England, Wales, and Northern Ireland (Sainsbury Centre for Mental Health,

2008a). While around 15% of the incidents dealt with daily are related to PMI, police receive very little training in this area.

Two pieces of legislation define the role of police in dealing with mentally ill offenders in England and Wales: the Police and Criminal Evidence Act (PACE) 1984 and the Mental Health Act 1983 (updated from November 2008 by the Mental Health Act 2007). Under PACE, police can arrest someone considered to be in need of police intervention, and where the person is suspected of having a mental illness and needs to be controlled and taken to a safe place, Section 136 of the Mental Health Act 1983 allows police to take him or her from a public place to a "place of safety" for up to 72 hours. An examination of, and guide to the use of, Section 136 of the Mental Health Act 1983 dealing with police custody as a place of safety was published by the IPCC (2008). In line with police experiences elsewhere in the world, it stresses the need for officer training in recognising and dealing with PMI, the need for alternative safe places where they can be taken, clarification as to who is responsible for the transportation of offenders to various destinations, and the problem faced by police where there are long delays at hospitals while an assessment is made. Sometimes, even where alternative safe places existed, they would not necessarily accept violent or extremely intoxicated individuals, who then reverted to police custody. Changes to the Mental Health Act 1983 included the amendment of Section 44 to allow the transfer of PMI from one place of safety to another (for example, the transfer of those who are no longer violent, to a hospital). Also included was the amendment to the definition of mental disorder so that it was uniform throughout the Act; however, this could potentially encompass those with a personality disorder and result in an increase in the numbers detained. Also allowed is "supervised community treatment," which may also lead to some being rearrested if they encounter problems out in the community once again. It is too early to tell what will be the result of these changes. The guide makes detailed recommendations and suggests helpful procedures for police that mainly relate to more funding of facilities (for example, to include adequate staff), more training for police in recognising mental disorders and continuing training over time, overcoming delays at hospitals, more detailed record keeping, more use of ambulances for transportation of nonviolent offenders, and obtaining feedback from "consumers."

A review by Kinderman and Tai (2008) of the international literature, human rights considerations, and psychological approaches to mental health care finds that the supervised community treatment orders provided for in the amendments to the 1983 Mental Health Act (Mental Health Act 2007) are "valuable, lawful, and compatible with the European Convention on Human Rights, providing certain specific conditions are met," namely, that the powers of the act are limited, as in Scotland, to persons whose ability to make decisions is significantly impaired, that each order has time limitations and is subject to review by a tribunal, and that the order should benefit the subject by providing more appropriate treatment or a less restrictive environment. New Zealand, most states of Australia and provinces of Canada, and many states in the United States have some form of such treatment orders (Kinderman & Tai, 2008).

The trend toward an emphasis on risk containment mentioned previously in the article by Priebe and colleagues (2005) is reflected in a form of sentence in the UK Imprisonment for Public Protection (IPP) known as created by the Criminal Justice Act of 2003 and implemented in 2005 (Sainsbury Centre for Mental Health, 2008b). This is an indeterminate sentence issued to offenders who are identified by the courts as dangerous but whose offences do not carry a life sentence. The sentence has been very controversial, leading to the Court of Appeal twice declaring it unlawful, with further appeals to come. Overuse of the sentence has created systematic problems for the criminal justice system. Due to the numbers of prisoners with mental health problems (up to 90% in England and Wales have at least one mental health problem) there are insufficient behavioural programmes for them—they often have complex needs, such as alcohol and drug addiction, sometimes in combination with mental health problems—and with no treatment, they have no hope of improvement and thus eventual release. This sentence has now been reconfigured in the latest Criminal Justice Act to try to reduce the frequency of use. The IPP has become the fastest growing custodial sentence in England and Wales, having a greater impact of the criminal justice system than any other sentence in recent times. Central to the debates relating to IPP and risk "is the hypothesis that the IPP sentence is conflating 'dangerousness' with 'mental illness', and that the IPP sentence is an example of 'reverse' diversion 'where offenders with mental illness are more likely than others to be detained in prison than diverted away'" (Rutherford, 2008, cited in Sainsbury Centre for Mental Health, 2008, pp. 54–55).

The issue of the detention of mentally ill offenders in police cells has attracted a lot of criticism and comment in the UK. In *The Independent* newspaper, the chair of the Association of Chiefs of Police (ACPO) Mental Health Group at that time, Commander Rod Jarman, complained that police who were not trained to look after the mentally ill were nevertheless increasingly left "holding the baby." He referred to the "national problem" of these people being held in police cells because there is nowhere else to take them. A Department of Health spokesman stated that the police station was sometimes the most appropriate or, indeed, only safe facility available. Despite a government allocation of 130 million pounds to health authorities to build appropriate centres, many areas did not take up the money because they could not afford to staff them. Detentions under section 136 of the Mental Health Act (persons arrested because they are a danger to themselves or others) rose in London alone by 50% between 2005 and 2006, and nationally the rise is thought to be around 25% (*Independent*, November 4, 2007). Commander Jarman claimed that the National Health Service was "not pulling its weight" in the care of such people. PMI who end up in police cells designed for criminals, where they can be held for up to 72 hours, are not only costly to police in terms of staffing, but can themselves be traumatised. As many as 200 such people a year commit suicide within two days of leaving police custody because they have not received the help they need (*Independent*, November 4, 2007). One consequence of this situation has been that Devon and Cornwall Police informed its health authority that the mentally ill would no longer be held in its cells.

At the present time, however, definite improvements are taking place. An indication of a continuing, positive direction being taken by police in the UK is summed up in the statement of Simon Cole, chief constable of Leicestershire Constabulory, and the new head of the Association of Chief Police Officers in "Responding to Mental Ill-Health and Disability," January 17, 2012 (the police chiefs' blog). He focusses on several issues facing the police that were raised in the Equality and Human Rights Commission (EHRC) report *Hidden in Plain Sight*, notably how police are supporting those experiencing disability harassment. A requirement to record disability hate crime was implemented in April 2008, and while different approaches to this have been taken by different forces, the most promising is that which engages with disabled members of local communities. The National Policing and Improvement Agency now ensures that disability hate crime is dealt with in core leadership training packages and that information about the EHRC is available and linked to other ongoing work on violence and situational vulnerability. Additionally, Cole reports that over 80% of mental health detainees are going straight to places of safety—police cells being only used in exceptional circumstances—and that all transport involving the mentally ill should be made by ambulance. Cole also refers to the Bradley Report of 2009, which reviewed the dealings of the criminal justice system with people with mental health problems and learning disabilities. He will be representing the ACPO on the review body to examine the progress made with Bradley's recommendations. He also mentions in the coming months a cross-government hate crime strategy as part of the government's mental health strategy. No doubt increased pressure is on police since the unanimous finding of the European Court of Human Rights in May 2012 that the detention of a mentally ill man in police custody for more than three days without medical care breached his human rights (European Court of Human Rights, 2012a). The UK government was ordered to pay him 3000 euros in respect of "non-pecuniary damage" and 8,150 "in respect of costs and expenses" (European Court of Human Rights, 2012b).

A further indication of advances in police practices in the UK was the recommendation that de-escalating techniques be part of police training with respect to managing the risks of restraint, and the implementation of mental health first aid training. The Metropolitan Police Authority identified these as part of police training, as there is evidence that certain groups, including PMI and those with learning disabilities, are more vulnerable to risks when restrained (Ministerial Council on Deaths in Custody, 2011).

Antistigma Programmes

Despite efforts since the 1950s to reduce prejudice toward the mentally ill, the issue persists today, affecting the self-esteem and well-being of this sector of the population and presenting one of the greatest obstacles to treatment (Warner, 2008). The "persistent and disabling nature of psychiatric stigma has recently led to the establishment of global mental health awareness campaigns" (Pinfold, Thornicroft, Huxley, & Farmer, 2005, p. 123). The World Psychiatric Association Program to Reduce Stigma and Discrimination Because of Schizophrenia, launched in 1996, established antistigma programmes in 20 countries and included local projects targeting criminal justice personnel. Based on a review of the literature on antistigma programmes, Pinfold and colleagues have examined the effectiveness of one such programme involving police officers in Kent in the UK. Their findings indicated that while mental health training workshops were useful, personal contact with PMI was the most important factor in changing officers' attitudes. The most effective component of this programme was, in the case of these officers, face-to-face contact with PMI recounting the stories of their contact with the police. It is important for such people to be part of the core presentation team in any such programme rather than just as guest speakers.

These findings are in line with those from a German antistigma project seminar entitled "Psychiatric Patients and Relatives Instruct German Police Officers—An Anti-stigma Project of 'Basta—The Alliance for Mentally Ill People'" (Wundsam, Pitschel-Walz, Leucht, & Kissling, 2007). The seminar was developed by a German antistigma organisation in cooperation with sociology teachers of the Bavarian police academy. The findings emphasised the importance of personal contact between police, the "patient," and the patient's relatives as the main focus in similar antistigma interventions.

Diversion Schemes

Since the early 1990s the government in the UK has worked on promoting diversion of mentally ill offenders from the criminal justice system. Developments in criminal justice and mental health policy over this period have been significant, such as the establishment of approximately 150 court-based diversion schemes across England and Wales and 40 police liaison schemes for which the main point of entry is the police station (Hartford,

Carey & Mendonca, 2006; McGilloway & Donnelly, 2004). A recent comprehensive report on diversion in the UK, published by the Sainsbury Commission (Sainsbury Centre for Mental Health, 2009), concluded that although the benefits are multiple (crime-related cost savings alone are conservatively estimated at 20,000 pounds per case), existing arrangements were not delivering these benefits. Lacking a clear national policy framework, diversion services have developed haphazardly, vary widely, and are insecurely funded. National coverage is "patchy"—only about one-fifth of the potential caseload is seen, with some cases of severe mental illness being missed by police or court staff. Opportunities were also being missed to influence decisions on charging, remand, or sentencing. Among 21 recommendations, the report lists first the establishment in every primary care trust area in England of a diversion and liaison team for PMI coming into contact with the criminal justice system. Specifically relating to police were recommendations that the government examine where improvements might be made in the identification of mental illness by police officers, court officials, and other criminal justice staff. All diversion and liaison teams should develop and agree on plans for training criminal justice staff in mental health issues.

Notwithstanding the problems identified in the Sainsbury report, there are police station diversion schemes in the UK that appear to be very effective. James (2000; James & Harlow, 2000) describes an effective comprehensive diversion service in London that was established to cover three police stations in Westminster: Charing Cross, West End Central, and Marylebone. These utilised the services of forensic community psychiatric nurses (CPNs) who were attached to the local community mental health and social services teams and had immediate access to the local forensic service for advice and support. Part of the logic of concentrating resources at the police station, and thus at the start of the process for the PMI, was that early identification of seriously ill people would prevent further offending. Variations of this model exist in Birmingham and North Humberside. James (1999) mentions that there have been successful experiences in areas with less population and in many local police stations, but in both cases there is little or no published information (for more discussion, see Laing, 1995; Etherington, 1996; Chung, Cumella, Wensley, & Easthope, 1998).

An additional benefit of the presence of CPNs was that it obviated the necessity for an appropriate adult to be present with the PMI and the concomitant problems associated with finding suitable candidates to fill this role. The issue of the role of the appropriate adult is discussed separately later in this chapter.

The most firmly established diversion services are in London and Birmingham—England's two largest cities; however, it is possible to adapt the model to a semirural or small-town environment where there are on-call CPN services to courts and police stations with the backup of a consultant psychiatrist (James, 1999). Birmingham has the largest court complex in the EC, and its forensic diversion service is not restricted to the courts, but also functions as a network of different agencies in the community, including the Community Services Department in the police force. The police divert from various police stations, like the court, under a system called diversion at point of arrest (DAPA), which is planned to eventually cover the whole of Birmingham (Riordan et al., 2000; Chung et al., 1998). DAPA started in 1992 in Birmingham as a pilot study. The crucial element in the success of this system was the amount of time spent building professional relationships between CPNs and police during the project's inception. Its success led to the extension of the scheme in other parts of the city.

Other diversion schemes in the UK exist in Scotland (Chung et al., 1998) and Northern Ireland (McGilloway & Donnelly, 2004)—the latter is discussed in more detail below.

The scheme implemented in Belfast, Northern Ireland, in 1998 is a multi-agency police liaison scheme designed to identify offenders with psychiatric illness or learning disabilities within the integrated health and social care system in Northern Ireland (McGilloway & Donnelly, 2004). It resembles the DAPA model in the West Midlands (see Chung et al., 1998) and the CPN police liaison scheme in London, involving rapid screening and assessment at the time of first contact with the criminal justice system, as well as a mechanism for appropriate referral or diversion to health and social services. The scheme is based in the largest of four police stations in Belfast, which operate under PACE Northern Ireland Order (1989) legislation and provide specialised settings for the questioning, identification, and treatment of mentally disordered suspects (McGilloway & Donnelly, 2004). Two community mental health nurses, liaising with forensic medical officers, police officers, court officials, probation officers, plus other health and social service professionals and voluntary agencies, provide the service. What is unique is that, in addition, the nurses coordinate follow-up care and ongoing advice and support to offenders, the police, and health care professionals. All users of the service expressed very positive views of the experience, particularly the success of the multiagency work between and within health and social services and the criminal justice system, as well as the valuable work of the community mental health nurses. The high demand for this service led to its being extended to include some other PACE stations throughout Belfast.

An important finding was that almost half of the mentally ill offenders were identified from the routine screening of custody record forms, as opposed to a recommendation from the forensic medical officer (FMO) or police or other criminal justice personnel. In addition, the FMOs missed a significant proportion of potentially more severe cases, suggesting that the detection rate in a criminal justice setting may be low, possibly due to masking effects of alcohol or drugs and the frequent clinical presentation of depression (McGilloway & Donnelly, 2004). Another possibility is that police were not thorough enough—a situation that may be improved by the mental health awareness training being implemented at the time in a number of local police stations. Such schemes as described above then can be effective in more accurately identifying mental illness than criminal justice personnel. The long-term impact of the scheme, however, was considered by no means certain in the absence of a fully integrated forensic mental health service in Northern Ireland. Birmingham (2001) makes the point that many initiatives set up in isolation from mainstream services often fail to achieve their long-term goals, particularly of nurse-led schemes that are most effective when fully integrated with local psychiatric services or staffed by (senior) psychiatrists (Birmingham, 2001).

The Appropriate Adult

Nemitz and Bean (2001) describe the situation that led to the introduction of provisions under the PACE Act for an appropriate adult (AA) to be present at police stations during interviews of adults with mental health problems. The vulnerability of the mentally ill in police custody not only increases the propensity for suicide and self-harm, but also increases the likelihood of false confessions, since many PMI are highly suggestible and likely to agree with anything that they feel will please their questioners (Laing, 1995; Cummins, 2006; Nemitz & Bean, 2001). Increasing prison rates and the numbers of PMI ending up in prison (despite diversion schemes) suggest that this is not happening. In many cases, the police fail to ensure that an AA is present, and this may be for a number of reasons. One is that the AA's role is full of contradictions, complex and demanding, appearing to be "somewhere in the middle of the conflict between the suspect and the [police] officers," and that there is a lack of suitable and trained people to fill such a role (Cummins, 2006, p. 273). Cummins also suggests that the presence of an AA has an important effect on police behaviour during an interview, increasing the likelihood that legal representation is sought so that evidence cannot be challenged at a later date. So while the role is important, it must be carried out by a suitably qualified person, or it can do more harm than good. Nemitz and Bean (2001) refer to certain moves in England and Wales to introduce training schemes for volunteers to act as AAs.

Research carried out between 2010 and 2011 focussing on medical examinations carried out by FMEs on mentally disordered or vulnerable detainees in police custody in England and Wales (both countries being governed by the 1984 PACE Act) resulted in changes to FME training, improved conditions in consultation rooms at custody suites, and changes in FME recording practises (Lowe, unpublished paper). FME qualifications were to be standardised and a list compiled of appropriately qualified FMEs on whom the police could call when needed. This should also assist court officials and lawyers should the case go to court. The research also revealed that over half the police forces in England and Wales contract out these medical services, possibly to reduce costs, resulting in health care professionals such as nurses or paramedics, whom FMEs viewed as less qualified than themselves, being called to attend examinations.

While PACE had improved the position of PMIs in police detention, this research found that mistakes were still being made and many detainees died at their own hands, and despite having shown warning signs, many were still being declared fit for either detention or interview (Sanders, Young, & Burton, 2010, cited in Lowe).

A Study of Police Practices and Attitudes in Some Western and Northern European Countries

Netherlands

In Rotterdam in the Netherlands community care networks, including the local police force, along with welfare services and housing corporations, in close cooperation with emergency psychiatric services, have been found to prevent the problems with the mentally ill from escalating, thus reducing the necessity of involuntary admission (Wierdsma, Poodt, & Mulder, 2007). These networks started in 1992, increasing to more than 25 a decade later, and were particularly important in underprivileged neighbourhoods in identifying at an early stage those with psychiatric problems.

Further information from the Netherlands (van Oijen, 2011), for which there was only a brief abstract available in English, indicates continuing concern regarding the interrogation of vulnerable "mentally retarded" subjects. There is no definition as to who is covered in the "vulnerable" category; however, it makes sense to assume that those with a mental illness are included too.

Also from the Netherlands, a study by Adang, Kaminski, Howell, and Mensink (2006) looking at the effectiveness of pepper spray (oleoresin capsicum) in "use of force" encounters by police, mentions that it was less effective on suspects under the influence of drugs and on violent suspects (this was similar to findings in a study by Kaminski, Edwards, & Johnson, 1999, cited in Adang et al.). While findings relating to mental state were reported as not significant, one wonders whether drug (or alcohol use) could have been masking mental illness in some subjects and resulted in them being made more aggressive and less incapacitated (thus more difficult to arrest) by the use of the spray.

Denmark

An article from Denmark (Sestoft, Rasmussen, Vitus, & Kongsrud, forth-coming) describes a new model of working practice between the local police department, social services, and psychiatry/mental health services (PSP), which was introduced in Frederiksberg, Denmark, and subsequently imple-mented by law throughout Denmark in 2009 due to its success. A qualitative study of four municipalities where the model was implemented was conducted by the Danish National Centre for Social Research to make recommenda-tions for future implementation of the model in other Danish municipalities (Vitus & Kjaer, 2011). The PSP cooperation was primarily initiated by the police in Frederiksberg in 2004 to assist in handling vulnerable persons who, due to substance abuse, psychiatric disorders, or other social problems, miss out on assistance because they get lost in the system due to not belonging solely to one of the above-mentioned three sectors. Amendments to the Judicial Code, Administration of Justice Act, and Processing of Personal Data Act eased exchange of information between sectors. To the knowledge of the authors of the Danish article there are no similar collaboration mod-els in other north European countries, and only a few studies on outcomes of systematic cooperation between the mental health system and other gov-ernmental sectors have been published, for example, in North America and Australia (those in Europe are already covered in this chapter). What is dif-ferent about the Danish PSP is that it is not a project but a "forum" in which cases are discussed, followed by responsibility/action being allocated to one of the cooperating organisations. Thus, there is no mobile or outreach team, and hence no extra operational costs, and therefore it is the first of its kind. The full evaluation of PSP Frederiksberg is published, but only in Danish (Vitus & Kjaer, 2011). The evaluation concluded that the aims of the PSP, to prevent social disruption and crime and improve assistance for vulner-able citizens, had been achieved, and the organisations were positive about the model but would prefer users to be more directly involved at an earlier stage to avoid further marginalisation. In addition, PSP cooperations have improved relationships between involved sectors through exchange of expe-rience and new constructive working relationships.

France

A promising example of a collaboration between a mental health outreach team and a police department endeavouring to respond to the clinical needs of homeless people in the streets of downtown Marseille, France, is that reported by Girard et al. (forthcoming). In 2006 and 2007, as a result of public pressure on politicians precipitated by the increase in homeless people with severe mental disorders, a right to housing became enforceable through the courts (Loison-Leruste & Quilgars, 2009, cited in Girard et al., forthcoming). Although over 60 mental health teams were created in France between 2005 and 2008 (Mercuel, 2008, cited in Girard et al., forthcoming), this appears to be the first report of collaboration with the police. Due to pressure regarding public safety, a new national central police station was created in the centre of Marseille in 2006, and the outreach team initiated a collaboration with the National Police Department of Marseille (they were unable to establish contact with the municipal police department) in the hope of fostering better relations and ongoing communication, leading to fewer arrests and incarcerations of homeless mentally ill. In addition to mental health outreach, this team runs a squat—a collective place to live that also serves for some as an alternative to psychiatric hospitalisation. As a result of a task force being set up consisting of police and the outreach team, practices common to both were identified, including negotiating to de-escalate conflict, although both had state powers to arrest or detain (police) or involuntarily hospitalise. The team members judged the presence of police during the involuntary hospitalisation process as helpful in reducing the potential for violence. Police felt that the social context of intervention was often more problematic than the intervention itself; for example, sometimes an insulting or critical crowd may be present probably due to negative public perceptions of police. They also noted that before the partnership they had frequently been unsuccessful in contacting mental health professionals—this was a key motivator for their participation during the pilot study period. Interestingly, the outreach team found the police reassuring for some patients, and for themselves as outreach workers, especially during involuntary hospitalisations. A notable aspect of the partnership was how ongoing communication and joint encounters between the partners led to a more successful collaborative process than was expected. When users were questioned in focus groups in the study, they stated that psychiatric coercion directly from the street, being a violent occurrence, was sometimes more frightening than police coercion. While the study had limitations, it does provide support for the possibility of partnerships between mental health outreach teams and police, despite big differences in professional culture, training, and practices, thus assisting the needs of the homeless mentally ill while simultaneously "recognizing and respecting the overlapping but different missions of outreach teams and the police" (Girard et al., forthcoming). Mention is also made of the testing of a new model of intervention to limit the violence of the police in working with people with schizophrenia (Compton et al., 2011, cited in Girard et al., forthcoming; see also Aiken et al., 2011).

Norway

A very recent study in Norway (Johansen, Morken, & Hunskaar, 2012a) that examined the role played by casualty clinics in the emergency care of people with mental health problems, including substance abuse, briefly mentions police involvement. This occurred in 148 of 887 cases examined. In the majority of these police brought a patient for examination, while in the remainder the police were called by casualty staff. Police were involved in 17 of 32 cases where there was threatening behaviour by the patient or relatives, including physical abuse of health personnel, 8 of these leading to involuntary admission of the patient to a psychiatric hospital. An earlier study (Johansen, Mellesdal, & Hunskaar, 2012b) found three times more police assistance in emergency psychiatric referrals from casualty clinics than referrals from other sources.

Greece

A small but valuable study of police attitudes toward mentally ill offenders carried out in Greece (Psarra et al., 2008) recommends changing attitudes through education and training. While laws vary according to the particular country, generally in Western Europe it is common practice for acutely mentally ill people to be involuntarily hospitalised. In Greece, where the law concerning involuntary hospitalisation was revised in 1992 (and included Law 2071/92 for the improvement of the health system), police are involved in the transfer of a person who has refused his or her legal obligation for psychiatric evaluation to the emergency department psychiatric section; his or her transfer to the proper psychiatric unit for involuntary admittance, after evaluation by two state psychiatrists, following a district attorney's order; and the management of violent offenders suspected as mentally ill, by appeal to the district attorney for psychiatric evaluation (Christodoulou et al., 2002, cited in Psarra et al., 2008).

While there has been a trend toward reinstitutionalisation in a number of Western European countries (Priebe et al., 2005), in Greece the mental health system was restructured based on de-institutionalised care, with a switch of government funding to enable more autonomous ways of living for the mentally ill, such as sheltered apartments and boarding houses, with a consequent reduction in hospital beds in all Greek psychiatric hospitals (Madianos, 2004, cited in Psarra et al., 2008). This may have resulted in more police encounters with PMI.

In the Psarra study multiple choice questionnaires were given to police officers who escorted people for psychiatric evaluation to a psychiatric hospital emergency department. Although the participating officers were not a representative sample (being mostly young and not very experienced), the findings are useful. These police officers reflected the attitudes often found in the general population, that is, that people with mental illness are unpredictable and dangerous. However, their experience in transporting mentally ill offenders probably compounded this since their contact would mainly be restricted to those in an agitated state and resisting apprehension and would not normally include those with insight into their illness, who adhere to their treatment, and are consequently less aggressive and rarely involuntarily hospitalised (Psarra et al., 2008). This suggests a need for education and training for those officers who appear not to have caught up with the principles of de-institutionalisation since a general population study in Greece indicated positive attitudes toward the social integration of the mentally ill and did not indicate a discriminatory attitude (Madianos, Economou, Hatjiandreou, Papageorgiou, & Rogakou, 1999, cited in Psarra et al., 2008).

Psarra and colleagues (2008) contrast Greek officers' attitudes that they did not consider it their responsibility to deal with the mentally ill with attitudes in the United States, where it is seen as part of the job of policing. For example, a survey in the United States found that police officers were interested in learning more about working with PMI and viewed it as an important part of their job—the more experienced of them rating mental illness training more highly than did those with less experience (Vermette, Pinals, & Appelbaum, 2005). Nevertheless, over 75% of the officers in the Greek study expressed a desire for more information about mental illness.

Another study (Douzenis et al., 2010) conducted in Greece in 2005 by psychiatrists from Athens University Medical School looked at over 2,000 mental health assessments for involuntary admission. They made the surprising finding that although in most of these cases the patient didn't offer resistance, the psychiatrists seemed to find it acceptable for the police officer to be present during the majority of mental health assessments, and the police considered it part of their duty to be present. The authors condemned this as undermining the psychiatrist's rapport with the patient and as a breach of the patient's confidentiality. However, they reported that it is not common practice in the greater Athens area and may occur mainly in rural areas, where there is a shortage of nursing staff, meaning the psychiatrist would possibly be working alone. Nevertheless, in the absence of any threat of violence from the patient, it suggests stigmatising attitudes may exist among some psychiatrists in Greece.

A comparison of police attitudes to mental illness can be made between the Greek officers and officers in a study carried out in southwest Scotland (Carey, 2001), where questionnaires were sent to all operational officers in a regional police service to ascertain the extent of their knowledge about, and attitudes toward, mental illness. It revealed that that while they were knowledgeable about the relevant legislation and accepted that mental illness is common and can be treated effectively in the community, they felt the need for and wished for more training in this area. Carey (2001) suggests that in a setting such as this, more effective liaison between sector psychiatrists and the local police would be beneficial in terms of earlier diagnosis and treatment of offenders with mental illness.

The situation in Greece can be contrasted with that in England and the United States, where there are education programmes to change police attitudes and help reduce stigmatisation (Pinfold et al., 2005). It has been shown that knowledge on the part of the police leads to less authoritarianism and discriminatory beliefs, and more positive views about the social integration of the mentally ill (Madianos, Priami, Alevisopooulos, Koukia, & Rogakou, 2005, cited in Psarra et al., 2008). Psarra and his colleagues recommend specialised training to improve attitudes and specific programmes to help police interact more effectively in encounters with the mentally ill.

Central and Eastern Europe

The political situation of any country determines the conditions in which the police must operate, and consequently the way they interact with the rest of society. The social upheaval produced by war and the stress of political and cultural change in Central and Eastern European countries, along with poverty, cannot fail to have increased the rate of mental illness among the general population in some of those countries, making interactions between PMI and police even more frequent and difficult.

In these areas of Europe where mental asylums have been the traditional solution for dealing with the mentally ill, 12 years after the establishment of democracy, the locus of psychiatric and social care remained largely institutional (Lewis, 2002). While community services have been developed in the richer countries like Italy, the Nordic countries, and the UK, there has been no such provision of alternative services in many poor Eastern European countries. A lack of qualified, trained staff compounds the appalling conditions for patients in some institutions in these poorer countries. Some attempts at reform have been linked to conditions of entry into the EU, and following the signing of the 2005 Helsinki Mental Health Declaration for Europe, many countries have also drafted improved policies for community-based mental health services. A recent article by Muijen (2008) indicates that some Eastern European countries are now creating diverse health care systems and developing mental health policies—partly driven by political and economic changes and partly through a growing awareness of the inability of the health system to address such conditions as depression and alcohol misuse (which are responsible for a large proportion of disability), and concerns about heavy reliance on asylums.

Republic of Croatia

Despite a lack of research on policing practises in Central and Eastern Europe with regard to the mentally ill, the attitudes and consequent practises of the police must reflect the authoritarian traditions to which they are accustomed. However, an article by Ljubin and colleagues (2000) describing the situation in the Republic of Croatia does provide some insight into attempts to change this traditional role for police. The article points out that the changing role of police within a newly democratic society parallels that of the society itself. Where the police role has traditionally been mostly repressive, now police must protect the individual's rights. Ljubin considers it as part of the role of Croatian police in collaboration with other institutions, such as the Ministry of Welfare and health institutions, to participate in programmes to promote the health of its citizens. He describes some recent activities of Croatian police in protecting citizens, particularly referring to the dangers posed from mines left over from war, and to the drug addiction problem.

Conclusion

The findings of the literature search suggest that either this is a relatively neglected area of study in most of Europe to date, or traditional academic databases do not capture the relevant policing literature—a quite likely scenario. Individual police departments, though, may possibly be conducting pilot studies (for example, on diversion) or programmes relating to police training in dealing with PMI that are either unreported or had not appeared in databases at the time of the search. Literature is now gradually emerging to indicate, however, that there are projects where police are collaborating with other agencies quite successfully and for the benefit of all parties involved, as in Marseille (France), Denmark, and the Netherlands.

Prison numbers are inexorably increasing, as is the representation of the mentally ill in the prison population (Sainsbury Centre for Mental Health, 2009). The literature reviewed suggests that improvements could be made in this situation through increased education and training of police to change attitudes (where necessary) toward mentally ill offenders, programmes to reduce stigmatisation of the mentally ill in the community and among police, and implementation of diversion schemes for offenders at the point of arrest to appropriate assessment and treatment in order to prevent further damage to the mental health of the offender and repeat offending on his or her part. Encouraging schemes involving police do exist, primarily in the UK, which may provide models for other countries to follow. From a humanitarian point of view and from a cost-benefit perspective, prisons are the least appropriate places for people with mental illness, but in many cases still the only option a police officer has that provides security, and in some cases treatment, for an offender.

References

Adang, O.M.J., Kaminski, R.J., Howell, M.Q., & Mensink, J. (2006). Assessing the performance of pepper spray in use-of-force encounters: The Dutch experience. *Policing: An International Journal of Police Strategies and Management, 29*(2), 282–305.

Aiken, F., Duxbury, J., Duxbury, C., & Harbison, I. Review of the medical theories and research relating to restraint related deaths. Caring Solutions (UK) University of Central Lancashire. Retrieved September 29, 2012, from http://iapdeathsincustody.independent.gov.uk/wp-content/uploads/2011/11/Caring-Solutions-UK-Ltd-Review-of-Medical-Theories-of-Restraint-Deaths.pdf

Birmingham, L. (2001). Diversion from custody. *Advances in Psychiatric Treatment, 7*, 198–207.

Bradley Report. (2009, April). Lord Bradley's review of people with mental health problems or learning disabilities in the criminal justice system. Retrieved September 29, 2012, from http://www.dh.gov.uk/prod_consum_dh/groups/dh_digitalassets/documents/digitalasset/dh_098698.pdf

Carey, S.J. (2001). Police officers' knowledge of, and attitudes to mental illness in southwest Scotland. *Scottish Medical Journal, 46*(2), 41–42.

Christodoulou, G.N., Angelopoulos, E., Alevizos, V., Anagnostopoulos, D., Vaidakis, N., Varsou, E., et al., (2002). *Psychiatriki: Psychiatry and the law*. Athens, Greece: Medical editions BETA.

Chung, M.C., Cumella, S., Wensley, J., & Easthope, Y. (1998). A description of a forensic diversion service in one city in the United Kingdom. *Medicine, Science and the Law, 38*(3), 242–250.

Cole, S. (2012, January 17). Responding to mental ill-health and disability. Retrieved September 29, 2012, from http://www.acpo.police.uk/ThePoliceChiefsBlog/201201SColeBlog.aspx

Compton, M.T., Bahora, M., Watson, A.C., & Oliva, J.R. (2008). A comprehensive review of extant research on crisis intervention team (CIT) programs. *Journal of the American Academy of Psychiatry and the Law, 36*(1), 47–55.

Compton, M.T., Demir Neubert, B.N., Broussard, B., McGriff, J.A., Morgan, R., & Oliva, J.R. (2011). Use of force preferences and perceived effectiveness of actions among crisis intervention team (CIT) police officers and non-CIT officers in an escalating psychiatric crisis involving a subject with schizophrenia. *Schizophrenia Bulletin, 37*(4), 737–745.

Cummins, I. (2006). A path not taken? Mentally disordered offenders and the criminal justice system. *Journal of Social Welfare and Family Law, 28*(3–4), 267–281.

Douzenis, A., Michopoulos, I., Economou, M., Rizos, E., Christodoulou, C., & Lykouras, L. (2010). Involuntary admission in Greece: A prospective national study of police involvement and client characteristics affecting emergency assessment. *International Journal of Social Psychiatry, 58*(2), 172–177.

Etherington, D. (1996). The police liaison community psychiatric nurse project. *Mental Health Review, 1*, 1–24.

European Commission. (2005). Placement and treatment of mentally ill offenders— Legislation and practice in EU member states (Final Report). Mannheim, Germany: Central Institute of Mental Health.

European Court of Human Rights. (2012a, March 5). Press release. ECHR 195.

European Court of Human Rights. (2012b, May 16). *Case of M.S. v. the United Kingdom.* Judgment.

Fazel, S., & Grann, M. (2004). Psychiatric morbidity among homicide offenders: A Swedish population study. *American Journal of Psychiatry, 161*(11), 2129–2131.

Fazel, S., & Grann, M. (2006). The population impact of severe mental illness on violent crime. *American Journal of Psychiatry, 163*(8), 1397–1403.

Girard, V., Bonin, J.P., Farnarier, C., Tinland, A., Pelletier, J.F., Delphin, M., Rowe, M., & Simeoni, M.C. (Forthcoming). Mental health outreach and street policing in the downtown of a large French city. *International Journal of Law and Psychiatry.*

Hartford, K., Carey, R., & Mendonca, J. (2006). Pre-arrest diversion of people with mental illness: Literature review and international survey. *Behavioral Sciences and the Law, 24*, 845–856.

Hartvig, P., & Kjelsberg, E. (2009). Penrose's law revisited: The relationship between mental institution beds, prison population and crime rate. *Nordic Journal of Psychiatry, 63*, 51–56.

James, D. (1999). Court diversion at 10 years: Can it work, does it work and has it a future? *Journal of Forensic Psychiatry, 10*(3), 507–524.

James, D. (2000). Police station diversion schemes: Role and efficacy in central London. *Journal of Forensic Psychiatry, 11*(3), 532–555.

James, D., & Harlow, P. (2000). Increasing the power of psychiatric court diversion: A new model of supra-district diversion centre. *Medicine, Science and the Law, 40*(1), 52–60.

Johansen, I.H., Morken, T., & Hunskaar, S. (2012a). How Norwegian casualty clinics handle contacts related to mental illness: A prospective observational study. *International Journal of Mental Health Systems, 6*(3).

Johansen, I.H., Mellesdal, L., & Hunskaar, S. (2012b). Admissions to a Norwegian emergency psychiatric ward. A prospective study of patient characteristics and referring agents. *Nordic Journal of Psychiatry, 66*, 40–48.

Johnson, A. (2007), Mental health campaign: Police should not have care of mentally ill, *The Independent*, November 4.

Kaminski, R.J., Edwards, S.M., & Johnson, J.W. (1999). Assessing the incapacitative effects of pepper spray during resistive encounters with the police. *Policing: An International Journal of Police Strategies and Management, 22*(1), 7–29.

Kinderman, P., & Tai, S. (2008). Psychological models of mental disorder, human rights, and compulsory mental healthcare in the community. *International Journal of Law and Psychiatry, 31*, 479–486.

Laing, J.M. (1995). The mentally disordered suspect at the police station. *Criminal Law Review*, 371–381.

Lewis, O. (2002). Mental disability law in central and eastern Europe. *Journal of Mental Health Law*. December 293–303.

Ljubin, T., Grubisic, M., Niksic, I., & Zarkovic-Palijan, T. (2000). *The role of the police in public health*. Paper presented at the 3rd Biennial International Conference on Policing in Central and Eastern Europe, September 21–23, Ljubljana, Slovenia.

Loison-Leruste, M., & Quilgars, D. (2009). Increasing access to housing: Implementing the right to housing in England and France. *European Journal of Homelessness, 3*.

Lowe, D. The medical examination of mentally disordered/mentally vulnerable detainees in police custody in England and Wales. Unpublished paper, Liverpool John Moores University.

Madianos, M. (2004). Clinical psychiatry: Psychiatric administration. Athens, Greece: Kastaniotis.

Madianos, M.G., Economou, M., Hatjiandreou, M., Papageorgiou, A., & Rogakou, E. (1999). Changes in public attiitudes towards mental illness in the Athens area (1979/1980–1994). *Acta Psychiatrica Scandinavica, 99*(1), 73–78.

Madianos, M.G., Priami, M., Alevisopooulos, G., Koukia, E., & Rogakou, E. (2005). Nursing students' attitude change towards mental illness and psychiatric case recognition after a clerkship in psychiatry. *Issues in Mental Health Nursing, 26*(2), 169–183.

McGilloway, S., & Donnelly, M. (2004). Mental illness in the UK criminal justice system: A police liaison scheme for mentally disordered offenders in Belfast. *Journal of Mental Health, 13*(3), 263–275.

Mercuel, A. (2008). Mobile psychiatric teams in France. In *Crisis intervention, social context, psychopathology, and deviance* [in French]. Paris: Furtos J (Masson).

Ministerial Council on Deaths in Custody, Independent Advisory Panel. (2011). Recommendations. Review of the medical theories and research relating to restraint related deaths.

Muijen, M. (2008). Mental disability services in Europe. An overview. *Psychiatric Services, 59*(5), 479–482.

Nemitz, T., & Bean, P. (2001). Protecting the rights of the mentally disordered in police stations: The use of the appropriate adult in England and Wales. *International Journal of Law and Psychiatry, 24*, 595–605.

Penrose, L.S. (1939). Mental disease and crime: Outline of a comparative study of European statistics. *British Journal of Medical Psychology, 18*, 1–15.

Pinfold, V., Thornicroft, G., Huxley, P., & Farmer, P. (2005). Active ingredients in anti-stigma programmes in mental health. *International Review of Psychiatry, 17*(2), 123–131.

Priebe, S., Badesconyi, A., Fioritti, A., Hansson, L., Kilian, R., Torres-Gonzales, F., et al. (2005). Reinstitutionalisation in mental health care: Comparison of data on service provision from six European countries. *British Medical Journal, 330*, 123–126.

Priebe, S., Frottier, P., Gaddini, A., Kilian, R., Lauber, C., Martinez-Leal, R., et al. (2008). Mental health care institutions in nine European countries, 2002–2006. *Psychiatric Services, 59*, 570–573.

Psarra, V., Sestrini, M., Santa, Z., Petsas, D., Gerontas, A., Garnetas, C., et al. (2008). Greek police officers' attitudes towards the mentally ill. *International Journal of Law and Psychiatry, 31*, 77–85.

Riordan, S., Wix, S., Kenney-Herbert, J., & Humphries, M. (2000). Diversion at the point of arrest: Mentally disordered people and contact with the police. *Journal of Forensic Psychiatry, 11*(3), 683–690.

Sainsbury Centre for Mental Health. (2008a). *Briefing 36: Police and mental health.* London.

Sainsbury Centre for Mental Health. (2008b). *In the dark. The mental health implications of imprisonment for public protection.* London.

Sainsbury Centre for Mental Health. (2009). *Diversion. A better way for criminal justice and mental health.* London.

Sanders, A., Young, R., & Burton, M. (2010). *Criminal justice* (4th ed.). Oxford: Oxford University Press.

Sestoft, D., Rasmussen, M.F., Vitus, K., & Kongsrud, L. (Forthcoming). The police, social services and psychiatry cooperation in Denmark—A new model of working practice between government sectors. A description of the concept, process, practice and experience. *International Journal of Law & Psychiatry.*

van Oijen, G. (2011, May). The mentally handicapped suspect interrogated [De verstandelijk beperkte verdachte verhoord] (English abstract only). *Process, 3.*

Vermette, H., Pinals, D., & Appelbaum, P. (2005). Mental health training for law enforcement professionals. *Journal of the American Academy of Psychiatry and the Law, 33*(1), 42–46.

Warner, R. (2008). Implementing local projects to reduce the stigma of mental illness. *Epidemiologia e Psichiatria Sociale, 17*(1), 20–25.

Wierdsma, A.I., Poodt, H.D., & Mulder, C.L. (2007). Effects of community-care networks on psychiatric emergency contacts, hospitalisation and involuntary admission. *Journal of Epidemiology and Community Health, 61*, 613–618.

Wundsam, K., Pitschel-Walz, G., Leucht, S., & Kissling, W. (2007). Psychiatric patients and relatives instruct German police officers—An anti-stigma project of "BASTA—The alliance for mentally ill people." *Psychiatrische Praxis, 34*(4), 181–187.

Vitus, K., & Kjaer, A.A. (2011). *The police, social service and psychiatry (PSP) cooperation. A survey of PSP Frederiksberg, Odense, Amager and Esbjerg* [in Danish]. Copenhagen, Denmark: The Danish National Centre for Social Research.

Zinkler, M., & Priebe, S. (2002). Detention of the mentally ill in Europe—A review. *Acta Psychiatrica Scandinavica, 106*(1), 3–8.

Developments in Australia

II

NSW Police Force Mental Health Intervention Team

4

Forging a New Path Forward in Mental Health and Policing in the Community

DAVID DONOHUE
GINA ANDREWS

Contents

Introduction

The NSWPF aims to ensure that we are not unnecessarily interacting with mental health consumers, or having consumers in our custody without cause. All NSWPF interactions with mentally ill and disordered persons need to be justifiable via legislative provisions. We do not want mentally ill persons becoming unduly "criminalised" because they have needlessly come under police notice and management. Research of the wider criminal justice system in NSW finds that over 40% of the persons in the criminal justice system have mental illness or mental disorder or cognitive disability (Baldry, 2012). From a NSWPF perspective this rate is too high. We need additional and better criminal justice diversion mechanisms for mentally ill and disordered persons. Such diversion mechanisms would see suitable consumers diverted by the police and courts into appropriate and integrated community-based clinical (such as adequate community mental health), forensic, and human service care that is tailored to manage consumers with serious mental illness to live supported and full lives in the community.

We state unapologetically that the police role is vital (yet relatively small) when it comes to managing the mentally ill and disordered in the community. Specifically, NSWPF's role is to manage acutely mentally ill persons in the community who are "high risk" and at direct risk of harm to themselves or others. High risk in this context is an incident where a mental health consumer poses a significant threat of harm to himself or herself or others. In these circumstances our police role is to safely, empathetically, and efficiently detain the mentally ill or disordered person under police statutory powers, as per the Mental Health Act 2007 (NSW), and transport the detained person via appropriate (and humane) transport to the nearest NSW Health emergency department or psychiatric facility for assessment, care, and treatment.

Throughout the NSWPF detention process we are proponents of the least restrictive methods for managing acutely mentally ill persons. Supporting this position are the Section 3 objectives of the Mental Health Act 2007 (NSW), and the fact that Australia is a signatory to the United Nation's Universal Declaration of Human Rights and the Convention on the Rights of Persons with Disabilities (CRPD) (NSW CAG, 2012). As party to these international treaties, Australian law at a federal and state level is required to enforce the principles contained in these treaties into relevant legislation, policy, and practise (NSW CAG, 2012). These treaties require that persons be treated with equal respect, irrespective of race, gender, age, and disability. An underlying drive in the CRPD is that it proscribes equal rights of all persons with disabilities to live in the community, with choices equal to others (Siska and Beadle-Brown, 2011). Further, these treaties aim to support the systems changes needed to ensure that persons with disabilities are treated equally. Australia's ratification of these treaties means that mental health consumers have equal and ready access to health care, managed with dignity, and have their human rights upheld. NSWPF upholds Australia's ratification of these treaties, and these instruments' principles guide our philosophical approach to mental health and policing.

Finally, and this is a point that we made in open forums and in our presentations at the 2011 32nd International Academy of Mental Health Law Conference to the policing and research fraternity present, the fraternity needs to be mindful to not unduly promote an industry for itself (Andrews, 2011; Donohue, 2011). The police role should remain a small, yet vital slice of the mental health service delivery sector, a role that is based on the presence of their being high risk and ensuring the safe apprehension and transportation of the consumer to the nearest suitable health facility for mental health assessment care and treatment. Unfortunately, there is still some resistance throughout the wider health sector with this position. Traditionally, as the result of archaic legislation and attitudes, police were disproportionately assigned responsibility to detain and transport persons under the Mental Health Act 2007 (NSW) from the community and between health settings. NSWPF has challenged this outdated and anticonsumer human rights approach, and aims to take policing and mental health into the twenty-first century. Despite this, some sectors still consider police must play a more significant role in managing mental health consumers in crisis.

Policing in New South Wales (NSW)

In 2011 Australia had a population of 22,696,000 (Australian Bureau of Statistics, 2012). NSW is the largest and most populous jurisdiction in Australia. NSW is one of seven states and territories in Australia. Finally, in Australia we have a federalist structure, whereby under the constitution the delivery of police and health services is devolved from the federal government, and is largely the remit of the states and territories.

Approximately one-third of Australia's population, or 7.2 million residents, reside in the state of NSW. Approximately 4.8 million of NSW's residents (63%) live in the capital city, Sydney (Business NSW, 2012). The remaining most voluminous subpopulation groups live in the regional cities on NSW's coastline. Sydney is also known as one of the world's most culturally diverse cities, due to its large migrant population. Finally, NSW is also a geographically diverse state with approximately 801,600 square kilometres, which covers the extremes of desert, a large coastline, and mountain terrain (NSW Police Force, 2012a). NSW is comparable in size to Texas in the United States, and is double the combined geographic areas of England, Scotland, and Wales (NSW Police Force, 2012a). Such sheer size results in one of the greatest policing challenges for the NSWPF—policing the vast distances between regional and rural centres. Such distances, combined with the distances between state-run NSW Health declared mental health facilities (the psychiatric facility premises subject to an order in force under Section 109 of the Mental Health Act (NSW) in regional and rural NSW), result in police resource pressure when managing mentally ill or disordered consumers in these areas.

NSW Police Force is 150 years old. It is the oldest and largest policing jurisdiction in Australia, and possibly in the English-speaking world. As of March 2012, the NSWPF has an actual authorised strength of 15,867 staff (NSW Police Force, 2012a). The NSW Police Force provides community-based policing in more than 500 police stations, to a wide range of culturally diverse communities speaking more than 30 languages throughout NSW (NSW Police Force, 2012a).

Mental Health and Policing in NSW

NSW Police Force's aim is to provide a world-class police response to those people in our community suffering acute mental illness. The NSWPF's Mental Health Intervention Team (MHIT) is at the forefront of community policing acute mental health in Australasia. Since the introduction of the NSWPF MHIT training model in 2008, NSWPF has made real achievements toward sustainable results for police, emergency services, and most importantly, consumers. As a result of the MHIT trial and implementation of MHIT, NSW Police Force has continued its close partnership with NSW Health, other government agencies, and consumer organisations. The MHIT model has already shown significant results in terms of policing, namely, in delivering quality mental health police education, and subsequently ensuring that the police are more confident in their skills and ability to interact with mental health consumers (Herrington, Clifford, Lawrence, Ryle, & Pope, 2009).

In 2011 the NSW Police Force responded to 36,583 mental health-related incidents. Within this number police attended 26,451 Mental Health Act unique incidents (NSW Police Force, 2012c). Figures 4.1 and 4.2 show that these annual police figures have been stable, with a slight steady increase

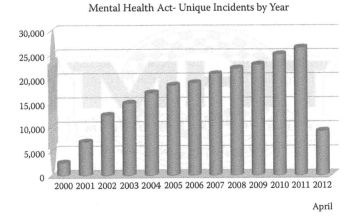

Figure 4.1 NSW Police Force Computerised Operating Policing System—total number of incidents under the Mental Health Act per annum.

Year	Unique Incidents
2000	2,659
2001	6,995
2002	12,499
2003	14,957
2004	17,089
2005	18.633
2006	19,138
2007	20,973
2008	22,121
2009	22,938
2010	25,063
2011	26,451
2012–April	9,175

Figure 4.2 NSW Police Force Computerised Operating Policing System—total number of incidents under the Mental Health Act per annum.

over recent years. Police management of mental health issues in the community represents a sizeable proportion of police business. In 2002, a survey of 131 Sydney-based police officers revealed that more than 10% of police time is spent managing persons with "mental health problems" (Fry, cited in Clifford, 2010). While such figures are debated, the data are an indication of the proportion of business that managing persons with mental health problems is for police. In a policing context, we would define a person suffering mental health problems as a person who is experiencing some form of mental illness or disorder that is affecting his or her rational decision-making process or when his or her culpability is affected. Complementing Fry's findings, it is our operational experience that police management of persons with mental health problems (as opposed to the narrow legislative definitions of mental illness (Mental Health Act 2007, s. 4) or disorder (Mental Health Act 2007, s. 15)) constitutes on average 10% to 15% of our operational work.

NSW Police Force: Mental Health Policing Priorities

Our corporate focus is to ensure police are involved in the safe and humane detention and transportation of high-risk mentally ill or disordered persons under police provisions in the Mental Health Act 2007 (NSW). We have prioritised three policy and legislative initiatives to support the progression of our philosophical position. First, in 2010 we implemented a policy directive that resulted in our police vehicles no longer being used in interhospital transport of mental health patients between mental health facilities. Second, we are negotiating at an interagency level the reassignment of police court-ordered transportation duties under Section 33, Mental Health Forensic Provisions 1990 (NSW). An amendment to this act allowed the Department of Corrective Services and Ambulance Service NSW new powers to transport persons who have been diverted from the criminal justice system, for the purpose of psychiatric assessment at a hospital. In reality, the continual reluctance of other agencies to take part in this process results in transportation responsibility falling back onto police. Our third priority is to ensure that there is a more balanced geographical cross section of Section 109 declared mental health facilities across NSW, enabling police to readily take persons they detain under the Mental Health Act 2007 (NSW) for assessment.

All three of these initiatives seek to minimise unnecessary police involvement with mental health consumers—and are in line with relevant human rights values (i.e., to minimise the unnecessary criminalisation of mentally ill persons due to police management of consumers) and the objectives of the Mental Health Act 2007 (NSW).

What the MHIT Delivers

The Mental Health Intervention Team is now an established name among Australasian police and the NSW mental health service delivery community. There are five facets to the MHIT model: the provision of training, policy development and advice, research, the provision of operational advice, and programme delivery.

First, the MHIT's premium training product is its four-day intensive training course. It trains on average one class of 30 police officers per month in a four-day training programme. Its goal is to train 10% of all NSWPF operational police by the end of 2015. Since its inception in 2007, by August 2012 it had trained over 887 NSW Police Force officers (including 18 health other police from across Australia and New Zealand) in its four-day MHIT course. NSWPF also provides a range of other mental health education and training products that are mainstreamed into existing police training courses (e.g., mental health is mainstreamed into the safe custody, domestic violence liaison, and police prosecutors training courses).

Second, the MHIT is involved in a diverse range of government policy development and coordination duties. For example, the NSW Police Force is a standing member on the NSW Mental Health Senior Officer Group and the NSW and Commonwealth Suicide Prevention Committees. Our main policy development and implementation responsibility is to ensure police are compliant with their responsibilities as outlined in the NSW Emergency Mental Health Memorandum of Understanding (MOU). The MOU is the key policy instrument that details police operational responsibilities, and other emergency services, as per the Mental Health Act 2007 (NSW).

Third, we are active in the research community. We value evidence-based policy research. We see our participation in research as contributing to the development of a strong evidence base to test and inform policing directions. We are currently managing four university-affiliated research projects. For example, we recently completed a NSW government quantitative research project with the University of NSW, "Mental Health Frequent Presenters to Police" (Baldry, Dowse, & Clarence, 2012a), and continue our involvement in a longitudinal piece of research with the University of NSW, "Mental Health Disorders and Cognitive Disabilities in the Criminal Justice System" (Baldry, Dowse, & Webster, 2012b).

Fourth, the MHIT provides 24-hour high-level operational advice to NSW police officers. This means that the manager of the MHIT is available 24/7 to operational staff to provide operational advice in cases of crisis.

Fifth, the MHIT provides a range of internal programmes tailored to police needs. For example, the MHIT manages a statewide network of 80 NSW Police Force mental health contact officers (one inspector in each of the 80 NSW local area commands). Each of the six police regions is represented by a superintendent. The MHIT manages the mental health contact officers network (i.e., 6 key superintendents and 80 inspectors of police) across NSW to ensure the streamlined implementation of the MOU and legislative compliance at a local level.

With four full-time staff and a part-time corporate spokesperson for mental health, the MHIT contains significant expertise in this complex area of mental health and policing.

Development of the Mental Health Intervention Team (MHIT), NSW Police Force

Today the way that NSW Police Force officers handle their interactions with high-risk mental health consumers has changed greatly due to our intensive MHIT police training programme (Laing, Halsey, Donohue, Newman, & Cashin, 2009). However, the impetus for MHIT training was sadly due to negative findings from a 2002 NSW parliamentary inquiry, and a growing number of adverse coroners' findings in NSW whereby coroners had recommended more comprehensive mental health training for our police officers.

The 2002 New South Wales Parliament Legislative Council's Select Committee on Mental Health

Inquiry into mental health services in New South Wales found that "police do a commendable job when encountering and assisting people with a mental illness" (NSW Parliament, 2002, p. 244). Police are not, however, trained to undertake the level of service they currently perform. It was identified at this inquiry that there was no specific mental health training for police. Rather, mental health training was a component of other training models (e.g., general recruitment training or in safe custody training) (NSW Parliament, 2002, p. 245). The police association indicated at the time that while training has improved, it did not go far enough (NSW Parliament, 2002, p. 244).

Echoing the parliamentary inquiry's findings, a 2004 NSW state coroner report entitled "Recommendations into Mental Health Issues" details a number of coronial reports with findings and recommendations that advocate additional mental health education and training for police. A typical example of such coroners' findings and recommendations during this time is encapsulated by Coroner Milledge:

> That the NSW Police Service urgently provides comprehensive training to all
> NSW Police Academy students and operational police officers in the appropri-
> ate dealing with the mentally ill. Such training should include issues such as
> the recognition of common and significant psychiatric problems, techniques
> for dealing with mentally ill persons and legal issues associated therewith.
> (NSW Coroner's Court, 2012)

As the NSWPF corporate spokesperson for mental health since 2008, David Donahue gave evidence at numerous coronial inquiries in the past five years where the consistent theme from these inquests has been ongoing recommendations for additional mental health training for frontline police.

On average over the last 10 years NSWPF has been subject to just under two adverse coroners' investigations annually, whereby police have shot or killed a mental health consumer during the course of operational duties. Such events deeply affect all those involved: police, other services, the wider community, and most importantly, the consumer's family. There are no winners in these scenarios, and the importance of adequate police training to be able to manage mental health consumers in acute situations is of increasing importance.

Following the findings of the 2002 Parliamentary Select Committee, and ongoing negative coroners' recommendations, in January 2006 an internal NSW Police Force working party was commissioned by the previous corporate spokesperson for mental health (David Owens) to review training for police on mental health. The working party identified three main areas of training delivery:

- NSW Police Force College—recruit training
- Field operations—continuing and mandatory training (safe custody, mandatory continuing police education (MCPE), internal publications)
- Specialist training—SPG negotiator training

Through a process of interview and audit, each NSWPF mental health training product was assessed and rated. A number of products were identified as outdated or too theoretical. While some products did have operational relevance, the key finding was that police had insufficient specialised training in mental health. Training that was delivered was typically ad hoc and lacked standardisation. This 2006 review also led to our research of North American mental health and policing solutions.

Background to the Development of the Mental Health Intervention Team (MHIT), NSW Police Force

The combination of the findings of the 2002 NSW Parliamentary Committee review, ongoing negative coroners' findings, lack of academic peer-reviewed publications on mental health and community policing training models, and the NSW Police Force review of mental health education and training products resulted in a NSW Police and NSW Health research tour of the United States in late 2006.

The objective of the research tour was to identify the best model of policing acute mental illness in the community setting for NSW. The reason the United States was selected for the research tour was that some of the jurisdictions within the United States are seen as world-leading experts when it comes to operational policing and managing acute high-risk mental illness in the community. Speculated causal factors for U.S. leadership in this field is primarily due to wider community access to guns, and the relatively higher numbers of police shootings of mental health consumers as a result of operational interactions. This has resulted in many U.S. jurisdictions having to scrutinise and refine their operational responses when it comes to policing the mentally ill in the community, and hence develop tailored policing training programmes.

In November 2006, David Owens (then an assistant commissioner and the NSWPF corporate spokesperson for mental health) and myself (in my capacity then as a NSWPF mental health contact officer) undertook a study tour on the status of mental health and community policing in the United States. Dr. Kevin Wolfenden, manager, Emergency Mental Health Care Program, NSW Health, also attended as our interagency research partner.

We visited five policing jurisdictions in the United States, and reviewed their response to policing and mental health. These included:

- Los Angeles Police Department—Systemwide Mental Assessment Response Team (SMART)
- Memphis Crisis Intervention Team (CIT)
- Chicago CIT
- New York
- Honolulu

These jurisdictions were chosen for a range of reasons. Memphis was chosen because its model was a collaboration with the University of Memphis and Professor Randolph Dupont (University of Memphis, 2012). Further, Memphis CIT is accepted as the home and leader of the original crisis inter-vention team (CIT) model. Chicago was chosen due to the similarity of its police force size to NSW's, as well as its then chief of police, Philip Cline, who was known as an innovative thinker. Los Angeles (ride-along model) was chosen because it would provide a comparative policing approach to the CIT. It was thought that New York may provide an alternative policing approach on the back of its former chief, William Bratton, being an innova-tive police commissioner leader. Honolulu was reviewed due to its reported "ice" (methamphetamine) epidemic at the time, and its possible parallels with NSW regarding ice use and mental health policing responses.

Each jurisdiction had either some similarity to NSW and the NSWPF in terms of socioeconomic status, population size, and policing issues, or known excellence in community policing and mental illness in the community.

Essentially the research presented two policing models adapted to pro-vide efficient policing responses to persons suffering mental illness. These two main models of innovation, developed in the United States, are the police-based specialised response, such as the Memphis Crisis Intervention Team (Cochran, Deane, & Borum, 2000; Hails & Borum, 2003), and adap-tations of a civilian officer ride-along model (Steadman, Williams-Deane, Borum, & Morrissey, 2000), which includes police-based specialised men-tal health response and the mental health-based specialised mental health response (Steadman et al., 2000; Hails & Borum, 2003; Reuland, 2004). Both models are reliant on interface with local health systems to ensure a receptive and efficient site to transfer care from police to health care services in appropriate cases (Cashin et al., 2006). What follows is an evaluation of our police research tour of the United States and the available literature review that informed the 2006 tour.

When evaluating each of these U.S. models we also considered the current legislative, resource, and geographic operating conditions within NSW. The model that we proposed to the NSWPF executive was considered to be what was achievable within these conditions. The proposed model for the NSW Police Force is informed heavily by the CIT model in Chicago. However, an innovation to this model is the employment of a NSW Health professional within the NSWPF MHIT.

Memphis—Crisis Intervention Team (CIT)

Our research tour started with the Memphis CIT model. The rationale to start with Memphis was that it is often accepted as the pioneer and standard when it comes to mental health and policing education and training. It is commonly accepted that the Memphis CIT model has had a profound effect on policing standards in North America, Canada, and Australasia.

Since commencement of the CIT programme in 1988, Major Sam Cochran (the Memphis police architect of CIT) and Dr. Randolph Dupont (key evaluator from the University of Memphis) have been pivotal in the development and success of CIT not only in Memphis, but internationally. They and their CIT officers have assisted in the training of officers and the development of CIT in many agencies throughout the United States.

The impetus behind the Memphis CIT model was the unfortunate death in 1987 of 27-year-old Joseph Dewayne Robinson, who was shot and killed during an incident with the Memphis Police Department. This shooting outraged the local community. Subsequently, in 1988, the Memphis (Tennessee) Police Department began working with members of the Local Alliance for the Mentally Ill and designed the crisis intervention team (CIT), in which specially trained officers respond to incidents involving people with mental illness.

The Memphis CIT training model is a joint initiative involving the Memphis Police Department, Memphis Chapter of the Alliance for the Mentally Ill, mental health providers, the University of Memphis and the University of Tennessee (Cable, 2013). These organisations work in partnership to train the specialised CIT unit. In addition to the initial 40 hours of CIT training, officers receive annual top-up training provided by mental health professionals. The CIT Memphis model works on a volunteer basis from within the Memphis Police Department, although candidates do have to apply to go through a selection process. According to the Memphis Police Department website, there are currently 225 Memphis PD-trained officers (Memphis Police Department, 2012). Putting this in perspective, the Memphis Police Department has an authorised strength of 2,977, which includes 288 civilian employees. CIT-trained officers make up approximately 8% of the Memphis uniformed police (Memphis Police Department, 2010).

The CIT model seeks to enhance and educate police response to people with mental illness in crisis; aims to prevent the mentally ill population from harming themselves, the community, or officers; and aims to prevent the police from harming people with mental illnesses in crisis situations.

The CIT training model is delivered in four stages. First, officers are educated on mental illness. Second, officers visit mental health centres and participate in group discussions with mental health consumers. Police are able to freely discuss with the consumer their experiences with law enforcement. Third, officers are assigned realistic scenarios regarding different mental illness crises, role-playing their responses. The final training session consists of discussing appropriate handling of various situations with individuals who have mental illness (Path Program Archives, 2001).

The CIT model promotes the dispatch of a CIT officer as soon as an incident has been categorised as possibly involving a person experiencing mental illness. The CIT officer is delegated as in charge of the incident involving a consumer, regardless of the rank or seniority of the other police at the scene.

Memphis police patrol as a single unit in a police car (i.e., one police officer per car), and in predetermined geographic areas known as sectors. Each officer knows his or her sector well, and typically the acute mental health consumers who reside within his or her area. CIT officers proactively attend the homes of local consumers who interact with police, ensuring they are taking medication and aiming to maintain a relationship with the consumer.

The CIT programme also aims to act as a jail diversion, keeping mental health consumers out of the criminal justice system and placing them into appropriate health care services. A CIT-trained officer is able to provide an eligible person a precharge criminal justice diversion option via prebooking programmes. This aspect of the CIT model aims to increase the care of the people with mental illness in the community setting, and reduce the inappropriate use of jails to house people with acute mental illness.

Evaluations of the CIT model have been positive. Key findings include reductions in injuries to individuals and police, reduction in downtime through waiting at hospitals for assessment, jail diversion, and improvements in consumer treatment and medication use. Importantly, the model has been assessed to be effective (e.g., cost-effective) and has improved police-community relations. The CIT model has been promoted as a best practise model for mental health policing (Dupont & Cochran, 2000).

A key finding worthy of discussion is that since the introduction of CIT training there has been a dramatic decrease in police use of lethal force. This has positively impacted the rate of injuries to Memphis police and individuals with mental illnesses interacting with police. Since the introduction of CIT training in 1988 there have been two deaths in custody of mental health consumers (both involved non-CIT-trained officers). Memphis police note that no CIT Memphis-trained officer has been associated with a death in custody of a mental health consumer since training was introduced. On top of this there has been a 40% reduction in reported injuries by police officers to individuals with mental illnesses (Dupont & Cochran, 2000; Reuland, Schwarzfeld, & Draper, 2009).

Another key finding worthy of discussion is that the CIT programme is also successful in goal diversion in Memphis. For example, jail custody of people with mental illness has dropped from 15% in 1988 (when the CIT was introduced) to 3% presently. The national average of imprisonment of individuals with mental illness in the United States is between 15% and 20%. Prior to the implementation of CIT, 20 arrests were made per 100 calls. In 2006 this decreased by 90% to 2 arrests per 100 calls (Dupont & Cochran, 2000). This finding shows the safety dividend of the CIT Memphis model (Reuland et al., 2009).

In summary, results from the CIT Memphis programme demonstrate lower rates of arrests (diversion), quicker response to emergency calls, enhanced safety of consumers and officers, and the training has left a positive impression on officers (Dupont & Cochran, 2000; Reuland et al., 2009).

CIT Memphis Application to the NSW Police Force

CIT Memphis strengths assessed by NSWPF include:

- Relevant to existing practises in NSW, the Memphis CIT programme implemented a memorandum of understanding between Memphis police and the local hospital emergency department. The effect of the MOU was that it reduced the time of officer involvement when seeking psychiatric involuntary assessment for a consumer. Lengthy hospital waiting times had been a major barrier for officers wishing to use the option of diversion (as opposed to arrest). CIT administrative efficiencies, and a reduction in police time spent at the emergency department, had relevance and appeal to the NSW situation.
- Strong knowledge within the community of the role of a CIT-trained officer. This was achieved through initial media coverage and recognition of the CIT badge police officers wear. Subsequently, CIT-trained police became known to consumers and carers, and members of the public started to ask for CIT officers.

- The CIT officer is able to determine that the consumer does not need psychiatric assessment. That is, if the original call consisted of a threat of self-harm or harm to another, the CIT officer is able to establish that the person is not in need of immediate care and establish appropriate diversion strategies. This is different from NSW, where the Mental Health Act (NSW) and common law duty of care issue places onus on police to have the person assessed by a delegated clinician.

However, we assessed three key challenges associated with the CIT Memphis model:

1. High resource investment and costs:
   - CIT training involves 40 hours (it is resource-intensive).
   - High training costs (training involves frontline police, course administrators, course instructors, and guest speakers).
   - The Memphis CIT model offers 24-hour community policing coverage (via four different overlapping fixed shifts).
2. Continued and unnecessary police involvement:
   - The CIT model advocates police as first responders (i.e., the primary agency responsible for the transportation of consumers for involuntary admission). However, NSWPF advocates that it is unnecessary for police to always be the first responder. Rather, police decisions on involvement should be based on high risk being present.
   - There is no ambulance involvement in the Memphis CIT model. This results in unnecessary pressure on police to undertake transports. Further, this means that consumers' clinical needs are not being addressed. Finally, this process runs contrary to our NSWPF human rights approach, in that many consumers who are not high risk are being unnecessarily criminalised due to police transportation involvement.
   - We have concern about CIT officers' proactive attendance of consumers' premises as part of follow-up. First, NSWPF does not see this as a core police function; rather, this is clinical or human services responsibility. Second, there is a risk that police presence can incite the person. This position was supported by Dr. Kevin Wolfenden (NSW Health), who accompanied NSWPF on our study tour to Memphis.
3. Police referral of involuntary persons for mental health assessment were not always accepted or processed quickly. The CIT model, as per the MOU, depends on 100% acceptance of all police referrals to the emergency department. This is key to the programme's evaluated success, that is, quick police officer release. The CIT programme may report

100% acceptance; however, our interactions with frontline Memphis police in 2006 disputed this assertion. This finding questions the credibility of the CIT Memphis model. Our site visits to the hospital reception provided us the opportunity to discuss the reception experience with mental health clinicians and police officers. While established MOU processes advocate the streamline reception and assessment of CIT officers' mental health referrals, a number of dislocations in the reception process were recognised. Process inefficiencies were attributed to the health insurance status of the consumer and the lack of availability of a psychiatrist or delegated medical officer at reception.

Los Angeles Systemwide Mental Assessment Response Team (SMART)

The Los Angeles Police Department employs 99,104 sworn officers and 2,827 unsworn staff (LAPD, 2012). Los Angeles is reported as the largest population in the state of California, with 3,792,621. It is the second most populous U.S. state after New York (U.S. Census Bureau, 2010).

The Los Angeles Police Department has a mental evaluation unit (MEU) that provides mental health and policing advice and service delivery. The MEU mission is to reduce the potential for violence during police contacts involving people suffering from mental illness, while also assessing available mental health services to refer the consumer to.

The MEU includes the Systemwide Mental Assessment Response Team (SMART). SMART is an operational arm of the MEU, in which mental health counsellors and police work together out of the LAPD premise side by side. This means that police officers and mental health clinicians are housed out of the same building and respond to calls as a team. The concept is that the SMART model frees up frontline police once they have come into contact with a mental health consumer. SMART officers work with police referrals to manage the assessment, diversion, and further referral process.

SMART officers attend incidents and make initial assessments. Depending on the nature of the offence, consumers can be released into police custody, not apprehended at all, or arrangements made with a receiving mental health provider.

The SMART team forms a central point of contact for all police information and advice for both police and mental health service providers. It is mandatory to notify the SMART section when a mental health consumer comes under LAPD notice. While a LAPD police or mental health worker can detain a mental health consumer, the placement of the consumer into the health system is done by the mental health worker (not the police).

SMART officers' recruitment is voluntary. It was apparent that police working in this area had prior mental health experience or a background in general nursing. We could not locate any publicly available data on the numbers of SMART-trained LAPD officers.

The SMART model employs a soft clothing (plainclothes) approach to facilitate the de-escalation of matters. It is accepted that consumers feel that the plainclothes option is less threatening than a uniformed approach.

Despite the fact that police and health officers work side by side, client case files from each organisation are separately managed. Typically, officers from each agency work together and exchange information about the consumer in preparation for a mental health assessment. Once the medical consult occurs, police take no further role.

High-risk consumers apprehended by SMART LAPD officers from the community setting are then taken to the nearest police station. Typically, LAPD transport from the field to the police station in police vehicles (a caged sedan is typically used as the first response vehicle). Transportation from the police station to a mental health facility is then by ambulance. Like NSW, LA ambulance can also use mechanical restraints for mental health consumers. Currently, the SMART team is located centrally and can provide operational and clinical advice via its police and clinicians, in each of the LAPD's four geographical commands, with a total of four car crews, 20 hours a day, 7 days a week, clinical (LAPD, 2011).

It is understood that in April 2008 the threat management team joined up with the MEU. This amalgamation enhanced the MEU's profiling capabilities. The threat management team profiles stalking suspects and workplace violence suspects. It is the LAPD experience that often such suspects experience some form of mental health crisis when they make threats and when they are engaging in acts of violence (RTBOT, 2012).

Also operating within the SMART model is the Case Assessment Management Program (CAMP). The more experienced detectives and health workers work in this area. This is where detectives and mental health workers follow up on what we in NSW refer to as mental health frequent presenters. The CAMP team also manages the high-risk cases, monitoring any changed patterns of behaviour. Proactive action is taken wherever possible. SMART officers take a proactive approach by analysing trends in the consumer or person of interest's behaviour. These data then inform a joint agency case management strategy, which aims to maximise the consumers' mental health and minimise the consumers' interactions with police.

CAMP officers do follow-up court visits, giving the judge assurance that mental health issues will be followed up. CAMP officers also do proactive follow-ups (home visits) and inquire if medication is being taken and doctors visits are being attended.

SMART Model Application to the NSW Police Force

The SMART model is a comprehensive mental health policing model. The SMART team is a central point of contact for both the entire LAPD and external agencies. The SMART team uses intelligence and court processes well to manage their frequent users, who are often a large drain on police resources.

There also seems to be adequate sharing of information between agencies for the betterment of the consumer.

The use of plainclothes and unmarked police vehicles is a positive. Police wearing plainclothes is a passive de-escalation technique. NSWPF consumer feedback has found that the police uniform and accompanying tactical appointments (e.g., firearms) are perceived to intimidate and threaten consumers. In some cases uniforms and appointments add to consumers' paranoia.

The SMART model is, however, resource-intensive. The cost of such a unit would be considerable in both setup and management. Our search of evaluations of the SMART model found that there were no independent academic or peer-reviewed evaluations of this model, or cost of the model.

SMART officers, while mobile and proactive in the majority of their work, were not always first responders. Accordingly, there was often some duplication in handling of jobs. If a SMART team was not dispatched to the job, the LAPD officer would then bring the consumer back to central division, where the SMART team would take over. In NSW it would not be considered best practise to convey a consumer, not under arrest, back to a police station for assessment by police and then await transport to a suitable institution. As identified earlier, such a situation would also undermine NSWPF's philosophical objective to decriminalise mental illness via minimising unnecessary consumer interactions with police.

Chicago CIT

Chicago Police employ approximately 12,244 sworn police officers, and approximately 1,925 other employees. Chicago has a population of 2,874,312 (U.S. Census Bureau, 2010). As a jurisdiction, it is slightly smaller in size than Sydney, NSW.

The Chicago Police have adopted a police model similar to that of Memphis CIT, with slight modifications to suit Chicago's policing environment. The Chicago CIT model is based on the Memphis CIT model.

The development and implementation of the Chicago CIT programme was driven by a small working group of advocates from the Chicago Police Department, National Alliance for the Mentally Ill of Greater Chicago (NAMI-GC), Illinois Department of Human Services, Office of Mental

Health, the Cook County Jail, and the Circuit Court of Cook County. Initial discussions began in 1999. The Chicago model aimed to address consumers needs with the following initiatives:

1. A voluntary consumer database. This can be accessed by first responders, treatment providers, the Cook County Jail, and the Circuit Court of Cook County. The database provides basic consumer information, including the nature of the illness, contact history, current medication, and so forth.
2. The establishment of a mental health court.
3. A prisoner reentry programme—linking persons leaving the corrections system with mental health services in the community.
4. Linkage of client database to inmate database at Cook County Jail to better identify mental health consumers upon entrance into jail.
5. Implement the CIT programme for the Chicago Police Department (NAMI, 2008).

In early 2004, Chicago Police began a CIT training trial with 80 police (supervisors and police officers). Forty police were trained in the two selected police districts. The two locations were selected because of the diversity of the community, health care services within these areas, and the two locations had the largest population of mental health consumers. Training began in October 2004, and the pilot programmes began in July 1, 2005. The CIT model was implemented in 2006 after the trial (Canada, Angell, & Watson, 2010).

A key aim for Chicago CIT is that most police divisions have 20% of their workforce trained in CIT. The Chicago CIT model includes a CIT supervisor (sergeant) on every three-person team. The rationale is because only the sergeants (supervisors) presently carry the taser appointment in the team. The taser provides a less lethal force option in crisis intervention. The CIT sergeant also has command and control of the scene, keeping untrained officers from interfering with CIT intervention, which they may not understand the complexities involved. The CIT sergeant understands that successful intervention may take time, and ensures the time investment necessary for nonforce options, reducing the risk of injury to officers and consumers in crisis.

As with the Memphis CIT, CIT supervisors and police officers must volunteer for the training.

Parallel initiatives to the CIT also need to be noted for their significance, as they all potentially positively impact consumer and agency outcomes. For example, in tandem with the implementation of CIT in the Chicago Police Department, the mental health court in Cook County was established. The Cook County Mental Health Court is the first felony mental health court in the United States, and the first court to directly link CIT-trained officers to the court. CIT officers involved in the mental health court project often are involved in locating and returning court-related clients safely back to programme service providers.

Chicago CIT Application to NSW Police Force

When compared to the Memphis CIT model, the Chicago CIT is a more comprehensive programme model for six reasons.

First, Chicago CIT has a strong involvement of health and other agencies. There is a heavy emphasis on consumer representatives having an active voice in the Chicago CIT programme.

Second, in contrast to Memphis, the Chicago CIT training model targets sergeants, alleviating the command and control issue that would arise with a junior officer attending the scene and taking command of a high-risk incident.

Third, there is a greater use of intelligence and integration with the Chicago CIT. The Chicago CIT is involved in a diverse range of consumer-related duties: the search for missing persons, investigation of patients under the control of the mental health court, and retrieval of these persons back to the court.

Fourth, there is a dedicated CIT office, and there is a CIT office coordinator to facilitate the CIT programme. A high-ranking lieutenant attends all meetings on behalf of the Chicago Police Department. All troubleshooting is handled by a central point, and intelligence and coordination of reporting are controlled at this central point.

Fifth, with regards to independent appraisal and evaluation, the Chicago CIT model has had strong analysis from the academic community. Several well-respected U.S. universities have appraised the CIT Chicago programme—enabling independent evaluation of the programme (Canada et al., 2010; Watson, Ottai, Draine, & Morabito, 2011).

Finally, the Chicago Mental Health Court is an ideal add-on to the CIT policing model. It provides the jail diversion required to keep the mental health consumers away from unnecessary incarceration.

New York Police Department (NYPD)

Disappointingly, in 2006 we found that the NYPD did not have any structured organisational approach for dealing with persons suffering mental illness. During our 2006 tour we interviewed a number of NYPD officers and found that police simply manage persons they perceive as experiencing acute mental illness by apprehending and then escorting them to the hospital for a psychiatric assessment. When we requested to speak to police who may be best equipped to deal with persons suffering acute mental illness, we were put in contact with the NYPD hostage negotiators. The NYPD's nonspecialised approach was not what we wanted for NSW.

In 2012 the NYPD still do not have a dedicated CIT or police mental health and policing unit, although in recent years there has been ongoing criticism from the media (Smith & Dougherty, 2010), consumer organisations (NYAPRS, 2012), and interagency colleagues (Montoya, 2008) calling for the establishment of such a unit due to NYPD's continuing history of officers shooting acutely mentally ill consumers. As recently as August 2012 the NYPD was being criticised by the local media for shooting a man with a history of mental illness in Times Square (WNYC News Blog, 2012) and police use of excessive force on an acutely mentally ill woman, resulting in her death in her mother's home (Pinto, 2012).

Honolulu

Our 2006 research visit established that Honolulu police had no specific strategy in place to deal with persons suffering a mental illness. It was clear that the Honolulu community had similar challenges to NSW concerning a surge in the use of the drug ICE (methamphetamine) and a subsequent surge in mental illness and policing issues. Although identified as a concern by Honolulu's health and community support agencies, there were no specific community policing initiatives at that time to deal with mental health and justice problems. In contrast, in 2012, Honolulu Police Department has a substantial mental health and policing unit—known as the Human Services Unit. This unit provides comprehensive 24-hour emergency psychological services to police officers in a personal capacity (e.g., counselling after a traumatic operational event) and advice in an operational capacity (e.g., providing professional consultation and assistance to police officers who handle critical incidents in the community to enable referral to crisis mental health teams) (Honolulu Police Department, 2012). However, it is apparent from media criticism that the unit does not provide general operational police staff with any specialist mental health training anywhere near the league of CIT (Vorsino, 2009). It is understood that the Honolulu police provide three hours of mental health and policing training (Vorsino, 2009).

Trial of the MHIT, 2007–2009

With the insights from the 2006 U.S. research tour, NSWPF set about developing a mental health and policing training model for NSW. Throughout 2007 the Mental Health Intervention Team training model was developed.

In January 2008, NSWPF commenced a trial of the MHIT programme with aim to provide enhanced mental health training to frontline officers (principally constables, senior constables, and sergeants) in three local area commands (LACs). The trial was delivered by a centrally located Mental Health Intervention Team command (referred to hereafter as the MHIT). The trial commenced in January 2008 and concluded in June 2009.

The NSW Police Force MHIT has four key aims:

1. Reduce the risk of injury to police and mental health consumers during mental health crisis events
2. Improve awareness by frontline police of risks involved in dealing with mental health consumers and strategies to reduce injuries to police and consumers
3. Improve collaboration with other government and nongovernment agencies in the response to and management of mental health crisis events
4. Reduce the time taken by police in the handover of mental health consumers into the health care system (NSW Police Force, 2012b)

Broadly, MHIT participants are trained to ensure its officers have enhanced skills to deal with individuals displaying mental health-related symptoms, namely, those in acute crisis.

The MHIT trial structure included five full-time staff: a superintendent commander, psychiatric clinical nurse consultant (CNC), sergeant education development officer, senior policy officer, and an analyst's position. The structure of the MHIT today remains similar, but with a slight reduction in staffing resources, with the commander's position being now filled by an inspector manager, and the analyst's position has been absorbed due to budget issues. The psychiatric CNC position and analyst's position were funded by NSW Health, and that funding contribution has been seen as a positive investment by police and stakeholders. The interagency focus of this initiative is a great strength of the MHIT model. The ability of the CNC nurse to give police clinical advice on operational and policy issues, liaise with NSW Health about operational issues involving consumers, and deliver MHIT training to police has been at times highly valued.

The NSWPF MHIT trial was held at three sites: Eastern Beaches LAC, Penrith LAC, and Tuggerah Lakes LAC. A control site at Campsie LAC was also monitored. Eastern Beaches, Penrith, and Campsie LACs are metropolitan Sydney sites, and Tuggerah Lakes LAC represents a busy regional NSW LAC. The trial and control sites were chosen with the following rationale:

- The sites were highly active according to numbers of police incidents managed under the Mental Health Act (NSW) (when compared to other LACs in NSW).
- Geographically, the three sites reflected regional and metropolitan diversity, and they could be readily serviced by the MHIT members.

Accordingly, over the course of the 18-month trial (January 2008 to June 2009) 121 police were trained and monitored in the 4-day MHIT model. Police participants from the trial and control sites were independently evaluated by the Charles Sturt University for the duration of the trial.

Today the MHIT training programme is essentially the same as the 2008 trial model. The MHIT training involves the delivery of intensive training by a wide range of subject experts over 4 days (totalling over 28 hours of face-to-face tuition). The MHIT training format includes lectures, a consumer panel, and interactive role-plays. A copy of the MHIT curriculum is shown in Table 4.1. MHIT participants are now sought from a wide cross section of operational police rank (constable through superintendents), specialist operational police rank, civilians with operational duties, and from geographically diverse local area commands across NSW. Operational police are still our key target participants.

CSU Independent Evaluation of the MHIT Trial

The Charles Sturt University (CSU)—via the Centre for Inland Health and the Australian Graduate School of Policing—independently evaluated the MHIT's 18-month trial period. The aim of the CSU evaluation was to assess the input, implementation, impact, and outcomes of the MHIT in the pilot LACs.

The CSU evaluated the MHIT at three points throughout the trial, examining process as well as outcomes. Research methodologies used by CSU included semistructured interviews, surveys, observational research, and analysis of official police data (e.g., NSWPF Computerised Operational Policing System data, which can be analysed as aggregate or as individual events and incidents) (Herrington et al., 2009, p. 13). The CSU evaluation of the MHIT trial concluded that the "NSW MHIT model compares favourably with established best practise for police training in interacting with mental health consumers" (Herrington et al., 2009, p. 2).

CSU's Evaluation Findings

The CSU had 19 findings about the MHIT trial. These 19 findings can be grouped into three categories: positive, neutral, and negative. Out of the 19 findings, 8 were positive, 7 neutral, and 4 negative. For full details of the 19 CSU findings, see Table 4.2.

Table 4.1 MHIT Curriculum

NSWPF Mental Health Intervention Team

	Day One	Day Two	Day Three	Day Four	Content Considerations
8.00 – 8.10am	Role Call	Role Call	Role Call	Role Call	Prerequisite: MOU On-Line module Progressive Scenario Verbal Judo/Negotiators Ambo involvement Mental Health Staff Feedback/interaction from MH patients and families (panel) Investigating/Interviewing people with Mental Health
8.10 – 8.30am	Introductions Housekeeping Ice breaker	OS Options OH&S Considerations	Legal Issues MOU Mental Health Act NSWPF Procedures Forensice Provisions	Crisis Intervention Skills Communication Tactical withdrawal	
8.30 – 9.00am	Opening – MHIT Commander Mental Health Spokesperson				
9.00 – 10.00am	Course Overview Questionnaire Experience/Expectations History	Child and Adolescent Disorders			
10.00 – 10.20am	Morning Tea	Morning Tea	Morning Tea	Morning Tea	
10.20 – 11.20am	Critical Incident Real life scenario	Geriatric Issues	Schedule 2/ Section 24 Writing for admissions	Crisis Intervention Skills Communication Tactical withdrawal	
11.20 – 12.20pm		Developmental Disabilities			
12.20 – 1.00pm	Lunch	Lunch	Lunch	Lunch	
1.00 – 2.00pm	Mental Illness: Signs and Symptoms	Family Perspectives and Consumer Panel	Psychotropic Medications	Role Plays	
2.00 – 2.45am			Substance Abuse and Co-occurring Disorders		
2.45 – 3.00pm	Afternoon Tea	Afternoon Tea	Afternoon Tea	Afternoon Tea	
3.00 – 3.45pm	Mental Illness: Signs and Symptoms	Family Perspectives and Consumer Panel ... continued...	Risk Assessment	Summary Evaluation Assessment	
3.45 – 4.00pm	Review of day Close	Review of day Close	Review of day Close	Review of day Close	

Table 4.2   Charles Sturt University: The Impact of the NSW Police Force Mental Health Intervention Team Trial: Analysis of Evaluation Key Findings

Findings	Positive	Neutral	Negative
1 The NSW MHIT model compares favourably with established best practise for police training in interacting with mental health consumers.	x		
2 One of the strengths of the MHIT has been the development of good relationships between the police and stakeholders in NSW Health, Ambulance Service NSW, and NGOs (such as the Schizophrenia Fellowship of NSW (SFNSW)). The value of engaging a senior police officer in the dual role of MHIT commander and corporate spokesperson from the outset assisted this, particularly in terms of brokering change at an executive level during the early stages of the programme.	x		
3 The MHIT Consultative Committee did not have the desired result of bringing together area health service directors, representatives from NGOs, and NSWPF.			x
4 Two years on from the implementation of the Mental Health Act 2007, the statewide memorandum of understanding (MOU) had yet to be amended to reflect the changes to the legislative framework. This limited the ability of NSWPF to effectively progress its interagency aims of limiting its involvement in mental health-related incidents			x
5 The pilot sites benefited from a great deal of oversight, which assisted the successful implementation of the MHIT in these LACs. The increase in the number of LACs receiving MHIT training as the programme expands across the state means there will likely be an increase in demands on the MHIT, which must be balanced against the team's resources, and its other project commitments.		x	
6 Qualitative data support the notion that the MHIT training led to an increased use of de-escalation techniques, with officers reporting that an increased understanding of mental health meant they were better able to deal with the situation. De-escalation techniques were also more likely to have been reported as being used in Mental Health Act incidents recorded on COPS events when an MHIT officer was present.	x		

Table 4.2 (continued)   Charles Sturt University: The Impact of the NSW Police Force Mental Health Intervention Team Trial: Analysis of Evaluation Key Findings

Findings	Positive	Neutral	Negative
7 Qualitative data from interviews with mental health consumers uncovered a perception that police were fearful of this group, and a belief that this fear inadvertently led to the escalation of events. This was supported by qualitative data collected from officers in the field, who noted increased confidence in dealing with these events and increased use of de-escalation techniques following the MHIT training.	x		
8 Most incidents attended by police do not require the use of coercive force, and comparison between the MHIT-trained cohort and frontline non-MHIT-trained colleagues found no differences in the use of force between these groups.		x	
9 Self-report data found a reduction in the number of times that medical attention was required for a member of the public (including a mental health consumer) as a result of a police officer using force during a mental health event following the introduction of the MHIT, although this did not differ between MHIT-trained and non-MHIT-trained officers, suggesting that factors other than training may have been responsible for the reduction over time. Consumers were more likely to receive injuries than other attendees at Mental Health Act events recorded on COPS; however, in most cases these injuries were self-inflicted.		x	
10 The sharing of information between NSWPF and NSW Health at a local level had improved through the course of the pilot programme, and some LACs had developed formalised care management plans for particular individuals, although there remained some concerns with the communication of this information to officers in the field.	x		
11 The MHIT training led to a significant and sustained increase in police officers' confidence in dealing with jobs involving individuals with a mental health problem, or a drug-induced psychosis.	x		

continued

Table 4.2 (continued)   Charles Sturt University: The Impact of the NSW Police Force Mental Health Intervention Team Trial: Analysis of Evaluation Key Findings

Findings	Positive	Neutral	Negative
12 Qualitative data from NSW Health staff working specifically in mental health were uniform in their perception of an improved understanding about mental health among the police officers they engaged with when a scheduled consumer was delivered to their care, and noted the flow-on effect that officers' increased understanding of mental health had on their engagement with consumers.	x		
13 While the LPCs in each of the pilot sites functioned well, it was difficult to come to effective interagency agreements when not all departments were represented. At one site intrahealth tension meant that representatives from the ED did not attend, and representatives from the ambulance service had only recently started to attend regularly. Police attending the hospital with a mental health consumer risked being caught between overlapping and contradictory interdepartmental agreements in such circumstances.			x
14 Self-rated data identified an improvement in the quality of the relationships between police officers and NSW Health representatives following the implementation of the MHIT, although no difference was found between trained and nontrained officers, suggesting that training contributed little to improved relations.		x	
15 Data suggest the widespread continuing practise of conveying mental health consumers in police vehicles, despite interagency guidelines that police vehicles are to be used as a last resort. Half of all Mental Health Act events recorded in July 2009 (which represents three-quarters of the events in which a mental health consumer was transported to the hospital) involved transportation by police. Only one-quarter of these involved police use of force, so it is hard to imagine that transportation by police vehicle was the most appropriate method in all of these cases.			x
16 Police attended significantly fewer Schedule 1 (involuntary medical practitioner schedules) calls following the implementation of the MHIT, although this reduction was global, and cannot be attributed to the training of individuals in the pilot sites per se.		x	

Table 4.2 (continued) Charles Sturt University: The Impact of the NSW Police Force Mental Health Intervention Team Trial: Analysis of Evaluation Key Findings

Findings	Positive	Neutral	Negative
17 A similar picture was evident with convey schedule incidents (i.e., absconded patients), and the reduction in the number of convey schedule events attended by officers in the MHIT LACs was greater than that in the non-MHIT LACs. However, this is largely a function of the MHIT-trained LACs attending considerably more convey schedules calls in the first place.		x	
18 There was a reduction in the average amount of time Schedule 1 and convey schedule incidents took; however, this reduction was global, and we hypothesise that improved interagency cooperation and associated path smoothing and local protocol agreements following the introduction of the MHIT resulted in quicker handover times for mental health consumers between police and NSW Health across LACs.		x	
19 Self-reported data revealed a reduction in the time reportedly spent at officers' last Mental Health Act event. MHIT-trained officers reported spending less time than non-MHIT-trained officers, suggesting that at the very least, the MHIT training had an impact on the perceived length of time that mental health events took.	x		
Total findings	8/19	7/19	4/19

A summary of the CSU evaluation findings when analysed in light of the MHIT's four aims established the following general outcomes:

1. A comparative analysis between MHIT-trained officers and non-trained officers found that there was no perceived reduced risk of injury to police and mental health consumers during mental health crisis events (Herrington et al., 2009, p. 9). This can be assessed as a neutral CSU finding.
2. MHIT-trained police officers noted a marked improved awareness and confidence in their dealing with mental health consumers and strategies to reduce injuries to police and consumers (Herrington et al., 2009, pp. 6, 11, 12). This can be assessed as a positive CSU finding.
3. One of the great strengths of the MHIT model was the improved collaboration with other government and nongovernment agencies in the response to and management of mental health crisis events

(Herrington et al., 2009, pp. 2, 10). This can be assessed as a positive CSU finding.

4. There was a real and perceived reduction in the time taken by police in the handover of mental health consumers into the health care system (Herrington et al., 2009, pp. 16–19). This can be assessed as a positive CSU finding.

Overall, the qualitative findings of the CSU's evaluation of the MHIT trial can be concluded as positive.

CSU Seven Recommendations

In addition to the evaluation findings in 2009, CSU made seven recommendations to NSWPF about the MHIT model. We concluded that while some of the CSU recommendations were applicable, some were not. We will now discuss the CSU's recommendations and NSWPF's responses to them. CSU recommendations are noted in italics and NSWPF's responses after:

1. *While the NSW MHIT model compares favourably with established best practise for police training in interacting with mental health consumers, we recommend that NSWPF consider expanding the MHIT training to include a module relating to mental health consumers as victims and witnesses to crime, prioritisation of training of police radio dispatchers, and addressing the issue of tasers explicitly.* NSWPF notes that it will integrate some new information on the respective topics of tasers and mental health consumers as victims in the 2012 revised content of the MHIT programme (due to be reissued in the middle of 2013). However, the detailed tactical training associated with tasers will continue as a separate course—as it has a heavy emphasis on tactics.

    There are three reasons for the separation of taser training from the MHIT training. First, at the time of the rollout of MHIT training, it was the opinion of the tactical trainers that while mental health consumers made up a disproportionately high number of interactions with police and taser releases, taser training should be based on the situation facing the officer, not the profile of the individual facing the officer (i.e., mental health consumer, indigenous, alcohol or drug effect, etc.). Second, the costs and timing associated with MHIT taser training would have delayed the trial and rollout of the MHIT trial and its implementation. Third, and of equal weight, the government of the day did not have the appetite to see the close correlation of mental health and policing training with taser training.

    With respect to the training of radio dispatchers, in 2011 we trained 20 of our radio dispatchers.

Finally, with respect to the recommendation that the MHIT model address the victimology aspect of the consumers that police manage, we note that the association of consumers and victimology is already addressed throughout the MHIT course. Accordingly, the topic does not warrant a separate module of training.

2. *While the MHIT has always been more than a training development and delivery programme, undertaking work that increases its scope beyond its core function must be balanced against the resources available to the team, particularly as the MHIT programme rolls out across the state.* We concede that resource pressure is a reality. The MHIT is currently a team of four full-time staff with a part-time corporate spokesperson. The full-time MHIT consists of an inspector manager, psychiatric clinical nurse consultant, sergeant project officer, and senior policy officer. Despite limited resources the MHIT is on target to roll out MHIT training to 10% (1,500 officers) of all operational staff by 2015, and it manages a broad range of research, policy development, and programme responsibilities. We concede that additional resources would be ideal. That said, our NSWPF MHIT has a combined relevant experience of 75 years in policing and mental health, and this expertise enables us to deliver on deadlines.

3. *Consideration should be given to reinvigorating the MHIT Consultative Committee, particularly as the MHIT rolls into new LACs and contact with area health services across the state increases.* While we concede that the MHIT Consultative Committee has not been reinvigorated, we note that the MHIT has been a standing agenda item for the NSW Emergency Mental Health Interdepartmental Committee (IDC) for bimonthly discussion since the MHITs implementation. The NSW IDC is a high-level state representative committee for interagency management of emergency mental health in NSW. The IDC has management-level representation from NSWPF, Ambulance Services NSW, and NSW Health. The IDC has been an appropriate operational substitute for the now defunct MHIT Consultative Committee.

4. *The revising of the statewide memorandum of understanding (MOU) should be progressed as a matter of urgency by the three signatory agencies.* The NSW Emergency Mental Health Memorandum of Understanding (MOU) between Ambulance Services NSW, NSW Health, and NSWPF provides the policy and operational framework for the management of people with emergency mental illness in the community (NSW Health, 2007). The CSU noted that a key difficulty with the existing MOU is that it has yet to be amended following the implementation of the Mental Health Act 2007. From a police perspective, the main reason that the MOU has not been reissued is that there is currently a negotiation breakdown between

NSWPF and NSWH over the issue of the respective agencies' transportation responsibilities under the act in regional and rural NSW. Today, there is a lack of declared mental health facilities (DMHFs) in regional and rural NSW, and under s. 22 police provisions in the act, police are required to take the detained person to the nearest DMHF for mental health assessment. In regional centres this may mean that police are transporting an involuntary consumer for hundreds of kilometres, bypassing functional emergency departments that could assist a consumer in crisis, in order to comply with the legislation (i.e., to take the apprehended person to the nearest DMHF). NSWPF sees our request for additional DMHFs in regional and rural NSW as a human rights issue, inappropriate use of police resources, and a safety and duty of care issue for NSWPF. To date, we have been unable to find interagency resolution on this issue, and have therefore not been in a position to sign off on a revised MOU. At the time of writing the issue has been referred to the respective agencies' executive for resolution.

5. *We recommend that the MHIT increase its interaction with nongovernmental organisations (NGOs) at a local as well as a state level.* The MHIT proactively considered CSU's recommendation, and we have involved ourselves with a diverse range of mental health consumer groups at a local and a state level. We have successful working relationships with the Schizophrenia Fellowship NSW, Richmond Fellowship, Suicide Prevention Australia, Mental Health Association NSW, and several smaller mental health NGOs. In addition, we have made it part of the job descriptions of each of the MHIT members, and our statewide network of 80 NSWPF mental health contact officers, to liaise with relevant consumer and affiliated NGOs at a local LAC level.

6. *As the MHIT rolls out across the state, it will increasingly involve police working in rural and remote communities, which poses some unique challenges.* The MHIT has aimed to train staff proportionately in all regions and remote areas across NSW. That said, some priority is given to assign training spots to LACs that have disproportionately high levels of police apprehension under the act, and some specialist operational units that manage disproportionately high mental health issues among their portfolio's population (e.g., aboriginal coordination team and youth liaison officers).

7. *We recommend that NSWPF consider revising the internal key performance indicators (KPIs) associated with the MHIT to ensure that it is able to monitor the programme.* The key KPIs for the MHIT have remained the same (primarily that 10% of all operational NSWPF

staff are trained in the MHIT model by 2015). As stated, our ability to deliver against these KPIs, with a small full-time team, is a reflection of the expertise and experience of the team. It is true, however, that forward management of MHIT staffing, proportionate to high levels of operational needs, is a resource challenge.

The CSU evaluation's findings and recommendations were welcomed by NSWPF, and we note that in the majority of cases we have implemented the recommendations and findings.

Implementation of the MHIT, June 2009 to Present

Following the success of the MHIT pilot programme and the positive evaluations by Charles Sturt University, in July 2009 the NSWPF Commissioner's Executive Team endorsed the MHIT as a permanent component of the NSW Police Force. NSW Health has continued to actively support the MHIT via funding the mental health CNC position from 2009 to today.

The MHIT model has achieved much, but we also concede that it is not without its challenges (internal and external). We will now discuss the model's achievements and challenges.

MHIT Model Achievements

Since the MHIT model has been implemented it has achieved much. The MHIT is on target to deliver its 2015 key performance indicator that a minimum of 10% of all operational police receive MHIT training. This equates to the training of approximately 300 officers per year as specialist mental health intervention officers. As of August 2012 we have trained approximately 6% of all operational staff—a total of 887 NSW police officers and stakeholders.

Since its implementation, the MHIT has received numerous awards affirming the merit of the MHIT training and team model. Some key awards received in 2011 included the Australasian Mental Health Services award and the Mental Health Association NSW Excellence in Service or Program Delivery Award.

The achievement of the MHIT model can be attributed to its structure, the specialist and unique skills mix of the MHIT staff, the MHIT's staffing continuity in the past two years, the NSWPF executive's support, and the focus on training operational staff who need and want to be trained. Most importantly, not one MHIT-trained police officer has been directly or indirectly involved in any adverse police coroners' events involving mental health consumers since we trialled the MHIT in 2008.

In a bid to promote a uniform and consistent approach when it comes to mental health and community policing across Australasia, we have proactively invited all the Australasian policing jurisdictions to participate in the MHIT programme (free of charge). To this end we have had 18 Australasian interjurisdictional police graduates. We have successfully licenced the MHIT model to the Australian Capital Territory (ACT) Police and Western Australian Police, and have assisted these jurisdictions with their implementation of the MHIT model. At the time of completing this chapter we have been leaders promoting a single policing model for mental health in Australia.

All MHIT students participate in a post-training qualitative evaluation survey to assess the MHIT training and its impact. It is clear from our internal NSWPF analysis of these semistructured questionnaires that the MHIT training is having an overwhelmingly positive impact on course participants. To test our assertion that the MHIT's implementation is having an ongoing positive impact in achieving the MHIT's four core objectives, we have contracted the Australian Institute of Policing Management and Charles Sturt University to independently evaluate the value of the MHIT's implementation to date.

Finally, it is important to reiterate that the MHIT model is more than training. In addition to the MHIT training programme, the MHIT administers comprehensive programme support and advice to the field (specifically our statewide network of 80 mental health contact officers), manages policy development and coordination and numerous university-affiliated research projects (e.g., mental health frequent presenters to police), and trialled a mobile MHIT response vehicle in the central Sydney metro region in 2011–2012. We assert that the success of the MHIT model is bigger than its training component (although this is key). The MHIT's success is also dependent on supportive legislation, policy and programme responses, regular liaison with the police at a local level in the field and liaison with key stakeholders (e.g., community mental health and NGOs), and finally, advocating and being research leaders on community policing and mental health issues where there is a dearth of evidence base. As you can see, there are many facets to the MHIT (beyond its training responsibilities).

MHIT Model Challenges

While the previous section reads as a glowing appraisal, we concede that the MHIT model, and the policing environment we work in, is not without challenges. These challenges impact the potential of the MHIT model. We will now address the challenges of the MHIT model in the context of external and internal factors.

External Challenges

There are five key external challenges that impact the MHIT capacity. First is the ongoing police role in lengthy and inappropriate transport of persons from community settings to DMHFs in remote and regional NSW. Until this issue is resolved at a legislative and policy level (i.e., an amendment to the Mental Health Act 2007 (NSW) and reissue of the MOU), both the consumer and NSWPF will continue to be on the back burner. For any legislative and policy changes to make practical inroads, additional DMHFs, or the reclassing of existing emergency departments to have additional powers to treat persons who are mentally ill or disordered, is needed. We reiterate that the existing situation (i.e., police managing lengthy transports of consumers to DMHFs in the main in police vehicles) does not comply with international human rights norms that Australia is signatory to, or the values that NSWPF upholds.

Second, the Ambulance Service NSW (ASNSW) has a legislated responsibility to apprehend and transport involuntary persons for the purpose of a mental health assessment. Practically, this means that ASNSW should be undertaking medium- to low-risk involuntary apprehensions and (in)voluntary transportations from community settings. Disappointingly, it is police experience that ambulance services undersubscribe their legislative powers when it comes to involuntary transportations. Police would like to see higher uptake of ASNSW powers than what is current.

Third, when it comes to mental health frequent presenters that police manage, there is a lack of response from mental health services. NSWPF define mental health frequent presenters as persons whom police detain under police powers in the Mental Health Act (2007) NSW three or more times per year. While mental health frequent presenters are small in overall number (7% of all individuals police deal with under police provisions in the Act), this population group is responsible for approximately 23% of all overall incidents police manage under provisions in the act (Baldry, 2012). As a cohort, they consume a disproportionately high amount of overall police resources. While some mental health services have strategic case management plans in place for mental health frequent presenters, the vast majority of health services either do not have ongoing case management plans in place or are reluctant to share these plans with police. It is our experience that police-referred mental health frequent presenters are seen by health as complex cases, treatment resistant, behaviourally hard to manage, clinically complex, and noncompliant with their treatment plans. Further, the majority have a forensic history and are subsequently perceived as threatening to health staff. It is our experience that police requests to NSW Health to have mental health frequent presenters proactively case managed requires intense lobbying, and often has limited success.

Fourth, there is the impact of alcohol and illegal drug abuse in the community and on policing. When illegal drug consumption grows, this has an adverse impact on policing resources, and a consumption spike tends to correlate with an increase in the number of mental health events police attend.

Finally, perhaps one of our biggest external challenges is to ensure interagency cooperation at a local level. Historically, we have found that most often the legislative and policy differences between the agencies can be ameliorated when there is interagency cooperation and productive working relationships in place. To support this, there needs to be better accountability measures via policy, and performance audits undertaken at the local level.

Ongoing Internal NSWPF Challenges

The NSWPF MHIT model faces five key internal challenges.

First, the proactive and reactionary nature of policing often means that resources are correlated (or diverted) to the portfolio of operational priority (e.g., domestic violence, child protection, etc.). This means that the MHIT has to justify with clear and verifiable data our business case for resources. Second, there are staffing resource issues that need to be managed. One of the reasons our small MHIT has succeeded to date is the stability and continuity of executive leadership. If staffing continuity became destabilised, this could prove an issue. Third, the MHIT is continually dealing with the everready cynicism from operational police that mental health is not part of core police duties. This means that police often don't see or understand the need to be trained in mental health. Junior police are less ready to embrace MHIT training. We often find it is the older, more experienced operational police who understand the complexities of community policing, that see training in mental health to have direct use. Fourth, there is the ongoing debate as to how much taser training we incorporate into mental health training. We recognise the need to have some representation of taser training in future MHIT training. Currently, taser release statistics in NSWPF demonstrate that approximately 23% of persons that police taser are known mental health consumers. A final internal challenge is the management of the surrounding political environment and its impact on the MHIT. The MHIT's political environment depends on the priorities of government, the political will of the Minister for Police, Commissioner, and available resources. All these factors impact organisational police priorities. It is also reality that competing police portfolio demands (e.g., domestic violence, mental health, child protection, alcohol, organised crime, etc.), and the politics of the day impact our ability to expand the MHIT program within NSW Police Force.

NSWPF Mental Health and Policing Vision

Our NSWPF community mental health policing vision is informed by our extensive experience in policing community mental health, evidence-based research, and academic literature on the topic. Our conclusion is that the management of acute mental health in the community lays firmly the remit of health and ambulance services, with limited strategic support from police in high-risk situations. Accordingly, this is our policing vision:

1. Conduct a trial of a dedicated mental health emergency response service unit. This unit would most appropriately work within health services and form a centralised dispatch area, that is, via a hospital facility attached to an inpatient unit or through a centralised ambulance station.

2. Decrease the overall role of police in managing persons with acute mental illness in the community, leaving the police role to management of high-risk and acutely mentally ill or disordered consumers. In turn, we need to better resource, train, and actively support ambulance services in taking on a more active role in the involuntary apprehension of mentally ill and disordered persons in the community.

3. A mental health emergency response service unit would consist of police, an ambulance-trained officer, and a clinical nurse consultant. This would provide a suitable platform to deliver quality services to the patient with the ability to effectively assess and medicate the patient when necessary.

4. A mental health emergency response service unit would provide mechanical restraints for transport and security of mental health patients. The clinical officers would be trained in the application of a suitable mechanical restraint device and the provision of rapid sedation.

5. A mental health emergency response service unit would have access to an appropriate vehicle that can safely and securely transport a patient. This vehicle would not be police marked (complying with our NSWPF human rights philosophy) and would provide the appropriate comforts to a person who is in mental health crisis, with access to necessary medical support.

6. Health service would provide a streamlined transitional process at hospital admission. This would mean that the mental health emergency response service unit would have immediate access to a doctor for psychiatric assessment, treatment, and any transport arrangements. Ideally, the receiving hospital would feed into the NSW psychiatric emergency care centres or declared mental health facility network.

7. A mental health emergency response service unit would amalgamate with any local mental health crisis team and provide a case management approach to mental health frequent presenters and other complex interagency mental health patients within the catchment. Such a strategy would provide duties for service downtimes.
8. In line with the above, the team could administrate relevant community orders and drug treatment programmes for consumers.
9. The team would be able to seek out and return absconded high-risk mental health patients.
10. Provide interhospital transportation for high-risk mental health patients.
11. Teams could be located in metropolitan and regional sites in NSW where there are the most voluminous numbers of mental health apprehensions. For example, there could be two separate teams in the Sydney metropolitan area (one servicing eastern Sydney and the other servicing western Sydney) and two teams in regional NSW (one servicing out of Newcastle and the other out of the Coffs Harbour area).

It is evident we need to continue to innovate our police approach to emergency mental health, and to provide appropriate and well-resourced mental health services in the community. NSW Police Force's position is clear: It will always assist the community and other services when it comes to protecting life and property, but it is not the NSW Police Force's responsibility to transport mental health patients between hospitals, engage in lengthy transports of consumers in police vehicles, retrieve routine mental health patients who have absconded, or apprehend people who are experiencing nonacute mental illness and disorder and transport them to hospital unless the level of risk is high enough to justify police involvement. All other functions are clearly the responsibility of ambulance and health services.

We will continue to train our police in emergency mental health in high-risk situations—with the aim to ensure a sensitive and safe police response to these situations. It is acknowledged that these strategies are resource-intensive. However, the consequences of not investing can be dire—whereby a police officer, in the course of his or her duties, has shot dead a consumer while managing the operational situation. The ripple effect of such fatalities is equally severe for the consumer's family and friends, police officers, and community involved. No one is a winner in such scenarios, and that it why NSWPF continues invest in MHIT training.

We advocate for more investment in community mental health for persons with mental illness and mental disorders. There is a business case for providing a proactive case management and community care model for acutely mentally ill persons in the community. It can be successfully argued that the costs associated with community care outweigh the long-term cost of a ballooning emergency mental health care service provision (Hickie, 2008).

Emergency mental health is a government issue; however, police should not be the lead agency in this area. Strategic thinking, resources, and the implementation of long-term plans enshrined in human rights norms are required to address the issue of persons suffering acute mental illness or disorder in the community.

References

Andrews, G. (2011). Mental health frequent presenters to NSW police. Paper presented at the 32nd International Congress of Mental Health Law, Berlin, July 19, 2011. Retrieved August 19, 2012, from http://www.ialmh.org/Berlin2011/Program%20Book%20-%20Berlin_Online%202.pdf

Australian Bureau of Statistics. (2012). Retrieved May 1, 2012, from http://www.abs.gov.au/ausstats/abs@.nsf/mf/3101.0

Baldry, E. (2012). *Enabling or disabling: Imprisoning people with mental and cognitive disability* (Right Now no. 155). Retrieved August 19, 2012, from http://rightnow.org.au/topics/disability/page/3/

Baldry, E., Dowse, L., & Clarence, M. (2012a). Mental health frequent presenters to police. Research paper, University of NSW. Retrieved August 26, 2012, from http://www.mhdcd.unsw.edu.au/mhdcd-projects-studies.html.

Baldry, E., Dowse, L., & Webster, I. (2012b). Mental health disorders and cognitive disabilities (MHDCD) in the criminal justice system (CJS). Australian Research Council study. Retrieved from http://www.mhdcd.unsw.edu.au/australians-mhdcd-cjs-project.html#Partners

Business NSW. Retrieved May 1, 2012, from http://www.business.nsw.gov.au/invest-in-nsw/about-nsw/people-skills-and-education/population-estimates

Canada, K., Angell, B., & Watson, A.C. (2010). Crisis intervention team training in Chicago: Successes on the ground. *Journal of Police Crisis Negotiations*, 10(1–2), 86–100. Retrieved September 2, 2012, from http://www.ncbi.nlm.nih.gov/pmc/articles/PMC2990632/

Clifford, K. (2010). A thin blue line. *Police Practice and Research: An International Journal, 11*(4), 355–370.

Connecticut Alliance to Benefit Law Enforcement (CABLE). (2013). Retrieved January 12, 2013 from http://www.cable.web.org/resources/the-mephis-model

Cochran, S., Deane, M.A., & Borum, R. (2000). Improving police response to mentally ill people. *Psychiatric Services, 51*(10), 1315.

Donohue, D. (2011, July 19). Implementing and evaluating a Mental Health Intervention Team program in the NSW Police Force: Better outcomes for police and consumers? Paper presented at the 32nd International Congress of Mental Health Law, Berlin. Retrieved August 19, 2012, from http://www.ialmh.org/Berlin2011/Program%20Book%20-%20Berlin_Online%202.pdf

Dupont, R., & Cochran, S. (2000). Police response to mental health emergencies—Barriers to change. *Journal of American Academy Psychiatry Law, 28*, 338–344.

Hails, J., & Borum, R. (2003). Police training and specialized approaches to respond to people with mental illnesses. *Crime and Delinquency, 49*, 52–61.

Herrington, V., Clifford, K., Lawrence, P.F., Ryle, S., & Pope, R. (2009, December). The impact of the NSW Police Force: Final evaluation report. Centre for Inland Health Australian Graduate School of Policing. Retrieved August 19, 2012, from http://www.police.nsw.gov.au/__data/assets/pdf_file/0006/174246/MHIT_ Evaluation_Final_Report_241209.pdf

Hickie, I. (2008). *A new model for delivering selected mental health services in Australia.* Brain and Mind Institute University of Sydney.

Honolulu Police Department. (2012). Honolulu Police Department Human Services Unit. Retrieved September 3, 2012 from http://www.honolulupd.org/hpd/hsu. htm

Laing, R., Halsey, R., Donohue, D., Newman, C., & Cashin, A. (2009). Application of a model for the development of a mental health service delivery collaboration between police and the health service. *Issues in Mental Health Nursing, 30*(5), 337–341.

Los Angeles Police Department. (2011, March 3). Interdepartmental correspondence: Executive Director Board of Police Commissioners to Board of Police Commissioners. Retrieved September 2, 2012, from http://www.lapdpolicecom. lacity.org/030811/BPC_11-0104.pdf

Los Angeles Police Department. (2012). Retrieved July 2, 2012, from http://www. lapdonline.org/

Mental Health Act 2007 (NSW).

Mental Health Forensic Provisions 1990 (NSW).

Memphis Police Department. (2010). Memphis Police Department 2010 annual report. Retrieved August 25, 2012, from http://www.memphispolice.org/2010% 20MPD%20Annual%20Report%20for%20web.pdf

Memphis Police Department. (2012). Crisis intervention team. Retrieved August 25, 2012, from http://www.memphispolice.org/Crisis%20Intervention.htm

Montoya, C. (2008, October 28). Testimony of the Legal Aid Society at a public hearing on the report and recommendations of the New York State/New York City Mental Health Criminal Justice Panel. Presented to the New York City Council Committee on Public Safety and the Committee on Mental Health, Mental Retardation, Alcoholism, Drug Abuse and Disability Services. Enhanced Defence-MICA (Mentally Ill-Chemically Addicted) Project. Retrieved September 9, 2012, from http://www.legal-aid.org/media/68692/edptestimonyfinal.pdf

National Alliance on Mental Illness (NAMI). (2008). Chicago crisis intervention team—Lt. Jeff Murphy. PowerPoint presentation. Retrieved September 2, 2012, from www.nami.org/.../Chicago_presentation-CIT_networking_session.ppt

New York Association of Psychiatric Rehabilitation Services, Inc. (NYAPRS). (2012, April 4). Did the NYPD suffocate a mentally ill woman to death while trying to cuff her? Retrieved September 9, 2012, from http://www.nyaprs.org/e-news-bulletins/2012/2012-04-04nypd.cfm

NSW Consumer Advisory Group (CAG)—Mental Health, Inc. (2012). Human rights. Retrieved August 19, 2012, from http://www.nswcag.org.au/human-rights.html

NSW Coroner's Court. (2012). Findings and recommendations relating to major incidents: Recommendations relating to mental health issues. Retrieved August 26, 2012, from http://www.coroners.lawlink.nsw.gov.au/coroners/ findings.html,c=y

NSW Health. (2007). Mental health emergency response memorandum of understanding 2007. Retrieved September 15, 2012, from http://www.health.nsw.gov.
au/pubs/2007/mou_mentalhealth.html

NSW Parliament. (2002). *NSW Legislative Council. Select Committee on Mental
Health Inquiry into mental health services in New South Wales* (parliamentary
paper no. 368, pp. 1–361). Retrieved August 25, 2012, from http://www.
parliament.nsw.gov.au/Prod/parlment/committee.nsf/0/f742b6b2e561abdeca2
56c73002b7f87/$FILE/fullreport.pdf

NSW Police Force. (2012a). About us. Retrieved May 1, 2012, from http://www.
police.nsw.gov.au/about_us

NSW Police Force. (2012b). Mental health. Retrieved September 9, 2012, from http://
www.police.nsw.gov.au/community_issues/mental_health

NSW Police Force. (2012c, April). Computerised Operating Policing System (COPS)
extracted data. Unpublished.

Path Program Archives. (2001). Police mental health provider service collaboration—
Major Sam Cochran. Retrieved August 25, 2012, from http://pathprogramarchive.
samhsa.gov/pdf/Sam_OutlineAndList.pdf

Pinto, N. (2012, August 15). A call to harm. The Village Voice, online community
news website. Retrieved August 18, 2012, from http://digitalissue.villagevoice.
com/article/A+Call+To+Harm/1144659/122275/article.html

RTBOT. (2012). Retrieved September 2, 2012, from http://www.rtbot.net/Los_
Angeles_Police_Department_Threat_Management_Unit

Siska, J., & Beadle-Brown, J. (2011). Developments in deinstitutionalisation and community living in the Czech Republic. *Journal of Policy and Practice in Intellectual
Disabilities, 8*(2), 125.

Smith, A., & Dougherty, M.C. (2010). NYPD must do the right thing by the mentally
ill. Business Wire—a Berkshire Hathaway Company. Retrieved September 9,
2012, from http://blogs.impre.com/latin_nation/tag/nypd

Steadman, H.J., Williams-Deane, M., Borum, R., & Morrissey, J.P. (2000). Comparing
outcomes of major models of police responses to mental health emergencies.
Psychiatric Services, 51, 645–649.

University of Memphis, Department of Criminology and Justice. (2012) Retrieved
August 25, 2012, from http://www.memphis.edu/cjustice/dupont.htm

U.S. Census Bureau. (2010). U.S. Census. Retrieved September 2, 2012, from
http://2010.census.gov/news/releases/operations/cb11-cn68.html

Reuland, M. (2004). *A guide to implementing police based diversion programs for people with mental illness* (pp. 1–45). Delmar, NY: Technical Assistance and Policy
Analysis Centre for Jail Diversion.

Reuland, M., Schwarzfeld, M., & Draper, L. (2009). *Law enforcement responses
to people with mental illnesses: A guide to research informed policy and practice* (pp. 1–36). New York, NY: Council of State Governments Justice Center.
Retrieved August 25, 2012, from http://consensusproject.org/downloads/le-
research.pdf

Vorsino, M. (2009). Honolulu police get training to better deal with the mentally ill.
Honolulu Advertiser. April 22, 2009. Retrieved January 12, 2013 from http://
www.the.honoluluadvertiser.com/article/2009/Apr/22/In/Hawaii90422404.
html

Watson, A.C., Ottai, V.C., Draine, J., & Morabito, M. (2011). CIT in context: The impact of mental health resource availability and district saturation on call dispositions. *International Journal of Law and Psychiatry, 34*(4), 287–294.
WNYC News Blog. (2012, August 14). After Times Square shooting, focus shifts to preventing violent confrontations. Retrieved September 9, 2012, from http://www.wnyc.org/blogs/wnyc-news-blog/2012/aug/14/times-square-shooting-prompts-analysis/

The Mental Health Intervention Program

5

Preventing and Resolving Mental Health Crisis Situations

QUEENSLAND POLICE SERVICE

Contents

Introduction

The *Fourth National Mental Health Plan* sets and guides the agenda and priorities for collaborative government action on mental health across Australia (Commonwealth of Australia, 2009). Under the plan, in the priority area of prevention and early intervention, a key action is to provide education about mental health and suicide prevention to frontline workers in the emergency services (including police), welfare, and associated sectors. Similarly, the

Queensland Plan for Mental Health 2007–2017 prioritises action to improve mental health literacy and access to mental health training for nonclinical workers in key government services (Queensland Health, 2008). The *Queensland Plan* also supports the continuing implementation and development of the Mental Health Intervention Program to improve collaborative responses between the Queensland Police Service (QPS), emergency services (including the Queensland Ambulance Service (QAS)), and public mental health services. This programme aims to provide better outcomes for individuals with a mental illness, their families, and their carers.

Police Powers in Queensland
Under the Mental Health Act 2000

The police response to mental health incidents in Queensland is largely determined by the requirements of the Mental Health Act 2000 (Qld). In Queensland the Mental Health Act 2000 defines mental illness as "a condition characterised by a clinically significant disturbance of thought, mood, perception or memory."

The Mental Health Act 2000 commenced on February 28, 2002, and replaced the Mental Health Act 1974, within the context of broader mental health reforms.

Under the act, police have the power to intervene in situations involving people with a mental illness. Generally this includes apprehending, detaining, or transporting a person believed to have a mental illness who is a danger to himself or herself or others, or a person who has failed to comply with assessment documentation or a treatment order, to the relevant mental health service for assessment or treatment.

The purpose of the act (Section 4) is to

provide for the involuntary assessment and treatment, and the protection, of persons (whether adults or minors) who have mental illnesses while at the same time:

a) Safeguarding their rights and freedoms; and
b) Balancing their rights and freedoms with the rights and freedoms of other persons.

The act (Section 8) also incorporates the *United Nations Principles for the Protection of Rights of People With Mental Illness*, including recognition that mentally ill people have the same basic human rights as others.

Section 33 allows police to apprehend a person who appears to be mentally ill, if they have reasonable grounds for believing that:

I. a person has a mental illness; and

II. because of the person's illness there is an imminent risk of significant physical harm being sustained by the person or someone else; and

III. proceeding under division 2 of this section of the legislation would cause dangerous delay and significantly increase the risk of harm to the person or someone else; and

IV. the person should be taken to an authorised mental health service for examination to decide whether a request and recommendation for assessment should be made for the person.

Under Section 30, police may detain a person who is believed to have a mental illness, for the purpose of examination under a justice's examination order, to determine if they should be taken to a mental health service for a mental health assessment.

Section 34 of the act applies to emergency examination orders (EEOs) and states that a police or ambulance officer must take the person to an authorised mental health service for examination to decide whether assessment documents for the person should be made.

Section 35 states that "immediately after taking the person to the authorised mental health service, the police or ambulance officer must make an EEO for the person." After making the order, the police or ambulance officer must give the order to a health service employee at the health service. The person may be detained in the health service while the order is being made.

In addition to this legislative framework, the QPS response is also supported by the operational procedures manual (OPM), local standard operating procedures, and the recording of information on the Queensland Police Records and Information Management Exchange (QPRIME). The OPM provides guidance and instructions in all aspects of operational policing. Although not exhaustive, it provides service policy, orders, and procedures in relation to most policing issues. Chapter 6 of the OPM contains procedures that are designed to ensure that contact between police and a person with a special need is conducted in a manner that is fair and does not place the person at a disadvantage. Section 6.6 of this chapter outlines policing procedures in relation to mental health incidents.

The Queensland Environment

The QPS developed a service delivery model for mental health incidents that was based on policing 24 hours a day, 7 days a week, to more than 4 million Queenslanders. The Mental Health Intervention Program (MHIP) model was based on population, demographics, land area, density, health services, and the rate of mental health incidences and police calls for service. It considered that Queensland is one of the most decentralised states in Australia. Covering 1.7 million square kilometres, it is Australia's second largest state and represents more than a quarter of the country's total land area. To put Queensland in perspective, it is more than seven times the size of the United Kingdom, more than five times the size of Japan, and more than two and a half times the size of Texas.

The QPS has more than 10,500 police officers and approximately 4,200 support staff working in a variety of conditions, from Cape York in the north, to the Gold Coast in the south and the remote far west, across 430 establishments, including police stations, neighbourhood police beats, and shop fronts. Any police officer across the state may come into contact with a person with a mental illness, in a crisis situation or otherwise. An important consideration for the model was the need to assist persons with a mental illness in remote and rural areas as well as metropolitan areas.

Background to the Mental Health Intervention Program

The QPS and Queensland Health (QH) have been working collaboratively through the Mental Health Partnership Project since 1998. It supported a range of reforms in service delivery, service management, and policy development across the two departments.

There were a number of key events and drivers that led to and shaped the formation of the MHIP in Queensland. These included:

- The *Final Report of the Mental Health Crisis Intervention Ad Hoc Advisory Group* to Australian police and health ministers, by Dr. Harvey Whiteford, the then commonwealth director of Health and Family Services, strongly supported the establishment of protocols and shared services between health and police in relation to addressing crisis situations with mentally ill persons (Whiteford, 1998).
- During 2002, in response to an increase in calls for service related to mental health incidents in the police district of Logan (an outer suburb of Brisbane, capital city of Queensland), a trial training project based on the Memphis Crisis Intervention Team model (United States) was run in partnership between the QPS and the local QH mental health service. Two hundred general duties officers received training. An evaluation of the programme conducted over a three-month period directly after the training reported an increase in officers' understanding of mental illness and capacity and willingness to approach and respond to people with a mental illness.

- In November 2003, QH and the QPS jointly sponsored a Policing and Mental Health Best Practice Conference on the Gold Coast where prominent experts from the U.S. Memphis Mental Health Crisis Intervention Team model provided information on the details of their model.
- In 2003–2004 the annual report of the Office of the Public Advocate recommended that "the Queensland Government, through QH and the QPS, fund the development and implementation of Crisis Intervention Teams that respond to crisis situations involving police and people with a mental illness" (Office of the Public Advocate, 2004).
- In 2005, the Office of the Public Advocate also made recommendations in a 2005 discussion paper, "Preserving Life and Dignity in Distress," that QH establish protocols for the provision of specialised mental health advice to police for the safe and humane resolution of critical mental health incidents (Office of the Public Advocate, 2005).
- In 2005–2006 the Queensland Government State Budget provided funding to the QPS, QH, and QAS to implement the MHIP. The QPS, as lead agency, partnered with QH and the QAS to design and implement an innovative response that would improve encounters involving people with mental illnesses.

Implementation of the Programme Across the State

The MHIP was established as a statewide project with a staged implementation schedule across the entire state of Queensland from 2006 to 2009.

The initial objective of the project was to train 1,200 general duties or first response officers. This number was determined based on modelling that suggested that training 1,200 police across Queensland would achieve a spread of at least one police officer at every station, on every shift, who had received specialised training in mental health. The QPS had already investigated the Memphis model in depth in 2003; however, it determined that the geographical spread and number of officers across Queensland would not allow for a specialised "team" response where only a select percentage of officers received training at one point in their career. The elements of the training provided through the Memphis model were integrated into a series of training packages that have now been developed for all QPS officers throughout their entire career.

A strong component of the training considered necessary for mental health awareness was tactical communications. The QPS identified existing training in this area and who within the service was most qualified to deliver this. It was determined that QPS negotiators were the most highly skilled police in this area and would be the most appropriate officers to facilitate training to general duties officers. The QPS trains and maintains a number of police throughout the state who are accredited as police negotiators. A police negotiator is a specialist communicator trained and equipped to respond and negotiate with people in diverse situations that are beyond the capabilities of normal policing, such as hostage and siege incidents and suicide intervention.

Train-the-trainer sessions were held for police negotiators to become facilitators of the first response officer training package. QPS regional and district mental health intervention coordinators (MHICs) were nominated, trained, and established within the particular police region scheduled for implementation, and this was followed by the rollout of first response officer training in districts where coordinators had been appointed. District MHICs from QH and QAS were established concurrently, through planned project information sessions and the coordinated rollout of training.

The progressive rollout to strategically selected districts in the first stages meant that positive feedback on the training and coordinator role spread to other districts. Although the training was not mandatory, senior management encouraged all staff, where practical, to attend the training. Because of the positive response to the training, in the first six months alone, over 1,500 police in southeast Queensland were trained. This was well over the initial statewide target of 1,200 police that had been identified.

A Tri-agency Approach

The MHIP is a statewide tri-agency partnership between the QPS, QH, and QAS. The programme is aimed at the prevention and safe resolution of incidents involving people with a mental illness who are involved in a mental health crisis.

Key benefits of the MHIP include:

- Appropriate responses to people with a mental illness experiencing a mental health crisis that result in:
  - A safer outcome for individuals
  - A safer work environment for QH, QPS, and QAS staff members
  - Increased public safety
- Rapid and accessible mental health responses for a person experiencing a mental health crisis
- Enhanced skill and knowledge levels of staff in the QPS, QH, and QAS
- Improved relationships and cooperation between the QPS, QH, and QAS
- Increased and improved community support networks and crisis prevention capacity

The MHIP's cohesive, continuous improvement framework has led to a number of collaborative responses across the state. It is widely regarded as having achieved significant outcomes against its original project objectives.

Components of the Mental Health Intervention Program

The programme relies heavily on the three agencies working together at a district level and building upon existing collaborative protocols, particularly information sharing arrangements.

The three main components of the MHIP are:

- Targeted, and where appropriate, joint training for mental health intervention (mental health literacy, response techniques, legislation, policies and procedures, roles and responsibilities of each agency)
- District MHICs in all three agencies (lead training and agency improvement, case management and problem solving at the local level)
- Information sharing guidelines and a memorandum of understanding (MOU) that allows the exchange of information between QH and the QPS for prevention, precrisis planning, and crisis intervention

Police, ambulance, and health staff work together at a district level to seek solutions to localised issues.

Targeted Training for Mental Health Intervention

The QPS, QH, and the QAS provide training for personnel on enhanced skills to de-escalate situations involving people with a mental illness. Under the programme, a typical intervention or response to a person with a mental illness in a crisis situation would involve trained general duties police officers, ambulance officers, and mental health staff providing a more timely and coordinated response. Each agency provides agency-specific training to staff, including participation of the partner agencies where relevant.

Training and information sessions are provided to QPS staff to:

- Understand and recognise signs of potential vulnerability arising from a person's mental illness
- Identify the most appropriate response—whether criminal justice, health care, or nongovernment response, or a combination of all
- Seek better outcomes for individuals with a mental illness, their families, and carers

The primary QPS training product, the first response officer (FRO) training, is a course facilitated by district QPS negotiators, is often attended by health and ambulance staff, and has a number of key topic areas, including:

- General mental health awareness and understanding—identifying behaviours, reducing stigma
- Tactical communications—personal space, listening skills, building empathy and rapport, influence model (aligns with existing threat assessment and officer safety concepts)
- Understanding legislation, policies, and procedures
- Presentations from local district mental health services or community support organisations

The last session in the FRO training is scenario based, with trained role-players and a built-in de-brief component. Typically there are 6 facilitators for every 18 participants. The QPS negotiators lead the training and mental health clinicians, and ambulance officers are also involved, where possible. All police attendees are required to participate in various role-playing scenarios. Individuals are then assessed to gauge the skills and competencies developed through the training.

FRO training is just one of the mental health training packages that is provided to QPS staff. A continuum of training is provided to police over the course of their career, from initial recruit training, to on-the-job competencies, and to specialist supervisor training. From recruit through to first-year constable, shift supervisor, and district duty officer, police will get over 100 hours of training on mental health. This training is fully embedded in existing training frameworks, ensuring sustainability and that packages are reviewed every three years.

A full list of the QPS mental health training packages, modules, and professional development courses offered across the training continuum for police is provided in the Appendix near the end of this chapter.

QPS Regional and District Mental Health Intervention Coordinators (MHICs)

The MHIP provides district MHICs with resources to enable police, ambulance, and health staff to work together, at a district level, to implement local solutions to local mental health issues. MHICs from the three agencies communicate on a regular basis to identify issues, discuss complex cases, develop preventative interventions (such as precrisis plans), and identify alternative pathways of referral. By working together at the local level, QH, the QPS, and

QAS are designing customised intervention strategies to manage individual mental health crisis situations.

The QPS has established and trained a statewide network of coordinators across the 8 police regions and 31 police districts. The functions and duties of the district MHICs include:

- Coordinating mental health policing strategies and monitoring the effectiveness of those strategies in dealing with mental health issues within the district
- Leading and coordinating the implementation of the MHIP within their district
- Providing direction, guidance, and advice to QPS members and the community regarding mental health issues
- Liaising with the regional MHIC in relation to strategies to deal with mental health issues
- Reporting quarterly on their MHIC functions to their officer in charge and regional MHIC
- Chairing district MHIC meetings
- Overviewing the development and standardisation of district standard operating procedures (SOPs) and protocols relating to mental health incidents
- Conducting precrisis planning, case management, and assisting in the preparation of crisis intervention plans outlined in the *Preventing and Responding to Mental Health Crisis Situations and Information Sharing Guidelines* arrangement between the QPS and QH
- Providing assistance to officers in the assessment of and response to mental health incidents according to local protocols and, where necessary, assisting with requests for information from QH and QAS

In addition to the district MHICs there are eight regional MHICs at senior commissioned officer rank who oversee:

- The implementation and ongoing effectiveness of the MHIP objectives within their region
- The development and maintenance of regional and district SOPs and protocols
- The training of first response officers in mental health intervention
- The management of allocated budget and operating costs
- The representation of the QPS, at a regional level, with other government and nongovernment agencies

Each agency also has a central coordinating area for managing MHIP across the state. The QPS state coordinator for MHIP is responsible for:

- Overviewing the implementation and ongoing effectiveness of MHIP and objectives within the regions
- Liaising and consulting with the regional and district MHICs as necessary
- Facilitating regional mental health intervention meetings on a regular basis
- Overviewing the development and existence of regional and district SOPs and protocols
- Overviewing and monitoring the training of first response officers in mental health intervention
- Coordinating the functions and activities of regional and district MHICs
- Representing the QPS, at the state level, with other government and nongovernment agencies
- Managing the programme evaluation response and consultation process with stakeholders
- Overviewing the management of allocated budget and operating costs

Recording of Mental Health Incidents

The MHIP has also been responsible for enhancing the Queensland Police Records and Information Management Exchange (QPRIME) system in relation to the recording of mental health-related incidents. A number of functionalities have been implemented to streamline and improve the accuracy of processes for recording mental health incidences. This includes from the initial call for service in the computer-aided despatch system, to the attending police officer's entry in the police database QPRIME. This has ensured greater consistency regarding the recording of individual incidents, enhanced intelligence for potential future police involvement, and more accurate statistical analysis of incident data. A particular focus has been implementing case management processes to assist in identifying at-risk individuals who have come into repeat contact with police for mental health-related incidents.

Information Sharing

Intervention at Time of Crisis

The QPS has a formal MOU agreement with QH that allows the sharing of specific information about a mental health consumer in a crisis situation that may involve risk to the consumer or others.

Under the MOU, QH can provide information to QPS in situations where there is a serious risk to life, health, or safety, and where disclosing confidential information will help to avert the risk. Where police are involved in such situations, the QPS and QH can communicate and coordinate at the earliest possible opportunity to resolve the situation.

Prevention and Precrisis Planning

A crisis intervention plan (CIP) allows consumers of mental health services to actively contribute to their treatment in times of crisis, and to maximise their health and safety in such circumstances. A CIP may be developed collaboratively between the consumer and the mental health service and police, or (when necessary) without the consumer's involvement. A CIP can assist in ensuring readily accessible information in times of crisis, particularly outside of business hours. The CIP is designed to outline relevant aspects of the person's illness, behaviour, disability, culture, history, and treatment that will help police understand the person and the situation.

The MOU also allows for cooperation and information sharing between police and mental health clinicians to resolve crisis situations involving a person with a mental health problem who is not known to QH mental health services. In these situations, mental health clinicians may provide advice to police either over the phone or at the forward command post at the scene.

Additionally, there is also an MOU between the QPS and QAS, "Mental Health Collaboration," which was endorsed in 2007. This MOU is in relation to transportation of people with a suspected mental illness, information provision, and identification of roles between the two agencies.

Current Status of MHIP in the QPS

In 2010, MHIP was transitioned from project status to a permanent QPS programme with dedicated staffing, including a state MHIP coordinator, research analyst, and administrative support. In that same year, the QPS hosted the first policing and mental health symposium in the southern hemisphere. A number of international and Australian mental health experts and practitioners from law enforcement, justice, and the human services sector came together to discuss mental health-related issues facing frontline response agencies like police and emergency services.

Since the staged implementation of MHIP between 2006 and 2009, and the establishment of the three core components of training, agency coordinators, and information sharing, the programme has continued to evolve. While the initial project focus was on the role of first response officers in dealing with mental health crisis situations, the programme has reviewed, developed, and implemented enhancements across all aspects of the system. These include call taker processes, police intervention at the scene, hospital and ambulance handover procedures, and case management of frequent mental health consumers. These have been achieved through the ongoing improvement of policies and procedures, the use of new technologies and systems, the expansion of training content and scope, collaborative interagency problem solving, and coordination and communication.

Subsequently, the achievements and successes of MHIP in improving responses in the mental health area have seen the programme portfolio expand to include other areas regarding vulnerable people, such as disabilities and suicide intervention and prevention.

External Recognition

In 2008 the Queensland state coroner stated in his findings of inquest into the deaths of four male persons that the QPS was to be "commended for the commitment it has demonstrated in responding to the training needs of officers who can be expected to interact with persons suffering from mental illness" (Barnes, 2008). And further:

> By April 2007, over 3,500 officers had undertaken specific training programs under the umbrella of the Mental Health Intervention Project. Further, the operational skills training which all officers undertake on a regular basis has complementary components such as the tactical communication skills course. This training fits within a suite of courses designed to equip officers to make decisions consistent with the situational use of force model adopted by the Service. (Barnes, 2008, p. 134)

The 2010 *Suicide and Suicide Prevention in Australia: Breaking the Silence* report acknowledges the QPS as the only Australian police service training all frontline police officers in mental health (Mendoza & Rosenberg, 2010).

Conclusion

It is likely that police will increasingly be required to respond to incidents in the community involving people with mental illness. Police have an important role in helping to facilitate people's access to appropriate health care and treatment. The QPS is committed to continually improving its response to people in the community who are experiencing mental health crisis situations through the collaborative approach of the MHIP. This is reflected in the current *QPS Strategic Plan 2012–2016* (Queensland Police Service, 2012) under the priority of reducing the overrepresentation of vulnerable people (including people with a mental illness) as both victims and offenders.

Appendix

The QPS Mental Health Training Continuum

Training Package	Audience
Police Recruit Training	
Initial recruit training, prior to induction, includes lectures, workshops, and practical scenarios. All recruits are assessed by competent officers in a combination of written exams, classroom questioning, and practical scenarios. There are also guest lectures from mental health consumer and carer groups.	All police recruits (Mandatory)
First-Year Constable	
This is on-the-job training where constables attend a number of mental health incidents under the supervision of a field training officer. The officer must be assessed as competent before he or she is permanently appointed. The assessment is based on practical experience, assessed by the field training officer, district supervisors, and then the district education and training officer.	All first-year constables (Mandatory)
First Response Officer	
This is face-to-face training to provide strategies, procedures, and advanced tactical communication skills to assist in the de-escalation of mental health incidents. The training is delivered by MHIP-trained facilitators (QPS negotiators) and includes lectures and scenarios. The assessment is competency based, and each officer must complete six different scenarios. Training is delivered together with ambulance and health personnel.	Mandatory training
Constable Development Program	
The Constable Development Program contains a mental health module normally commenced in the third year of service. This is a self-paced assignment based at a university undergraduate level of study. The assessment is competency based and conducted by police and health facilitators.	All police between years 3 and 5 of their service (Mandatory)
Competency Acquisition Program	
This is a self-paced learning book, containing information on mental disorders—cognitive, personality, mood, schizophrenia, and others, including treatment and crisis intervention. The training reinforces tactical communication skills to assist in the de-escalation of mental health incidents. It contains instruction on information sharing provisions and incident command protocols. Assessment is competency based and completed by the officer's immediate supervisor and then the district education and training officer.	Staff members and police at all ranks

continued

The QPS Mental Health Training Continuum (continued)

Training Package	Audience

Online Learning Product

This is an online learning training product that is scenario based and assists officers to apply the Mental Health Act 2000 and QPS policies and procedures in relation to people with a mental illness, in particular, forensic and classified mental health patients. It contains instruction on handling mental health incidents and explanation of the mental health assessment process. It also contains assessment on providing assistance to victims of crime where the offender is a mental health patient.

Audience: Staff members and police at all ranks

District Duty Officer

Aimed at on-road supervisors (sergeants and senior sergeants)—the operational decision makers at mental health incidents. A one-day workshop provides the participant with skills to supervise general duties patrol crews who attend incidents involving crisis situations with people with a mental illness. The training also covers information sharing, precrisis planning, and intervention strategies.

Audience: Since 2010 has been incorporated into mandatory training for all district duty officer courses.

District Mental Health Intervention Coordinator

Provides the participant with the knowledge and skills to fulfil the roles and responsibilities of a district mental health intervention coordinator—including a broader understanding of legislation, policies and procedures, case management, community engagement, strategies to address repeat calls for service, risk management, and research and analysis.

Audience: DMHICs

Communications Centre Staff

This training provides strategies, procedures, and advanced tactical communication skills for call taker staff, including telephonic skills to assist de-escalation of incidents. Delivered by trained QPS negotiators; includes lecture and scenarios and competency-based assessment.

Audience: Civilian and police communications centre staff

Mental Health First Aid (MHFA): Youth, Adult, and Aboriginal and Torres Strait Islander

This programme provides participants with the ability to:

- Recognise the signs and symptoms of various adult/youth/indigenous-related mental health problems
- Know where and how to get help
- Know what sort of help has been shown by research to be effective

Audience: Targeted police across the state

A trial of the Mental Health First Aid (MHFA) training course was conducted in 2009–2010 in Brisbane and Cairns with 100 police receiving training. An evaluation of the trial was extremely positive. In September and October 2010 Queensland Health provided training to nine QPS staff to become trained MHFA facilitators. The QPS commenced targeted delivery of these products across Queensland in 2011.

The QPS Mental Health Training Continuum (continued)

Training Package	Audience

Applied Suicide Intervention Skills Training (ASIST)

The ASIST workshop develops participants' skills to recognise and reduce the immediate risk of a suicide, and increase the support to a person at risk. A trial of this training was conducted in 2010 in Brisbane, Toowoomba, and Mackay. Evaluation of the trial was positive, and rollout commenced in 2011 focussing on all QPS negotiators and QPS peer support officers (PSOs). PSOs are police and staff members who volunteer their time to assist and support colleagues experiencing personal and work-related difficulties.	QPS negotiators Peer support officers (civilian and police)

Certificate in Mental Health Awareness

This course provides participants with an awareness, appreciation, and understanding of: • Mental health and mental illness • Common mental illnesses • Stigma in a mental health context • Recovery model for mental health • Complexity of mental illness	Policelink—nonurgent call centre staff (police and civilians) Communication centre operators Detectives and plainclothes officers

Understanding Suicide Contacts

This training provides information around the signs of suicidal behaviour and gives call takers an insight into the internal thinking processes of someone who presents as possibly suicidal. It also covers the important area of the call takers' natural responses, how to overcome any unhelpful reactions, how to follow standard operating procedures to keep the caller safe, and how to use effective self-care strategies.	Policelink—nonurgent call centre staff (police and civilians)

References

Barnes, M. (2008). *Office of the state coroner: Findings of inquest into the police shootings of Thomas Dion Waite, Mieng Huynh, James Henry Jacobs and James Michael Gear* (Coronial findings delivered on March 17, 2008). Brisbane, Australia: Queensland Courts. Retrieved July 18, 2012, from http://www.courts.qld.gov.au/__data/assets/pdf_file/0004/86728/cif-waite-td-huynh-m-jacobs-jh-gear-jm-20080317.pdf

Commonwealth of Australia. (2009). *Fourth national mental health plan: An agenda for collaborative government action in mental health 2009–2014*. Canberra: Commonwealth Department of Health and Ageing.

Mendoza, J., & Rosenberg, S. (2010). *Suicide and suicide prevention in Australia: Breaking the silence*. Sunshine Coast, Australia: Connetica Consulting Pty Ltd.

Office of the Public Advocate—Queensland. (2004). *Annual report 2003–04*. Brisbane, Australia: Department of Justice and Attorney-General, Queensland Government.

Office of the Public Advocate—Queensland. (2005). *Preserving life and dignity in distress: Responding to critical mental health incidents.* Brisbane, Australia: Department of Justice and Attorney-General, Queensland Government.

Queensland Health. (2008). *Queensland plan for mental health 2007–2017.* Brisbane, Australia: Queensland Government.

Queensland Police Service. (2012). *QPS strategic plan 2012–2016.* Brisbane, Australia: Queensland Government.

Whiteford, H. (1998). *Final report of the Mental Health Crisis Intervention Ad Hoc Advisory Group: An examination of mental health crisis intervention practices and policies regarding the fatal use of firearms by police against people with a mental illness.* Canberra: Commonwealth Department of Health and Family Services.

Core Requirements of a Best Practise Model for Police Encounters Involving People Experiencing Mental Illness in Australia

A Victorian Perspective

STUART THOMAS

Contents

Introduction

Concerns about the frequency and nature of police contact with people experiencing mental illness are longstanding, with commentary now spanning some 45 years (Bitner, 1967; Lurigio & Watson, 2010). The idea that a best practise model of policing when it comes to these encounters can be (1) conceptualised, (2) articulated, and (3) realised is therefore clearly a highly seductive one and something that scholars and practitioners alike would obviously aspire toward. The challenge faced is that trying to propose a model that can be generalised to all situations and jurisdictions runs the real risk of being overly generic, and therefore of only limited practical utility to policy makers and operational members. On the other hand, suggesting something too specific could mean that the idiosyncrasies and diversity of different settings/environments render the model pretty much impotent outside of those narrowly defined parameters. This chapter sets out to describe some of the key findings that have arisen in the context of a programme of research exploring police encounters with people with mental illness across the state of Victoria in Australia, and considers how this evidence base could help inform best practise.

How Frequently and In What Context Do Police Encounter Mental Illness?

One of the most commonly asked issues at this interface is the quite fundamental question of just how commonly police members are coming into contact with people experiencing mental illness. Anecdotal evidence, both internationally and in the Victorian context, suggests that these encounters are commonplace (e.g., Wylie, 1990), but until recently there has been very little in the way of hard evidence with which to back up such claims.

Briefly, by way of context, like many Westernised societies, and as discussed in the chapter by Tamsin Short (see Chapter 7), Victoria went through a somewhat protracted period of deinstitutionalisation whereby mental health services made the fundamental shift toward a community-based service delivery model, culminating in the late 1990s. This coincided with a similar shift in core police practise to a more community-oriented policing model (Brogden & Nijhar, 2005) that necessitated the adoption of broader social welfare roles and responsibilities (Stenning & Shearing, 2005). With a greater community engagement mantra and assertive outreach models adopted in order to engage with community members and resonate with their needs, the accessibility of police to the general public has been enhanced greatly. Quite laudably, these processes have been a contributing factor to the increasing rate of contact between police members and people experiencing mental illness. Blame has been firmly directed at the scarcity of mental health services, to the extent, some have argued, of police becoming "street corner psychiatrists" (Teplin & Pruett, 1992). Indeed, this argument has strong empirical support if the arrest rate (e.g., Klein, 2010) and occurrence and overrepresentation of mental disorders in the remand and sentenced prison populations are considered (Fazel & Danesh, 2002). This has led scholars and practitioners alike to argue that police are essentially being forced to arrest people experiencing mental illness due to an absence of other (more appropriate) mental health disposal options (Lamb, Weinberger, & de Cuir Jr., 2002).

The Situation in Police Custody

Findings from research that considered the prevalence of psychiatric symptoms, histories of mental health contact, and psychiatric medication usage among a large sample of over 600 police cell detainees across the state found that over half of the sample had previously had contact with the public mental health services in Victoria, and that a third of them exhibited psychiatric symptoms according to a well-established psychopathology scale. Furthermore, a third of those included were in treatment for mental disorders at the time of their arrest (Ogloff, Warren, Tye, Blaher, & Thomas, 2010). Adding to this, more focussed research carried out in two busy police stations in the metropolitan area of Melbourne in 2008–2009 found similarly that over half of the 150 police cell detainees interviewed had previously been in contact with the public mental health service in Victoria (Baksheev, Thomas, & Ogloff, 2010). However, quite remarkably, three quarters of this sample met diagnostic criteria for at least one major mental disorder; the most common mental disorders found were mood disorders (32%), drug and alcohol disorders (alcohol dependence, 21%; opioid dependence, 21%), and post-traumatic stress disorder (13%). Of note, when compared to estimated rates in the general community, the odds of meeting diagnostic criteria for psychotic disorders were more than 15 times higher among police cell detainees than the estimated rates in the general community (the latter typically being around 1% to 1.5%; Short, Thomas, Luebbers, Ogloff, & Mullen, 2010). What was interesting with this study, and in response to the potential criminalisation hypotheses posed by others previously (e.g., Holley & Arboleda-Florez, 1988), was that just over two-thirds of the detainees interviewed had been detained for nonviolent offences; however, virtually all of them had a prior criminal record that, two-thirds of the time, was for violent offences.

In the context of a recent Victorian Office of Police Integrity (OPI) report, which described deficiencies in the provision of health care services coupled with overcrowding and unacceptably long length of stays in police cells, the core concern raised was that the police role had become partly a custodial one, despite not being considered a core function of policing (Brouwer, 2006). While there are a number of broader systemic issues centred around the availability of suitable accommodation in remand centres, for example, the situation faced raised a number of significant concerns from a human rights perspective in relation to the detention of people in police custody (Strong, 2010). Indeed, this situation is further complicated by findings that those being detained who met criteria for mental disorders presented as having a number of needs (mostly unmet needs, thus representing ongoing difficulties) across a range of psychiatric, social, and welfare domains

(Baksheev et al., 2010). While this is perhaps not surprising (e.g., Cummins, 2007; Heffernan, Finn, Saunders, & Byrne, 2003), it does raise vitally important concerns about the need for interagency collaborations that enable these additionally vulnerable individuals to be linked in with community health and welfare services to help facilitate timely access to support services post-release. Furthermore, while senior police members in watchhouses may well be committed to the welfare of the people detained in custody, issues pertaining to core competencies in duty of care and the custodial role are still brought into question by critics and represent ongoing training priorities (Strong, 2010).

The Broader Context of Community Policing

Victoria Police is a centralised statewide armed police force of around 11,250 sworn members (Victoria Police, 2009; cited in Kesic, Thomas, & Ogloff, 2012). A large-scale survey of operational police across the state of Victoria, incorporating the views of over 3,500 respondents, demonstrated that police reported they were coming into contact with a person experiencing mental illness on a frequent basis, estimating that approximately one-fifth of people they come into contact with in a week are mentally ill, and that these contacts were consuming a significant amount of their time (Godfredson, Thomas, Luebbers, & Ogloff, 2011). What was perhaps most interesting, though, in this context was the wide range of circumstances under which this contact was actually occurring. Most commonly, the outcome of the encounters was listed as a "mental health apprehension" (under powers set out in the Mental Health Act 1986 (Vic)) or "arrest," but commonly "no further action" was also reported. This finding is perhaps salient here in providing evidence in support of the social welfare role of contemporary community policing, as well as helping to partially dispel populist beliefs about the perceived dangerousness of people with mental disorders (e.g., Kesic, Ducat & Thomas, 2011). Our findings from the police survey bring into question the manner in which police members are identifying instances of mental illness, and also raise the additional issue of how good police members actually are at identifying signs and symptoms of mental illness.

Police Completing a Mini Mental Status Examination

The police surveyed in the study by Godfredson and colleagues (2011) reported that members most frequently considered the content of speech, behaviour and actions of the person, his or her appearance, the presence of aggression or violence, and body language or movements to be associated with mental illness. Consistent with this, they reported most commonly relying on "person-based information" gleaned from the nature of their contact with the person and behaviours observed on scene, but also made use of previously recorded contacts with the person on their police database. Furthermore, when shown a video vignette of a scenario that, due to the nature of the situation presented, potentially provided ample scope for members to use their discretionary powers, police participants were more likely to identify a preference for a mental health-related outcome as presenting signs and symptoms of mental disorder across the three scenarios became more apparent/severe (Godfredson et al., 2011).

What is really quite interesting, therefore, is that police essentially inferred that they are completing what really boils down to an abbreviated mental status examination (MSE), akin to that of a mental health practitioner, covering areas including appearance, behaviours, speech/communication, and levels of cooperation or resistance (e.g., Schwecke, 2003). These MSE skills were advanced and point to the accumulated practical wisdom inherent in police members learned, in great part, through repeated exposure to vulnerable people in the community. The contradiction here, of course, is that despite the Mental Health Act legislation, both in Victoria and in other jurisdictions, not requiring police to "exercise any clinical judgment as to whether a person is mentally ill," the expectation is still there from the general public's perspective (Lurigio & Watson, 2010). Indeed, recent case law in Victoria (*Stuart v. Kirkland-Veenstra* [2009] HCA 15) indicates that police should be considering risks in relation to what would be considered a reasonably foreseeable risk of harm, and where there is doubt perhaps to err on the side of caution (Scott, 2010). As such, the requirements of the requisite, albeit perhaps still informal, clinical assessment abilities of the operational police officer become blurred within the parameters of his or her *parens patriae* role.

What is very clear is that pockets of best practise between police and community agencies exist, at the very least, on a local level. It would appear that these essentially individualised initiatives have come about through relationships that have been forged between particularly proactive senior operational police members and members of community agencies; informal agreements and common understandings commonly form the backbone of the success of the creative partnerships that we have found. A recent initiative set up by Victoria Police, for example, called the Police and Community Triage (PACT) initiative, seeks to facilitate increased opportunities to divert vulnerable groups (such as people with mental illness, substance use, and homelessness) away from the criminal justice system by linking individuals with a wide range of community-based health, social and welfare organisations providing support, advice, and advocacy services. A large number of health and nongovernmental organisation service providers have signed a memorandum of understanding with the police to help facilitate these referrals that the PACT team then follow up to see if the client has taken up support services. The initiative is currently being piloted for a 12-month period and independently evaluated.

Focussing on Improved Outcomes

Arguably one of the biggest challenges for the police is addressing community perceptions of their role, function, and value. Much of the information community members base this on comes from the mass media, which can have its positives as well as some potential drawbacks (Kesic, Ducat, & Thomas, 2011). Also dominant at this interface are the perceptions that members of the community form based on their encounters with police. Of concern, therefore, are findings discussed by Tamsin Short (see Chapter 7) that highlight that people with severe mental disorders are much less likely to have an official record of having reported being the victims of crime to police than general community members. These findings contrast with a number of previous, mainly self-report studies, which have suggested substantially raised rates of victimisation (Maniglio, 2009), thereby suggesting that unless victimisation experiences are severe (i.e., involving third parties through violent or sexual offences), people with severe mental illnesses are not bringing these incidents to the formal attention of police.

A procedural justice framework for considering encounters between police and community members has the potential to be informative in this context, as it places particular emphasis on the perceived quality of the interaction between the operational member(s) and citizen (e.g., Thibaut & Walker, 1975). The argument follows that improving the perceptions of fairness by community members of the methods used by the police in achieving policing-related outcomes impacts on community members' assessments of procedural justice. Tyler has argued that this can not only serve to increase police legitimacy and levels of compliance with the law, but also lead to improved cooperation by community members with the police (Tyler, 2000, 2005). It is likely that people experiencing mental illness, especially with more severe disorders, are perceiving lower levels of procedural justice in their encounters with police members, but this remains unclear at this time.

Previous research in this area suggests that there are four relational dimensions forming key antecedents to procedural justice: (1) participation, (2) quality of interpersonal treatment, (3) neutrality of decision making, and (4) trustworthiness (Tyler & Wakslak, 2004). When considered alongside indices of legitimacy, sensitivity to justice, and fairness of the outcome, recent research with victims of crime suggests that higher perceived levels of procedural justice are reported when victims perceive the police to be acting more legitimately, when they consider the outcome of the encounter to be fair, and when they are more satisfied with the process overall. Perhaps most importantly, from a policy and practise level, a recent Victorian study found that victims of crime valued process-oriented assessments of procedural justice over outcome-oriented assessment (Elliott, Thomas, & Ogloff, 2011a). These findings suggest that victims are placing most weight on the process of the encounter at two levels: the individual and policing levels. First, at an individual level, higher levels of procedural justice were most overwhelmingly associated with the victim feeling like a valued member of the community. Additionally, victims reported getting some therapeutic gain from the encounter, centred on giving them a sense of closure, helping them to recover, and enabling them to move on with their lives. Interestingly, these gains were reported regardless of the actual outcome of reporting their victimisation experience to police. In addition, those participants who had previously had contacts with police as offenders were more likely to indicate that the nature of their contacts with police as victims could impact upon (and improve) their sense of legitimacy and trust in the police, thus motivating them to go on to be law abiding (Elliott et al., 2011a).

These findings suggest the real significance of procedural justice in community members' interactions with the police and highlight some quite simple, practical guidance for police members when engaging with victims of crime generally (Elliott, Thomas, & Ogloff, 2011b). First, participants valued police members' unacceptance of the crime and feeling that police were taking the case seriously. Related to this, participants also reported the importance of police members having nonblaming attitudes. A common fear among victims of crime was their concern that their case wouldn't be considered serious enough, so the fact that police took action as a result of the victim reporting the crime validated their experience. An additional area of focus from the victim's perspective was evidence that police have followed up on the case and passed on information about their actions and investigations to the victims, primarily so as to reassure the victim that the police had not given up on the case. The other main area of note from the victim's perspective was police members' interpersonal and communication skills. This was articulated by victims in relation to police members' ability to relate to the victim, allowing him or her to tell his or her story of what happened, giving him or her options about whether to proceed, and perhaps most importantly, normalising the experience for the victim. It is argued that gathering this kind of information on police processes with victims could be an important conduit for more formally validating the experience of victims of crime. Furthermore, this could serve to improve community perceptions of procedural justice as well as providing a measure of police outcome beyond the traditional indices of crime statistics and clear-up rates that starts to acknowledge the breadth of the community policing role (Elliott et al., 2011b). The degree to which these findings relate to and resonate with people who are experiencing mental illness, and especially perhaps those with severe mental disorders like schizophrenia, remains unclear at this time. Short (see Chapter 7) makes the very practical suggestion that clinicians should include routine questions about crime victimisation in their clinical assessments to help understand its commonality in this population. This would have the added advantage of helping us to understand the underlying mechanisms that may encourage, inhibit, or dissuade mental health clients from reporting victimisation incidents to police.

Implementation of a Screening Tool for Identifying Mental Illness

Thinking back to the overrepresentation of severe mental illnesses in police custody and the limited opportunities police have to identify mental illness, another significant practical solution for the police could be the implementation of a screening tool to be used upon reception to police custody. The process of screening for the presence of mental illnesses at this juncture could potentially have a number of significant positive implications for both the police and those in need of health or welfare service supports. Current uptake or use of such methods appears somewhat piecemeal, with our research finding that while some police stations had implemented some form of proxy screening methods with the assistance of custodial nurses, others had no such processes in place (Baksheev, Ogloff, & Thomas, 2012). This is again in contrast with policies and practises in different Australian jurisdictions, some of which have instigated comprehensive screening at the court and even the holding cell level.

The Custody Risk Assessment Form, which was used on one of the sites sampled, is essentially a simple tick box list recording the presence of a number of different risk factors or concerns, with items including "depressed or suicidal," "currently on medication," and "mentally ill or been diagnosed with mental illness." We found that it correctly classified just over half of the participants at that site as having a current mental illness or not, and of note, we found that it was better at identifying those without mental illness than those with a mental illness. Of concern, though, it had a high false negative rate, thereby missing a significant proportion of those who had a current mental disorder according to the SCID-I assessments conducted (First, Spitzer, Miriam, & Williams, 2002).

Clearly, this "hit rate" is not acceptable for a screening tool whose purpose, one would argue in this context, should be to be overly inclusive. As essentially the first step in a psychiatric triage process, the aim of such a screen would be to make sure that all cases (i.e., those with mental illness) are identified at the expense of introducing a small number of false positives (i.e., those who screen as having a current mental illness who in fact do not). The trialling of two screening tools in the police cell setting found that the use of a standardised tool improved the predictive accuracy to moderately good levels, with correct predictions (in these cases being rated as requiring further mental health assessment or not) for between 70% and 80% of the detainees interviewed (Baksheev et al., 2012). While overall there were no statistically different differences between the two tools trialled (the Brief Jail Mental Health Screen (BJMHS), Steadman, Scott, Osher, Agnese, and Robbins, 2005; and the Jail Screening Assessment Tool (JSAT); Nicholls, Roesch, Olley, Ogloff, & Hemphill, 2005) when considering the identification of serious mental illness, the JSAT was significantly better at predicting Axis 1 disorders (excluding substance use disorders).

In sum, the results suggest a significant advantage to introducing a standardised screening tool into practise in police custody settings. Due to the deleterious nature of the police cell environment on mental health and wellbeing, and the high level of unmet needs evident in this additionally vulnerable population, there are clearly a number of immediate "here and now" benefits brought about by the early identification of those with mental illnesses. These would include, but are not restricted to, identifying the need for crisis intervention in high-need situations and facilitating access to the timely provision of treatment opportunities for those in need of follow-up mental health care and support services. The challenge, however, is to balance the need to meet what amounts to a significant public health need with the other practicalities and procedural burdens already placed on police members working in extremely busy police custody environments. What this research does suggest is that ad hoc solutions are not providing sufficient protection for those presenting to police cells with significant psychiatric distress. As well as identifying and piloting an appropriate standardised screening tool, the other significant implication here, both in the custodial setting and more generally in the context of community encounters, surrounds the perceived need for increased and improved training for police in identifying and responding to mental illness.

Training

You will see a never-ending call for the need for training to help resolve the current skills/knowledge deficits of police in improving their encounters with people with mental illness. Such statements are, however, deceptively straightforward. The problem with this kind of conclusion is that very little attention is given to the "what actually works" criterion and translating this perceived, measured, or otherwise determined knowledge or skills-based deficit into practise. While jurisdictions across Australia and internationally differ with their models of training, recent research suggests that a combination of classroom-based knowledge acquisition sessions with scenario-based training may offer the optimal training medium—especially when it comes to resolving encounters with people experiencing mental illness. This reflects what Borum (2000) describes in relation to the key to training police not being so much on the acquisition of knowledge, but more on how to embed that knowledge and apply it routinely in practise. There also appears to be a distinct benefit to tapping into the expertise of clinicians/experts in conjunction with the experience of seasoned police members who can help translate this knowledge into a more practical and palatable format. Perhaps quite understandingly, the latter is considered particularly important for members in validating and ultimately valuing the content of the training being delivered, thereby increasing the propensity for cultural change (Brouwer, 2009).

This approach to training has been specifically focussed upon in Victoria in relation to police use of force. The police survey data presented by Godfredson and colleagues (2011) found that police considered one of the main challenges when resolving encounters with people experiencing mental illness to be avoiding using force. Interestingly, this was also a criticism recently applied to the training provided to Victorian Police members by the Office of Police Integrity in relation to currently recommended approaches still being predominantly focussed on hands-on tactics as opposed to being verbal and communications based (Brouwer, 2009). Furthermore, detailed analyses of use of force data in the Victorian context, reported in this text in Chapter 8 by Dragana Kesic, reinforced police concerns and supported OPI criticisms by demonstrating that police were using more severe levels of force on people that they had reported as "appearing to be mentally ill." The same was true for those who had documented mental health histories with public mental health services. Some have speculated that this is because police members are misattributing the behaviours of mentally ill people as dangerous when they may not be (Brouwer, 2009) in a significant proportion of instances.

An internal review of police shootings that occurred between July 2005 and December 2008 suggested that there was something inherently flawed with the police approach style, stating "there is a tendency to revert to the 'must resolve quickly' style accompanied with a communication style that may inflame the situation, particularly those involving vulnerable people" (Victoria Police Corporate Management Risk Division, 2009, cited in Brouwer, 2009, p. 28). Anecdotally speaking, that does not appear to be the case, however, with operational members interviewed reporting very advanced communication and de-escalation skills. In fact, the skills demonstrated are akin to those set out as best practise guidelines for frontline mental health workers working in inpatient psychiatric services (National Institute of Clinical Excellence, 2005). What is interesting about the latter is that these guidelines were in fact developed from the collective clinical wisdom of the guideline development group, as opposed to being derived from theoretically based empirical research evidence (Roberton, Daffern, Thomas, & Martin, 2011). Therefore, in lieu of a substantiated evidence base to underpin the parameters and focus of the suggested police approach style in such instances, one could argue that a similar model of guideline development to that utilised in psychiatry could be readily adopted with operational police members. Indeed, such a proposition is intuitively appealing in that police have very limited opportunities for classroom-based training, so for the majority of operational members, learning occurs on the job through repeated exposures to different situations, risk, and vulnerabilities. As such, there is a significant practical policing wisdom that can potentially be tapped into and utilised as an invaluable learning tool for others. This is certainly a model evident in the scenario-based training initiatives currently adopted in the Victorian context, with peer-based learning, review, and reflection high on the agenda with all activities undertaken during training.

Future Directions: Moving Beyond the Abstract Into the Concrete

One of the principal limitations and barriers with translating research findings into policy and practise remains the discord between initiating compliance checking and embedding change into practise. The main challenge is that what the research undertaken in Victoria is suggesting needs to happen actually amounts to a need for significant cultural change in policing. While there are a number of small easy gains that can be achieved in the short term, the broader systemic issues, especially those around interagency partnership initiatives, will need to be considered as a much longer-term proposition. Other jurisdictions have considered this by adopting other service models.

Currently in Victoria, as with most jurisdictions, police and psychiatric crisis services operate in parallel. It is often the case that only one service is available to attend a crisis situation, and police often face significant pragmatic barriers when attempting to resolve situations involving mentally ill persons (Owen, Fischer, Booth, & Cuffell, 1996). Ideally, it would seem that police and mental health services need to join forces to manage the relatively small, but highly significant, number of people with severe mental illness who come into contact with the criminal justice system. This idea has certainly been at the forefront of policing policy and development internationally over the past two decades.

In 1988, police in Memphis, Tennessee, collaborated with the National Alliance on Mental Illness to develop a new approach to crisis intervention that became known internationally as the Memphis model. Essentially, the Memphis model is a programme of prearrest jail diversion for people with mental illness, in which specialised police units (crisis intervention teams) are deployed to crisis situations in which there is some suggestion of mental disturbance among the participants. The crisis intervention teams are staffed by police officers who have received specialised mental health training, and who can make appropriate mental health referrals as required. Critical to the model is the availability of a 24-hour crisis drop-off service in the hospital emergency department, which is mandated to have a 100% acceptance rate for police referrals (Cochran, Deane, & Borum, 2000).

Evaluations of the Memphis model have demonstrated positive outcomes for police, offenders, and the community, with a reduction in police officer injuries and an increase in the number of specialised mental health response calls (Steadman, Deane, Borum, & Morrissey, 2000). However, not all jurisdictions have the capability or resources to support the specifics of the model (especially in relation to the mandated acceptance of all police referrals to the emergency department), so this limits the generalisability of the concept quite considerably. Indeed, it could be argued that the success of the Memphis model is largely attributable to the guaranteed availability of a mental health crisis drop-off service, rather than police officer training per se. Nevertheless, its success clearly advocates for a collaborative working partnership between police and mental health services (Steadman et al., 2000).

Since the inception of the Memphis model, other programmes have been developed that are similarly based on collaboration between police and mental health services. In 2007, Victoria conducted a three-month trial of a policing/mental illness model that involved collaboration between police, mental health, and ambulance services. The Police, Ambulance, and CAT (crisis assessment and treatment team) Emergency Response (PACER) programme is a secondary response unit comprising both a uniformed police officer and a mental health clinician who are called to attend crisis situations in which there are suspected mental health issues. The PACER programme was initially trialled in a single police division in Victoria, with further funding recently allocated to continue the trial for a further 12 months (Pearson, 2009).

The research considered here provides further evidence that such a collaborative, interagency model between the police and health services is warranted; this clearly needs to be a real focus in the development of a best practise model. While this is by no means a straightforward proposal to enact, with significant privacy and information sharing issues needing to be considered alongside many other practical issues, common sense and the shared vision of all those working at (and affected by) this complex interface surely need to be the common catalyst for initiating change.

Results from this programme of research in Victoria, Australia, highlight a number of practical markers for change in the context of police encounters with people experiencing mental illness and define some of the parameters indicative of a best practise model at this interface. Perhaps most fundamentally, police members need to consider that encounters with people experiencing mental illness are in fact the norm, as opposed to being the exception. This in itself potentially necessitates the need for significant cultural change, but it is clearly a significant step toward helping police members carry out their duties more effectively and efficiently. While achieving cultural change is a longer-term, somewhat abstract proposition, a series of more discrete initiatives can be initiated in tandem to help provide measurable gains at this interface. Proactive engagement with members on these discrete initiatives should be considered fundamental in relation to both maximising the uptake of the initiatives and sustaining their momentum over time. Ultimately, these more practical steps need to contribute to facilitating more timely identification of those experiencing mental illness, and then prioritising access to supports and health care for those identified as being in need. Previous research has found that this identification can be as straightforward as simply asking every person if they have any special needs (Gudjonsson, Clare, Rutter, & Pearse, 1993). The translation of the growing evidence base into actual policing practise will require significant thought as well as time to implement and then measure any changes. What is vital is that we need to move beyond proposing what amounts to abstract concepts, inherent in many best practise models, to the development of a practical toolkit for members that is actively supported and reinforced by a service structure that is receptive to the needs of its community.

References

Borum, R. (2000). Improving high risk encounters between people with mental illness and police. *Journal of the American Academy of Psychiatry and the Law, 28*, 973–976.

Baksheev, G.N., Ogloff, J., & Thomas, S. (2012). Identification of mental illness in police cells: A comparison of police processes, the Brief Jail Mental Health Screen and the Jail Screening Assessment Tool. *Psychology, Crime and Law, 18*, 529–542.

Baksheev, G.N., Thomas, S.D.M., & Ogloff, J.R.P. (2010). Psychiatric disorders and unmet needs in Australian police cells. *Australian and New Zealand Journal of Psychiatry, 44,* 1043–1051.

Bitner, E. (1967). Police discretion in emergency apprehension of mentally ill persons. *Social Problems, 14,* 278–292.

Brogden, M., & Nijhar, P. (2005). *Community policing: National and international models and approaches.* Cullompton, Devon: Willan Publishers.

Brouwer, G. (2006). *Conditions for persons in custody.* Melbourne: Ombudsman Victoria and Office of Police Integrity.

Brouwer, G. (2009). *Review of the use of force by and against Victorian Police.* Melbourne: Office of Police Integrity.

Clayfield, J.C., Fletcher, K.E., & Grudzinkas, A.J. (2011). Development and validation of the mental health attitude survey for police. *Community Mental Health Journal, 47*(6), 742–751.

Cochran, S., Deane, M.W., & Borum, R. (2000). Improving police response to mentally ill people. *Psychiatric Services, 51,* 1315–1316.

Cummins, I. (2007). Boats against the current: Vulnerable adults in police custody. *Journal of Adult Protection, 9,* 15–24.

Elliott, I., Thomas, S.D.M., & Ogloff, J.R.P. (2011a). Procedural justice in contacts with the police: The perspective of victims of crime. *Police Practice and Research: An International Journal,* in press.

Elliott, I., Thomas, S.D.M., & Ogloff, J.R.P. (2011b, May). Procedural justice in contacts with the police: Testing a relational model of authority in a mixed methods study. *Psychology, Public Policy and the Law.*

Fazel, S., & Danesh, J. (2002). Serious mental disorder in 2300 prisoners: A systematic review of 62 surveys. *Lancet, 359,* 545–550.

First, M.B., Spitzer, R.L., Miriam, G., & Williams, J.B.W. (2002). *Structured clinical interview for DSM-IV-TR axis 1 disorders, research version, patient edition (SCID-1-P).* New York: Biometrics Research, New York State Psychiatric Institute.

Godfredson, J.W., Thomas, S.D.M., Luebbers, S., Ogloff, J.R.P. (2011). Police perceptions of their encounters with individuals experiencing mental illness: A Victorian survey. *Australian and New Zealand Journal of Criminology, 44,* 180–195.

Gudjonsson, G.H., Clare, I., Rutter, S., & Pearse, J. (1993). *Persons at risk during interviews in police custody: The identification of vulnerabilities.* London: Royal Commission on Criminal Justice, HMSO.

Heffernan, E.B., Finn, J., Saunders, J.B., & Byrne, G. (2003). Substance-use disorders and psychological distress among police arrestees. *Medical Journal of Australia, 179,* 408–411.

Holley, H.L., & Arboleda-Florez, J. (1988). Criminalisation of the mentally ill. Part 1. Police perceptions. *Canadian Journal of Psychiatry, 33,* 81–89.

Kesic, D., Ducat, L.V., & Thomas, S.D.M. (2011). Australian print media depictions of contacts between the police and persons experiencing mental illness. *Australian Psychologist,* in press.

Kesic, D., Thomas, S.D.M., & Ogloff, J.R.P. (2012). Estimated rates of mental disorders in, and situational characteristics of, nonfatal use of force incidents in Victoria. *Social Psychiatry and Psychiatric Epidemiology.*

Klein, G.C. (2010). Negotiating the fate of people with mental illness: The police and the hospital emergency room. *Journal of Police Crisis Negotiations, 10,* 205–219.

Lamb, H.R., Weinberger, L.E., & de Cuir Jr., W.J. (2002). The police and mental health. *Psychiatric Services, 53,* 1266–1271.

Lurigio, A.J., & Watson, A.C. (2010). The police and people with mental illness: New approaches to a longstanding problem. *Journal of Police Crisis Negotiations, 10,* 3–14.

Maniglio, R. (2009). Severe mental illness and criminal victimisation: A systematic review. *Acta Psychiatrica Scandinavica, 119,* 180–191.

National Institute of Clinical Excellence. (2005). *Clinical practice guidelines on the short-term management of disturbed/violent behaviour in in-patient psychiatric settings and emergency departments* [full guideline]. London: Royal College of Nursing.Nicholls, T.L., Roesch, R., Olley, M.C., Ogloff, J.R.P., & Hemphill, J.F. (2005). *Jail screening assessment tool (JSAT): Guidelines for mental health screening in jails.* Burnaby, BC: Simon Fraser University.

Ogloff, J., Warren, L., Tye, C., Blaher, F., & Thomas, S. (2010). Psychiatric histories and symptoms and histories among people detained in police cells. *Social Psychiatry and Psychiatric Epidemiology, 46,* 871–880.

Owen, R.R., Fischer, E.P., Booth, B.B., & Cuffell, B.J. (1996). Medication noncompliance and substance abuse among patients with schizophrenia. *Psychiatric Services, 47,* 853–858.

Pearson, D.D.R. (2009). *Responding to mental health crises in the community.* Melbourne, Australia: Victorian Auditor-General's Office.

Roberton, T., Daffern, M., Thomas, S.D.M., & Martin, T. (2012). De-escalation and limit setting in forensic mental health units. *Journal of Forensic Nursing, 8*(2):, 942–1101.

Schwecke, L.H. (2003). Nursing process. In N.L. Keltner, L.H. Schwecke, & C.E. Bostrom (Eds.), *Psychiatric nursing* (4th ed., pp. 111–119). St. Louis, MO: Mosby.

Scott, R. (2010). The duty of care owed by police to a person at risk of suicide. *Psychiatry, Psychology and Law, 17,* 1–24.

Short, T.B.R., Thomas, S.D.M., Luebbers, S., Ogloff, J.R.P., & Mullen, P.E. (2010). The epidemiology of psychosis: Prevalence and use of mental health services in a random community sample. *Australian and New Zealand Journal of Psychiatry, 44,* 475–481.

Steadman, H.J., Deane, M.W., Borum, R., & Morrissey, J.P. (2000). Comparing outcomes of major models of police responses to mental health emergencies. *Psychiatric Services, 51,* 645–649.

Steadman, H.J., Scott, J.E., Osher, F., Agnese, T.K., & Robbins, P.C. (2005). Validation of the Brief Jail Mental Health Screen. *Psychiatric Services, 56,* 816-822.

Stenning, P.C., & Shearing, C.D. (2005). Reforming police: Opportunities, drivers and challenges. *Australian and New Zealand Journal of Criminology, 44,* 167–180.

Strong, M. (2010). *Update on conditions in Victoria Police cells.* Melbourne: Office of Police Integrity.

Teplin, L.A., & Pruett, N.S. (1992). Police as streetcorner psychiatrist: Managing the mentally ill. *International Journal of Law and Psychiatry, 15,* 139–156.

Thibaut, J., & Walker, L. (1975). *Procedural justice.* Hillside, NJ: Erlbaum.

Tyler, T.R. (1990). *Why people obey the law.* New Haven, CT: Yale University Press.

Tyler, T.R. (2005). Policing in black and white: Ethnic group differences in trust and confidence in the police. *Police Quarterly, 8,* 322–342.

Tyler, T.R., & Wakslak, C.J. (2004). Profiling and police legitimacy: Procedural justice, attributions of motive, and acceptance of police authority. *Criminology, 42,* 253–281.

Victoria Police. (2009). *Victoria Police annual report 2008/2009.* Melbourne: Victoria Police.

Wylie, J. (1990). Deinstitutionalisation of the mentally disabled and its impact on police services. *Australasian Centre for Policing Research, 63.*

Suggested Reading

Godfredson, J., Ogloff, J.R.P., Thomas, S.D.M., & Luebbers, S. (2010). Police discretion and encounters with people experiencing mental illness: The significant factors. *Criminal Justice and Behavior, 37,* 1392–1405.

Lipson, G.S., Turner, J.T., & Kasper, R. (2010). A strategic approach to police interactions involving persons with mental illness. *Journal of Police Crisis Negotiations, 10,* 30–38.

Ogloff, J.R.P. (2002). Identifying and accommodating the needs of mentally ill people in gaols and prisons. *Psychiatry, Psychology and Law, 9,* 1–33.

Pogrebin, M.R., & Poole, E.D. (1987). Deinstitutionalisation and increased arrest rates among the mentally disordered. *Journal of Psychiatry and Law, 15,* 117–127.

Vatne, S., & Fagermoen, M.S. (2007). To correct and acknowledge: Two simultaneous and conflicting perspectives of limit-setting in mental health nursing. *Journal of Psychiatric and Mental Health Nursing, 14,* 41–48.

Watson, A.C., Corrigan, P.W., & Ottati, V. (2004). Police officers' attitudes toward and decisions about persons with mental illness. *Psychiatric Services, 55,* 49–53.

Policing and the Mentally Ill

Victimisation and Offending in Severe Mental Illness

7

TAMSIN SHORT

Contents

Overview

This chapter will review two important types of police interactions with the mentally ill: criminal offending and crime victimisation. For clarity, the chapter will focus on severe mental illness, rather than mental illness more broadly, which encompasses a much larger section of the population. Severe mental illnesses typically affect 1% to 2% of the population, and include diagnoses such as major psychotic and mood disorders.

It is well recognised that the vast majority of people with severe mental illness do not engage in violent or criminal behaviour, and that mental illness is generally less predictive of violence than other factors, such as substance abuse, gender, or psychopathy (Angermeyer, 2000; Swanson, Holzer, Ganju, & Jono, 1990; Swartz et al., 1998; Tengstrom, Grann, Langstrom, & Kullgren, 2000). However, there is now good evidence to show a modest but significant increase in the risk of both violence perpetration and violent victimisation in people with severe mental illness, as compared to others in the community (Douglas, Guy, & Hart, 2009; Maniglio, 2009; Walsh, Buchanan, & Fahy,

2002). As the frontline workers of the criminal justice system, it is the police who usually make the first contact with these mentally ill victims and offenders. The remainder of this chapter will examine these interactions in more detail, summarising recent research and examining the implications for the Australian context. Given that the mentally ill are, by definition, a vulnerable population, the reasons how and why they become involved with the criminal justice system, and how the police respond to these interactions, are certainly worthy topics for discussion.

Police Contacts With the Mentally Ill: The Impact of Deinstitutionalisation

While severe mental illness affects relatively few individuals, it accounts for a disproportionately large volume of mental health resources in the community (Short, Thomas, Luebbers, Ogloff, & Mullen, 2010). In addition to this increased use of clinical and support services, people with severe mental illness are also more likely to come into contact with the police, whether through offending, victimisation, family violence, welfare checks, substance abuse, or other "on the street" contacts. The type and frequency of contacts between police officers and mental health patients have changed considerably since the deinstitutionalisation movement of the 1960s to 1980s, which saw almost all mental asylums and institutions in Australia closed down in favour of community-based mental health care (MacKinnon & Coleborne, 2003). As a consequence of this reform, the majority of Australian mental health patients now reside, and are primarily treated, within the community, where they are more likely than ever to come into contact with police. Despite the apparent success of the deinstitutionalisation movement in improving patient independence and autonomy, some have expressed concern about the potential risks that people with severe mental illness may pose to, and face from, the general community (Brekke, Prindle, Bae, & Long, 2001; MacKinnon & Coleborne, 2003). It has been argued that policing services have had to pick up the slack, acting as a sort of triage service for psychiatric facilities, apprehending unwell individuals, transporting patients to the hospital, and conducting welfare checks in homes and on the streets. Discussions with police officers about their interactions with the mentally ill reveal that these are neither uncommon nor brief encounters (Godfredson, Thomas, Ogloff, & Luebbers, 2011). While it is hard to quantify exactly how much time police spend with mentally ill people, one Australian study reported that approximately 10% of police time was spent in contact with people experiencing mental illness. Two of the most commonly discussed interactions between police and mentally ill people involve criminal behaviour and crime victimisation. The following sections will now discuss two key elements of policing practise: police responses to mentally ill offenders and mentally ill victims.

The Mentally Ill as Offenders

The idea that mental disorder may be related to violence dates back centuries, and is far from a recent, or uniquely Australian, concept (Monahan, 1992; Porter, 2002; Rosen, 1968). There are numerous references in ancient Greek and Roman literature to the potential dangerousness and violent tendencies of the mentally ill. For example, in *The Laws*, Plato wrote: "If a man is mad, he shall not be at large in the city, but his family shall keep him in any way they can" (cited in Porter, 2002, p. 89). Similarly, Roman philosopher Philo Judaeus described a subsection of the mentally ill as being "dangerous to both the madmen themselves and those who approach them" (cited in Rosen, 1968, p. 89).

Over the years, opinions have fluctuated about whether people with severe mental illness are more or less violent than the average person. In the early twentieth century, it was thought that mental illness may protect against offending, and that people with severe mental disorder would actually be *less* likely to commit an offence than others in society. It was not until the early 1990s that consistent evidence for the increased risk of violence and crime among mentally ill populations began to emerge (see Monahan, 1993; Mullen, 1997, for a review). After decades of research, there is now robust evidence of a moderate, but significant, association between severe mental illness and violent crime, particularly for persons who also abuse illicit drugs or alcohol (Angermeyer, 2000; Douglas et al., 2009; Wallace, Mullen, & Burgess, 2004). A recent Australian study concluded that people with severe mental illness were somewhere between three and five times more likely than the average person to commit a violent crime. Epidemiological studies have consistently found that roughly 10% of severely mentally ill patients have a record of criminal violence (Walsh et al., 2002). Interestingly, the prevalence of severe mental disorders seems to be even higher among homicide offenders (Asnis, Kaplan, Hundorfean, & Saeed, 1997; Fazel & Grann, 2004; Moskowitz, Simpson, McKenna, Skipworth, & Barry-Walsh, 2006). Homicide offences, because of their serious nature and fatal consequences, tend to have higher detection rates by police. As a result, research on known homicides is generally thought to be a fairly good representation of all homicidal behaviour. In Australia, schizophrenia disorders are 13 times more common among homicide offenders than in the general population (Bennett et al., 2011).

Unsurprisingly, the presence of substance abuse in combination with severe mental illness greatly augments the risk of violence and criminal behaviour (Tiihonen, Isohanni, Rasanen, Koiranen, & Moring, 1997; Wallace et al., 2004), and it is this group who are likely to occupy most policing and clinical resources. However, the evidence also indicates that substance abuse alone cannot account for the association between mental illness and violence, and that even people with severe mental disorder *without* a co-morbid substance use disorder are more likely than the general population to act violently (Brennan, Mednick, & Hodgins, 2000; Tiihonen et al., 1997). Similarly, people with co-morbid substance misuse and severe mental illness are more likely to engage in crime and violence than those with substance misuse alone, indicating that there is something particular about severe mental illness that increases the risk of violent behaviour, above and beyond that caused by substance misuse (Arseneault, Moffitt, Caspi, Taylor, & Silva, 2000; Smith & Trimboli, 2010).

In addition to criminal behaviour, the research indicates that people with severe mental illness are also more likely than others in the community to experience interpersonal conflict and family violence (Solomon, Cavanaugh, & Gelles, 2005). Perhaps unsurprisingly, research has demonstrated that people with severe mental illness often experience significant tensions in their familial and interpersonal relationships, and moreover, that family members are particularly likely to be the targets of violent behaviour (Estroff, Swanson, Lachicotte, Swartz, & Bolduc, 1998; Estroff & Zimmer, 1994). This contrasts with the common public perception that mentally ill violent offenders are unpredictable individuals who roam the streets, liable to lash out violently at any moment. In actual fact, it is families and carers who are far more likely than strangers to be attacked by a mentally ill person (Estroff et al., 1998; Solomon et al., 2005). Less research has been conducted on police responses to family conflict in the mentally ill, but policies for intervening, apprehending, and preventing family violence incidents have become increasingly commonplace in police forces in Australia and around the world.

Taken together, the research conducted to date strongly supports the argument that severe mental illness significantly increases the risk of criminal violence, but it also highlights that most mentally ill patients are not violent, and that most violent offences are committed by persons who have not been diagnosed with severe mental illness (Arseneault et al., 2000; Douglas et al., 2009; Fazel & Grann, 2006). Indeed, mental disorder is less predictive of violence than other factors, such as personality disorder, criminal history, and substance misuse (Elbogen & Johnson, 2009; Walsh et al., 2002). Nevertheless, mentally ill offenders occupy a notable proportion of both academic and police attention, and it is important to characterise the risks of offending in this population.

Severe Mental Illness and Crime Victimisation

Until recently, researchers and clinicians have focussed almost exclusively on the mentally ill as perpetrators, rather than victims, of violence. Indeed, there are relatively few studies examining the prevalence and risks of criminal victimisation among the mentally ill, especially in comparison to the vast number of studies on mentally ill offenders. This neglect is concerning, given that people with preexisting mental disorders may be especially vulnerable to the social, emotional, and financial effects of crime (Macmillan, 2001). However, over the past two decades, there has been a small but increasing number of studies that have focussed their attention on crime victimisation in people with severe mental illness (see Maniglio, 2009, for a systematic review). Overwhelmingly, this research has indicated that crime victimisation is a serious problem for people with mental illness, with self-reported victimisation rates of up to 97% being reported (Goodman, Dutton, & Harris, 1995). Moreover, comparisons with the general population have shown that people with severe mental illness are significantly *more* likely than others in the community to become the victim of a violent crime (Hiday, Swartz, Swanson, Borum, & Wagner, 1999; Teplin, McClelland, Abram, & Weiner, 2005).

Consistent with the literature on offending, substance abuse dramatically increases the chances of victimisation among both mentally ill individuals and others in the community (Stevens et al., 2007; Walsh et al., 2003). Having a history of criminal offending also increases the likelihood of victimisation among individuals with schizophrenia, suggesting a degree of reciprocity in the relationship between offending and victimisation (Hiday, Swanson, Swartz, Borum, & Wagner, 2001). However, neither offending history nor substance misuse can fully account for the increased rate of victimisation in severe mental illness, as even patients without co-morbid substance misuse or a history of criminality report increased rates of victimisation compared to the general community (Van Dorn, Volavka, & Johnson, 2011).

Importantly, the victimisation incidents reported by persons with severe mental illness include both violent and nonviolent crimes, and do not appear to comprise only minor or trivial offences. For example, people with severe mental illness have reported high rates of serious crimes, such as rape, robbery, aggravated assault, personal theft, and household burglary (Teplin et al., 2005). They are also at greater risk of homicide than others in the community (Hiroeh, Appleby, Mortensen, & Dunn, 2001). It has been suggested that deficits in decision making and judgement ability, combined with a disadvantaged lifestyle and active symptomatology, leave people with severe mental illness particularly vulnerable to violent crime (Teplin et al., 2005).

Most of the studies to date have used self-report methods to explore victimisation in the mentally ill. A much smaller number of studies, however, have looked at official rates of crime victimisation as recorded by police. Although official crime statistics are known to be an underrepresentation of the actual crime rate, it is nevertheless important to consider these in tandem with self-report experiences. In terms of policing policy and practise, it is the official rates of victimisation that provide an indication of police interactions with mentally ill crime victims, and official police statistics that are used to guide funding and resource allocations.

Crime Reporting by People With Severe Mental Illness

Despite the potentially serious consequences of crime victimisation for people with mental illness, the evidence suggests that many crimes against this population are undetected by, or unreported to, the police. While it is well known that many crimes are not reported to the police, this pattern of under-reporting may be especially true in the mentally ill population (Carcach, 1997; Coleman & Moynihan, 1996). Unfortunately, there is relatively little research on this topic, and comparisons with reporting behaviours in the general population are severely limited. However, in one study examining reporting behaviour of schizophrenia patients, Brekke and colleagues found that 59% of victimisation incidents were not reported to the police (Brekke et al., 2001). In a similar self-report study that questioned mentally ill victims of violent crime about their disclosure to police and other persons, it was found that almost half of all mentally ill crime victims interviewed had not reported their experience to the authorities (Marley & Buila, 1999). This was despite the fact that these victims described serious physical and sexual violence, including rape and aggravated assault. Interestingly, however, 70% of these crime victims had disclosed the crime to another party (such as a friend or worker), but not to the police. This suggests that victims with mental illness may be particularly reluctant to report crimes to the police, as opposed to family members or others, even in cases of traumatic and violent assault.

The decision to report a crime to police is thought to be influenced by a number of interrelated factors, including the type and perceived severity of the offence, the victim's past experiences with the police, and the potential consequences of reporting the crime (such as access to insurance or compensation payouts) (Carcach, 1997; Skogan, 1984). Personal characteristics of the victim and his or her past experiences with crime also have a significant impact on crime reporting behaviour. For example, repeat victims of crime are less likely than those with no history of victimisation to report to the police; this is possibly due to them having had prior negative experiences with the police, or assuming that nothing will be done. Worryingly, persons who are socially disadvantaged are also less likely to report crimes to the police, which may reflect strained relationships between this population and the police force (Carcach,

1997). While there is currently no research comparing reporting patterns in people with and without mental illness, these findings certainly suggest that people with mental disorder may be less likely than the average person to engage with policing services after being victimised. When one considers the constellation of psychiatric symptoms that may be experienced in severe mental illness, including paranoia, persecutory beliefs, and auditory hallucinations, it seems reasonable to think that this group may be less trusting of police and authority figures, and therefore less likely to turn to them for support.

The reduced reporting of crime victimisation among persons with mental illness may also relate to their daily life experiences and perceptions of what constitutes crime or abuse. It is reasonable to assume that persons who are exposed to high levels of violence and antisocial behaviour may have a higher threshold for deciding to report such behaviour to police. In support of this hypothesis, it has been shown that most mentally ill people who are victims of regular physical abuse from partners or family members do not consider their experiences to qualify as abuse, nor do they report these experiences to doctors and clinicians (Cascardi, Mueser, DeGiralomo, & Murrin, 1996).

Of further concern, there is some evidence that police officers are significantly less likely to take action in response to a complaint from a victim with schizophrenia, compared to an identical complaint from a person without schizophrenia (Watson, Corrigan, & Ottati, 2004). In this vignette study, police officers were also less likely to perceive a witness with schizophrenia as being credible, lending support to the hypothesis that people with severe mental illness experience stigmatisation within the criminal justice system (Frese, 2009; Teplin, 1983).

Thus, the available evidence suggests that people with mental illness may be both less likely to report crime to authorities and less likely to have their reports acted upon. This could have serious implications for both victims and the community at large. Unfortunately, individuals with a preexisting mental illness are already a vulnerable population, and they may be particularly susceptible to the adverse effects of crime victimisation (Macmillan, 2001). By not reporting crimes to the authorities, victims with mental illness may also be denied access to victim compensation and support schemes. Furthermore, official crime statistics are used to determine funding and resource allocations for police and victim services. Thus, the underreporting of crimes against the mentally ill may ultimately lead to reduced resources for this population, which could increase the harms that they experience as a result of crime.

Pathways to Violence and Crime Victimisation

In many ways, violence and victimisation are opposite sides of the same coin, and researchers have started to consider how the two behaviours are related

(Silver, Piquero, Jennings, Piquero, & Leiber, 2011). For example, Hiday and colleagues (2001) suggested that victimisation may mediate the relationship between mental illness and violent crime. They demonstrated that violent behaviour is significantly associated with crime victimisation, and went on to conclude that this relationship cannot be attributed to the spurious association with either substance misuse or socioeconomic factors. That is, victimisation exerts an independent effect on violence above and beyond the influence of common variables that have an effect on both. Silver and colleagues support this hypothesis, suggesting in a recent publication that the link between violence and victimisation may be due to interrelated psychosocial processes, such as interpersonal conflict (Silver et al., 2011). In other words, they speculated that interpersonal conflict may predispose an individual to both violence *and* victimisation, although it may exert different influences on these outcomes.

There is already considerable evidence to demonstrate that people with severe mental disorder have problems with interpersonal and family relationships (Chan, 2008; Estroff & Zimmer, 1994; Silver, 2002). Hiday and colleagues (2001) have also suggested that exposure to violence, through either victimisation experiences or offending behaviour, leads to a greater acceptance of violent behaviour, which in turn increases the likelihood that the individual will encounter or utilise violence in the future. Thus, the social context in which people with severe mental illness reside, and in particular their interpersonal relationships, may be an important predictive factor for their involvement in violence. If this is the case, then interpersonal relationships could also be seen as an important area for possible intervention and risk management, which could have a beneficial effect on both crime perpetration and victimisation.

At this stage, it is not known whether combinations of victimisation, offending, interpersonal conflict, and substance misuse have cumulative or additive effects on the risk of violence in severe mental illness. However, it is unlikely that such complex social and psychological variables would interact in a simple additive fashion, particularly given the considerable overlap between them. Instead, it seems likely that many of the associations between violence and victimisation will be reciprocal. For example, crime victimisation can be seen as both a precursor to and consequence of violent offending and severe mental illness. It seems most plausible, therefore, that there are many pathways to violence, and that any association between severe mental illness and crime is likely to be complex and multifactorial.

Implications for Policing Policy and Practise in Australia and Beyond

What are the implications of these research studies for policing policy and practise? Police, who often act simultaneously as a last resort and a point of first contact, have been referred to as the gatekeepers of both the mental health and criminal justice systems (Fukuroda, 2005; Lamb, Weinberger, & DeCuir, 2002). In Australia, the recent shift toward a community policing model, in combination with the deinstitutionalisation of the mental health system, has seen the police engage in a more visible social welfare role in the community, with a particular focus on meeting the needs of minority and vulnerable populations (Putt, 2010; Segrave & Ratcliffe, 2004). As such, there is an increasing recognition and consideration of the issues that police face on a day-to-day basis when dealing with mentally ill offenders, victims, and community members.

As frontline workers, police need to be cognisant of the risks and vulnerabilities associated with severe mental illness. People with severe mental illness are overrepresented not only in criminal violence, but also in instances of family and interpersonal conflict that may not result in criminal charges (Chan, 2008; Solomon et al., 2005). Having information about the risk of violence in people diagnosed with severe mental illness has the potential to facilitate a more effective police response, thereby improving outcomes for the police, as well as offenders, victims, and the broader community. In Australia, the Victoria Police *Code of Practice for the Investigation of Family Violence* clearly dictates that "police receive operational safety training and are aware of the risk factors when attending any incident" (Victoria Police, 2004, p. 8). Despite this, the *Code of Practice* does not specifically refer to mental disorder as a risk factor for family violence, nor does it highlight this as a relevant issue to be aware of in potential perpetrators. The research reviewed in this chapter suggests that such information may be warranted in the management of both family and criminal violence.

However, information about the risks associated with mental illness and substance misuse should not be provided in isolation, but rather accompanied by appropriate police training and an understanding of the inherent limitations in predicting human behaviour. It would be incorrect, for example, to make an overgeneralised statement that mental illness leads to violence, or to insinuate that all—or even most—people with severe mental illness will engage in violence. It should be emphasised to both police and community members that the presence of a violence risk factor does not inevitably lead to a violent outcome (Borum, 1996; Hart, Michie, & Cooke, 2007). Rather, it can be said that people with severe mental disorders are *statistically more likely* to engage in violent crime than others in the community, particularly if they have a history of substance misuse, offending behaviour, or crime victimisation. Furthermore, and contrary to popular perception, it is family members and carers, rather than strangers, who are most at risk of being on the receiving end of violent behaviour by mental health patients (Chan, 2008; Solomon et al., 2005).

In addition to responding to violent situations involving people with severe mental illness, police also have a duty to protect this vulnerable population from victimisation. Indeed, identifying and supporting victims is a key mandate of policing practise in Australia and around the world. Thus, it is important for police to recognise that people with severe mental illness are a vulnerable group who are likely to experience higher levels of violent victimisation than the general population, and that this victimisation may be both chronic and severe in nature. Despite the apparently widespread crime victimisation of the mentally ill, police should be aware that people with severe mental illness may be deterred or discouraged from reporting their victimisation experiences to authorities, perhaps especially so if they are suffering from paranoid symptoms, have a history of offending, or have otherwise perceived their interactions with police to be negative (Carcach, 1997; Skogan, 1984). While there is currently very little research examining perceptions of police among people with mental illness, the available literature does suggest that mentally ill crime victims, particularly those who are repeatedly victimised, may have more difficulty reporting their experiences to police (Carcach, 1997; Watson et al., 2004). In other words, this is a population who may be more likely to experience victimisation, but less likely to report it to authorities or otherwise seek supportive services.

One of the most concerning implications of a low reporting rate of crime among the mentally ill is that unidentified or unofficial crime victims are largely unable to access specialised victim services and compensation or restitution schemes. For example, most jurisdictions have some form of victims of crime compensation, particularly for serious violent crimes, but this sort of restitution is inaccessible to individuals who do not identify themselves as being victims. This is a particular problem given the preexisting vulnerabilities of victims with serious mental disorder and the serious adverse outcomes of victimisation in this population (McFarlane, Bookless, & Schrader, 2004). Moreover, a lack of response to the victimisation by clinical or police services may strengthen the victim's perception that his or her victimisation experience is normative, insignificant, or unworthy of attention, which in turn further discourages him or her from future disclosure. In this era of community policing, it seems pertinent that the police actively address this issue and endeavour to foster more positive relations with individuals experiencing severe mental disorder to encourage the reporting of crime victimisation. While much progress has been made in recent years, further efforts and reform are needed to improve relations between police and mentally ill victims, and to encourage people with severe mental illness to disclose their victimisation experiences so that they may access appropriate treatment and support services, and allow police to identify and prosecute the offenders.

Conclusion

Major mental illnesses, although rare, continue to represent a major public health concern in our society. Less than one in every 100 individuals can expect to be diagnosed with a severe mental disorder in their lifetime, yet it is this group who consume the vast majority of intensive public mental health services (Short et al., 2010). People with severe mental illness are also overrepresented in the criminal justice system as both perpetrators and victims of violent crime. The increased prevalence of violent behaviour is evident even in the absence of co-morbid substance abuse, although patients with substance misuse or a history of offending are particularly susceptible to violence, and these factors undoubtedly heighten the risk of criminality. Recent research shows that the significant association between severe mental illness and crime cannot be attributed solely to the influence of co-morbid substance misuse (Van Dorn et al., 2011). Thus, there appears to be something particular to major mental illness that increases the likelihood of both violent behaviour and crime victimisation.

The research presented in this chapter emphasises that people with severe mental illness are a vulnerable population, who, in an era of deinstitutionalisation, may face a number of potential risks and harms in our society. In Australia, as with many other jurisdictions, this has significant implications for the broader community who have traditionally viewed the mentally ill as a dangerous, rather than vulnerable, population. It also has particular implications for the police, who are charged with the difficult task of managing not only perpetrators and victims with severe mental illness, but also all other mentally ill individuals who come into contact with police during periods of crisis or distress.

References

Angermeyer, M.C. (2000). Schizophrenia and violence. *Acta Psychiatrica Scandinavica*, *102*(Suppl. 407), 63–67.

Arseneault, L., Moffitt, T.E., Caspi, A., Taylor, P.J., & Silva, P.A. (2000). Mental disorders and violence in a total birth cohort: Results from the Dunedin Study. *Archives of General Psychiatry*, *57*(10), 979–986.

Asnis, G.M., Kaplan, M.L., Hundorfean, G., & Saeed, W. (1997). Violence and homicidal behaviors in psychiatric disorders. *Psychiatric Clinics of North America*, *20*(2), 405–425.

Bennett, D.J., Ogloff, J.R.P., Mullen, P.E., Thomas, S.D.M., Wallace, C., & Short, T. (2011). Schizophrenia disorders, substance abuse and prior offending in a sequential series of 435 homicides. *Acta Psychiatrica Scandinavica*, *124*(3), 226–233.

Borum, R. (1996). Improving the clinical practice of violence risk assessment: Technology, guidelines, and training. *American Psychologist, 51*(9), 945–956.

Brekke, J.S., Prindle, C., Bae, S.W., & Long, J.D. (2001). Risks for individuals with schizophrenia who are living in the community. *Psychiatric Services, 52*(10), 1358–1366.

Brennan, P.A., Mednick, S.A., & Hodgins, S. (2000). Major mental disorders and criminal violence in a Danish birth cohort. *Archives of General Psychiatry, 57*(5), 494–500.

Carcach, C. (1997). Reporting crime to the police. *Trends and Issues in Criminal Justice, 68*, 1–6.

Cascardi, M., Mueser, K.T., DeGiralomo, J., & Murrin, M. (1996). Physical aggression against psychiatric inpatients by family members and partners. *Psychiatric Services, 47*(5), 531–533.

Chan, B.W.-Y. (2008). Violence against caregivers by relatives with schizophrenia. *International Journal of Forensic Mental Health, 7*(1), 65–81.

Coleman, C., & Moynihan, J. (1996). Haunted by the dark figure: Criminologists as ghostbusters? In M. Maguire (Ed.), *Understanding crime data: Haunted by the dark figure* (pp. 1–23). Buckingham, UK: Open University Press.

Douglas, K.S., Guy, L.S., & Hart, S.D. (2009). Psychosis as a risk factor for violence to others: A meta-analysis. *Psychological Bulletin, 135*(5), 679–706.

Elbogen, E.B., & Johnson, S.C. (2009). The intricate link between violence and mental disorder: Results from the national epidemiologic survey on alcohol and related conditions. *Archives of General Psychiatry, 66*(2), 152–161.

Estroff, S., Swanson, J.W., Lachicotte, W., Swartz, M.S., & Bolduc, M. (1998). Risk reconsidered: Targets of violence in the social networks of people with serious psychiatric disorders. *Social Psychiatry and Psychiatric Epidemiology, 33*(Suppl. 1), S95–S101.

Estroff, S.E., & Zimmer, C. (1994). Social networks, social support, and violence among persons with severe, persistent mental illness. In J. Monahan & H.J. Steadman (Eds.), *Violence and mental disorder: Developments in risk assessment* (pp. 259–298). Chicago: University of Chicago Press.

Fazel, S., & Grann, M. (2004). Psychiatric morbidity among homicide offenders: A Swedish population study. *American Journal of Psychiatry, 161*(11), 2129–2131.

Fazel, S., & Grann, M.C. (2006). The population impact of severe mental illness on violent crime. *American Journal of Psychiatry, 163*(8), 1397–1403.

Frese, F.J. (2009). Criminalization of mental illness: Crisis and opportunity for the justice system. *Psychiatric Services, 60*(11), 1561–1562.

Fukuroda, M.L. (2005). *Murder at home: An examination of legal and community responses to intimate femicide in California*. Los Angeles, CA: California Women's Law Center.

Godfredson, J.W., Thomas, S.D., Ogloff, J.R., & Luebbers, S. (2011). Police perceptions of their encounters with individuals experiencing mental illness: A Victorian survey. *Australian and New Zealand Journal of Criminology, 44*(2), 180–195.

Goodman, L.A., Dutton, M.A., & Harris, M. (1995). Episodically homeless women with serious mental illness: Prevalence of physical and sexual assault. *American Journal of Orthopsychiatry, 65*(4), 468–478.

Hart, S.D., Michie, C., & Cooke, D.J. (2007). Precision of actuarial risk assessment instruments: Evaluating the 'margins of error' of group v. individual predictions of violence. *British Journal of Psychiatry, 190*(Suppl. 49), s60–s65.

Hiday, V.A., Swanson, J.W., Swartz, M.S., Borum, R., & Wagner, H. (2001). Victimization: A link between mental illness and violence? *International Journal of Law and Psychiatry, 24*(6), 559–572.

Hiday, V.A., Swartz, J.A., Swanson, J.W., Borum, R., & Wagner, H.R. (1999). Criminal victimisation of persons with severe mental illness. *Psychiatric Services, 50*(1), 62–68.

Hiroeh, U., Appleby, L., Mortensen, P.B., & Dunn, G. (2001). Death by homicide, suicide, and other unnatural causes in people with mental illness: A population-based study. *Lancet, 358*(9299), 2110–2112.

Lamb, H.R., Weinberger, L.E., & DeCuir Jr., W.J. (2002). The police and mental health. *Psychiatric Services, 53*(10), 1266–1271.

MacKinnon, D., & Coleborne, C. (2003). Introduction: Deinstitutionalisation in Australia and New Zealand. *Health and History, Special Issue: Histories of Psychiatry After Deinstitutionalisation, 5*(2), 1–16.

Macmillan, R. (2001). Violence and the life course: The consequences of victimization for personal and social development. *Annual Review of Sociology, 27*(1), 1–22.

Maniglio, R. (2009). Severe mental illness and criminal victimization: A systematic review. *Acta Psychiatrica Scandinavica, 119*(3), 180–191.

Marley, J.A., & Buila, S. (1999). When violence happens to people with mental illness: Disclosing victimization. *American Journal of Orthopsychiatry, 69*(3), 398–402.

McFarlane, A., Bookless, C., & Schrader, G. (2004). *The prevalence of victimization and violent behaviour in the seriously mentally ill*. Canberra, Australia: Criminology Research Council.

Monahan, J. (1992). Mental disorder and violent behavior: Perceptions and evidence. *American Psychologist, 47*(4), 511–521.

Monahan, J. (1993). Mental disorder and violence: Another look. In S. Hodgins (Ed.), *Mental disorder and crime* (pp. 287–302). Thousand Oaks, CA: Sage Publications.

Moskowitz, A., Simpson, A.I.F., McKenna, B., Skipworth, J.J., & Barry-Walsh, J. (2006). The role of mental illness in homicide-suicide in New Zealand: 1991–2000. *Journal of Forensic Psychiatry and Psychology, 17*(3), 417–430.

Mullen, P.E. (1997). A reassessment of the link between mental disorder and violent behaviour, and its implications for clinical practice. *Australian and New Zealand Journal of Psychiatry, 31*, 3–11.

Porter, R. (2002). *Madness: A brief history*. New York: Oxford University Press.

Putt, J. (2010). *Community policing in Australia*. Canberra, Australia: Australian Institute of Criminology.

Rosen, G. (1968). *Madness in society*. Chicago: University of Chicago Press.

Segrave, M., & Ratcliffe, J. (2004). *Community policing: A descriptive overview*. Canberra, Australia: Australian Institute of Criminology.

Short, T.B., Thomas, S., Luebbers, S., Ogloff, J.R.P., & Mullen, P.E. (2010). Utilization of public mental health services in a random community sample. *Australian and New Zealand Journal of Psychiatry, 44*(5), 475–481.

Silver, E. (2002). Mental disorder and violent victimisation: The mediating role of involvement in conflicted social relationships. *Criminology, 40*(1), 191–212.

Silver, E., Piquero, A.R., Jennings, W.G., Piquero, N.L., & Leiber, M. (2011). Assessing the violent offending and violent victimization overlap among discharged psychiatric patients. *Law and Human Behavior, 35*(1), 49–59.

Skogan, W.G. (1984). Reporting crimes to the police: The status of world research. *Journal of Research in Crime and Delinquency, 21*(2), 113–137.

Smith, N.E., & Trimboli, L. (2010). Comorbid substance and non-substance mental health disorders and re-offending among NSW prisoners. *Crime and Justice Bulletin, 140*, 1–16.

Solomon, P.L., Cavanaugh, M.M., & Gelles, R.J. (2005). Family violence among adults with severe mental illness. *Trauma, Violence, and Abuse, 6*(1), 40–54.

Stevens, A., Berto, D., Frick, U., Kerschl, V., McSweeney, T., Schaaf, S., et al. (2007). The victimization of dependent drug users. *European Journal of Criminology, 4*(4), 385–408.

Swanson, J.W., Holzer, C.H., Ganju, V.K., & Jono, R.T. (1990). Violence and psychiatric disorder in the community: Evidence from the Epidemiologic Catchment Area Surveys. *Hospital and Community Psychiatry, 41*, 761–770.

Swartz, M.S., Swanson, J.W., Hiday, V., Borum, R., Wagner, R., & Burns, B.J. (1998). Taking the wrong drugs: The role of substance abuse and medication noncompliance in violence among severely mentally ill individuals. *Social Psychiatry and Psychiatric Epidemiology, 33*(Suppl. 1), S75–S80.

Tengstrom, A., Grann, M.C., Langstrom, N., & Kullgren, G. (2000). Psychopathy (PCL-R) as a predictor of violent recidivism among criminal offenders with schizophrenia. *Law and Human Behavior, 24*(1), 45–58.

Teplin, L.A. (1983). The criminalization of the mentally ill: Speculation in search of data. *Psychological Bulletin, 94*(1), 54–67.

Teplin, L.A., McClelland, G.M., Abram, K.M., & Weiner, D.A. (2005). Crime victimization in adults with severe mental illness. *Archives of General Psychiatry, 62*, 911–921.

Tiihonen, J., Isohanni, M., Rasanen, P., Koiranen, M., & Moring, J. (1997). Specific major mental disorders and criminality: A 26-year prospective study of the 1966 Northern Finland birth cohort. *American Journal of Psychiatry, 154*(6), 840–845.

Van Dorn, R., Volavka, J., & Johnson, N. (2012). Mental disorder and violence: Is there a relationship beyond substance use? *Social Psychiatry and Psychiatric Epidemiology, 47*(3), 487–503.

Victoria Police. (2004). *Code of practice for the investigation of family violence: Supporting an integrated response to family violence in Victoria.* Melbourne, Australia: Victoria Police.

Wallace, C., Mullen, P.E., & Burgess, P. (2004). Criminal offending in schizophrenia over a 25-year period marked by deinstitutionalization and increasing prevalence of comorbid substance use disorders. *American Journal of Psychiatry, 161*(4), 716–727.

Walsh, E., Buchanan, A., & Fahy, T. (2002). Violence and schizophrenia: Examining the evidence. *British Journal of Psychiatry, 180*(6), 490–495.

Walsh, E., Moran, P., Scott, C., McKenzie, K., Burns, T., Creed, F., et al. (2003). Prevalence of violent victimisation in severe mental illness. *British Journal of Psychiatry, 183,* 233–238.

Watson, A.C., Corrigan, P.W., & Ottati, V. (2004). Police officers' attitudes toward and decisions about persons with mental illness. *Psychiatric Services, 55*(1), 49–53.

The Role of Mental Disorders in Use of Force Incidents Between the Police and the Public

8

DRAGANA KESIC

Contents

Introduction

In the role of serving and protecting the public, and enforcing the law, police are given broad legal powers. Perhaps the most contentious of these are their right to use physical force to effect compliance from the public and the right to use lethal force in order to protect their own or another's life. There is no doubt that a police officer's decision to fire his or her weapon and potentially take someone's life is the most important he or she is faced with. A topic of some contention has been police use of fatal and nonfatal force on people who have a mental disorder. This chapter begins with a broad overview of the contacts between the police and people experiencing mental disorders. Following is the review of the findings regarding police use of nonfatal and fatal force on people who experience mental disorders, paying specific attention to the emerging research from Victoria, Australia. Finally, the chapter will conclude with describing some of the initiatives currently being undertaken to assist the police in working at this interface.

Due to the many societal, legal, and population changes, the contact between police and people with mental disorders has increased in recent decades (Cotton & Coleman, 2010). Apart from deinstitutionalisation lead-ing to the increase of persons with mental disorders in the community, policing changes in the 1970s and 1980s also brought the police out into the community on foot patrols and other types of visual presence (Sced, 2006). Police contact with people with mental disorders can occur in a wide variety of contexts, including being witnesses of crimes, victims of crime, alleged offenders, offenders, or persons in need of assistance.

A number of studies have considered the issue of the frequency of con-tact between police and persons experiencing mental disorders. Findings indicate that these encounters are commonplace in many countries around the world: the United States (Deane, Steadman, Borum, Veysey, & Morrissey, 1999; Ruiz & Miller, 2004), Australia (Fry, O'Riordan, & Geanellos, 2002), Canada (Hartford, Helsop, Stitt, & Hoch, 2005), and the United Kingdom (Moore, 2010). Fry and colleagues conducted a survey of 131 police officers in Sydney, Australia, and found that police reported spending 10% of their time dealing with people they perceived to be mentally disturbed. Around 74% of officers reported to have dealt with persons with mental health problems in the past month, and 70% had encountered suicidal behaviour. Given this frequency of contacts with people who appear to be experiencing mental dis-orders, it is not surprising that the police are their primary referral sources to emergency departments, being responsible for almost a third of such refer-rals internationally (Klein, 2010) and in Australia (Knott, Pleban, Taylor, & Castle, 2007; Lee, 2006). Recent research from Victoria has found that mental disorders are common among detainees in police cells (Baksheev, Thomas, & Ogloff, 2010); this notion is consistent with substantial literature on the over-representation of mental disorders in offending populations (see Chapter 7 by Tamsin Short for a review of this literature).

Despite the frequency of their contact, a common assertion has been that the police are reluctant to deal with people who are experiencing men-tal disorders (Borum, 2000; Fry et al., 2002, Ruiz & Miller, 2004), although this sentiment, others assert, is changing in recent times (Chappell, 2010). It has become apparent that some of this reluctance may be attributable to two main issues: (1) there are a lack of functional partnerships between the police and the mental health services (Brouwer, 2005; Fry et al., 2002), and (2) there is a lack of appropriate training for police on how to successfully manage people who appear to be experiencing a mental disorder (Brouwer, 2005; Chappell, 2008; Fry et al., 2002; Moore, 2010).

One of the main issues at this interface has been the use of force, more specifically, the use of fatal force, between police and people experiencing mental disorders. The International Association of Chiefs of Police (IACP) defined *force* as "that amount of effort required by police to compel com-pliance from an unwilling subject" (IACP, 2001, p. 1). Internationally, it is legally permissible for police officers to use force in execution of their work. However, the rights of the public must also be protected against use of excessive or inappropriate police force. To these ends, many countries around the world have adopted the United Nations Code of Conduct for Law Enforcement Officials, which stipulates that "law enforcement officials may use force only when strictly necessary and to the extent required for the performance of their duty" (United Nations, 1979, Article 3). The use of firearms is considered appropriate only when "strictly unavoidable in order to protect life" (United Nations, 1990, Provision 9).

Fatal force (also termed lethal force or deadly force) is defined as that force intended to cause death or serious injury, or the force that a reasonable person would perceive would cause death or serious injury (e.g., Police Commissioners' Policy Advisory Group, 1992). Due to their lethality, discharges of police firearms are generally considered as police use of fatal force. On the other hand, nonfatal use of force is generally considered as all other physical force used to restrain or control the citizen (Smith, 2004).

Research on use of force had been mostly conducted in the United States, and originally tended to concentrate more on fatal force encounters than nonfatal force encounters (Hickman, Picquero, & Garner, 2008). Despite the fact that the research of both fatal and nonfatal force has been numerous over the past five decades, there is a lack of research that has specifically examined the role of mental disorders in these encounters.

Fatal Force and Mental Disorders

Police use of fatal force is, fortunately, a very rare occurrence (Clifford, 2010; Fyfe, 2000). Only a limited number of studies have examined the potential role of mental state at the time of the incident, most commonly through considering whether the citizens appeared, or had evidence of, substance intoxication. Dealing with individuals who appear to be under the influence of substances or to be mentally ill is particularly problematic for the police (Kaminski, DiGiovanni, & Downs, 2004).

The studies that have considered a history or a presence of symptoms of mental disorder have also revealed significant implications. The Police Complaints Authority (2003) reported that just under half of the people involved in fatal shootings in England and Wales had mental health problems. Additionally, in half of these cases there was evidence of suicidal intentions and self-harming behaviour during the incident. Parent (1996) also reported that a third of the police fatalities that occurred in British Columbia between 1980 and 1994 had a recorded mental illness history, most frequently a diagnosis of schizophrenia. However, if the officers' perceptions of the decedents' behaviour at the time of the incident were taken into account, behaviours indicating the presence of mental illness were present in about half of the cases. Klinger (2001) asserted that proper analysis of a decedent's mental state, more specifically suicidal ideations and intent, at the time of the critical incident is very important because these factors can dramatically affect the outcome of the incident.

Suicide by Police

The mental state of the decedent has most consistently been examined and found to be a serious consideration in a subsample of police fatalities, mainly referred to as *suicide by cop** incidents. Although there are a number of oper-ationalised definitions of this phenomenon, in short, suicide by cop occurs when persons who are intent on committing suicide do so by provoking the police to shoot them. There are approximately 1 million suicides a year world-wide (World Health Organisation, 2010), and while most common methods of suicide differ across countries, the phenomenon called *victim-precipitated homicide* has been studied as an alternative method of suicide as long ago as 1959 by Marvin Wolfgang. The notion that people who intend to die sometimes choose to effect this by provoking another to kill them has been reported in many different societies and historical time periods (Lindsay & Lester, 2004). In their series of guidelines on prevention of suicide, the World Health Organisation (2009) recognises the importance of this phenomenon for police officers and advises that their recognition of signs of serious mental disorder and an ability to de-escalate these events will help to minimise fatal outcomes.

Suicide by police appears to be an international phenomenon, most commonly reported and studied in the United States (e.g., Lord, 2000), Canada (e.g., Parent, 1996), and recently the United Kingdom (Best, Quigley, & Bailey, 2004). Despite the fact that the research is still in its infancy, there are a number of different labels and definitions of the phenomenon: *suicide by cop* (e.g., Mohandie, Meloy, & Collins, 2009), *law enforcement assisted suicide* (e.g., Lord, 2000), *law enforcement officer forced assisted suicide* (e.g., Hutson et al., 1998), *police-involved victim-provoked shooting* (e.g., McKenzie, 2006) *victim-precipitated homicide* (e.g., Parent & Verdun-Jones, 1998), and *suicide by police* (e.g., Homant & Kennedy, 2000).

Additionally, the studies tend to use different definitions of the phenomenon. The differences between the various definitions of suicide by police seem to centre on how specifically, and conversely, how broadly, the phenomenon is defined. Consequently, estimates of how frequently this phenomenon

---

* *Suicide by cop* and *suicide by police* are used interchangeably in this review to account for the preferences of original research; however, the term *suicide by police* is preferred in the remainder of the chapter.

is potentially encountered in all incidents of police shootings differ accordingly, with research estimates of between 10% and 50% being reported (Best et al., 2004; Hutson et al., 1998; Mohandie et al., 2009; Parent 1996).

Despite the differences in definitions and research methodologies, a number of consistent factors emerge from this research. Namely, mental disorders, substance abuse/dependence, past suicide attempts, and the presence of criminal history occur frequently in the suicide by police cases (e.g., Hutson et al., 1998; Lord & Sloop, 2010; Mohandie & Meloy, 2011; Mohandie et al., 2009; Parent, 1996; Wilson et al., 1998). Studies found that during these incidents a significant number of decedents had alcohol, and to a much lesser extent, drugs in their system (Lord, 2000, Mohandie et al., 2009). The vast majority possessed weapons and engaged in violent behaviours such as threatening the police or members of the public with harm (Lord, 2000; Mohandie et al., 2009; Wilson et al., 1998).

When considering the extant findings of this limited literature, there seems to be much similarity in historical characteristics between suicide by police cases and suicides as reported in the general suicide literature, therefore lending some validity to this largely research concept. Namely, the presence of certain types of mental disorders, past suicide attempts, alcohol intoxication, and stressful life events have been found to be common factors associated with suicide (e.g., De Leo, Bertolote, & Lester, 2002).

Nonfatal Force and Mental Disorders

There is a significant lack of published studies examining mental disorders in nonlethal use of force encounters. The majority of the studies that have examined the interface have looked at the presence of mental disorders among many other situational factors, with only a handful of published studies examining the issue more directly.

The studies that examined the prevalence of mental disorders in nonfatal force incidents suggest variable estimates of the rates. Johnson (2011) reported that 7% of 208 police–suspect encounters where police used any physical force (defined as any physical touching, excluding searches and handcuffs) involved a suspect whom the police perceived to be "mentally unstable." In their analysis of oleoresin capsicum spray in the Netherlands, Adang, Kaminski, Howell, and Mensink (2006) found that 28.4% of citizens on whom the police discharged the spray were perceived to have clear signs of "mental confusion or disturbance." Furthermore, a number of studies reported that mental disorders are exceedingly common in incidents of police use of tasers (O'Brien, McKenna, Thom, Diesfeld, & Simpson, 2011; White & Ready, 2010).

Of the studies that peripherally examined the effect of mental impairment on use of force on and by police, the results are again mixed. Terrill's examinations (2005; Terrill & Mastrofski, 2002) of police–suspect encounters found that the observer-rated behavioural indications of mental disorder (rated as "mentally impaired") did not influence the severity of police use of force. McCluskey and colleagues (1999) found that higher levels of citizen's irrationality were associated with lower levels of citizen compliance. However, their measure of irrationality related to observed behavioural effects of alcohol intoxication, mental illness, and presence of fear, anger, or depression. Without making a distinction between mental illness and the rest of the indicators, it is not known whether citizen noncompliance was influenced by mental illness or by alcohol intoxication and emotional distress. More recently, Lawton (2007) found, through an examination of 747 official use of force reports from the Philadelphia Police Department, that police officers reported using more severe force on those citizens whom they perceived to be "mentally unsound," regardless of their behaviour at the time.

The four published studies that have examined the issue more closely present interesting findings. Ruiz and Miller's (2004) self-report study of officers in Pennsylvania found that police use of physical force when dealing with people with mental illness was not as common: 78% of respondents stated they "seldom" have to resort to physical force in these incidents. Injuries were reportedly very rare in these encounters. Despite these results, almost 43% of the respondents "agreed" or "strongly agreed" that persons with mental illness were dangerous, with the vast majority (88%) stating that these calls were as dangerous as those involving a fight and an armed robbery.

Others have also found that injuries rarely occur at this interface (Kaminski et al., 2004; Kerr, Morabito, & Watson, 2010). Kerr et al. (2010) found that 131 police officers, who recalled having at least one interaction with a person perceived to be experiencing mental illness in the past month, reported that injuries very rarely occurred in those incidents, and when they did, the vast majority were of mild severity that did not require medical care. Kerr and colleagues (2010) also found that the most likely highest level of force police used were verbal commands, followed by physical control (e.g., holding and open hand strikes). Additionally, police officers reported that in the vast majority of these cases the citizen was cooperative, and that equal numbers of these calls involved the persons with mental illness resisting officers passively (ignoring their demands) and actively (running away or pulling away from the officers) (Kerr et al., 2010).

Morabito and colleagues, on the other hand, interviewed 216 officers who recalled the most recent interaction with a person whom they perceived to be mentally ill (Morabito et al., 2010). When force was conceptualised as a dichotomous variable that included verbal threats in its definition, these researchers reported that around 70% of officers used force in their interactions with persons whom they perceived to be mentally ill. Additionally, in around 60% of these incidents persons who appeared mentally ill displayed resistive demeanour, and in almost half they reportedly engaged in physical resistance.

Another published study of 2,060 police arrests made during a seven-month period aimed to examine whether impairment (drug or alcohol intoxication, or mental illness) was associated with the use of force during arrest (Kaminski et al., 2004). The main finding was that drug intoxication, rather than alcohol intoxication or mental illness, affected police use of force during arrests. On the other hand, Johnson (2011) recently examined the effect of mental disorder on officer use of force through considering police self-report data on 619 police interactions with suspects they perceived as "mentally unstable" at the time. Johnson found those perceived to have been mentally unstable were more likely to receive severe force (17.2% of mentally unstable vs. 5% of mentally stable received serious force). However, further analyses suggested that more severe force was not used on those perceived to be mentally unstable because of their mental instability; rather, they were more likely to engage in violent behaviour, the consequence of which was police use of more severe force.

Therefore, the existing research is only in its beginning, and must be continued to ensure that the issues at this interface are understood and consequently improved.

Victorian Findings

Use of fatal force by police in Australia had been the topic of many formal investigations and much vocal social commentary. Between 1990 and 2004, there were 76 police shooting deaths across Australia, with the majority of these occurring in Victoria ($n = 29$), followed by New South Wales ($n = 18$) (Brouwer, 2005). The number of fatal shootings is very significant when considered in the context of the population size at the time.

Due to the increase in the number of police shootings in Victoria from 1988 to 1994, the Victoria Police launched five independent reviews to identify the reasons behind these incidents and ways of reducing the number of police shootings. One review, the Task Force Victor (1994), found that police were not adequately prepared to manage situations involving people with mental illness who were also violent.

Dalton (1998) found that a third of the 41 fatalities that occurred between 1990 and 1997 had a psychiatric history or were reported to have been depressed. In addition, half were under the influence of drugs or alcohol at the time of the incident. More recently, the Office of Police Integrity commissioned a review of fatal shootings by Victoria Police. Brouwer (2005) reported that since 1990, more than half (53%) of 32 people fatally shot by the police in Victoria had a mental disorder, and that since 1996, the proportion of victims experiencing a mental disorder increased from 31% to 44% (Brouwer, 2005).

In light of the reports regarding the commonality of mental disorders in fatal incidents, a number of studies were conducted in Victoria to examine the rates of mental disorders in fatal and nonfatal encounters with the Victoria Police. The findings of these sets of studies will be described below.

The first study, by Kesic, Thomas, and Ogloff (2010), was a data linkage study between three databases: the Use of Force Database (UoF), the Redevelopment of Acute and Psychiatric Information Directions (RAPID), uniformly called the Victorian Psychiatric Case Register (VPCR), and the Law Enforcement Assistance Program (LEAP). The study by Kesic et al. set out to examine the mental health and criminal justice characteristics of 48 decedents, the first of whom was fatally wounded in November 1982 and the last in February 2007 by Victoria Police. The majority of the decedents were known in some capacity to either the criminal justice system or the mental health system; most of them had been convicted of, or charged with, criminal offences, and nearly a quarter had been victims of crime. More than half had an Axis I mental disorder, and more than a third of these had more than one disorder. Collectively, all of the major mental disorders were significantly overrepresented in the fatalities sample as compared to the estimated treated prevalence rates of these disorders in the general community. Interestingly, and of particular note, although the number of fatalities halved after Project Beacon was initiated in late 1995, Axis I disorders were 6.5 times more likely to be found among the fatalities after 1996.

The second study of the fatalities analysed 45 of the 48 finalised coronial reports aiming to extend our understanding of these incidents by specifically examining the context in which they occurred (Kesic, Thomas, & Ogloff, 2012). Of interest here are the findings regarding possible suicidal motivations during these incidents.

Suicide by police was investigated by applying strict criteria in order to overcome some of the key limitations of the existing research. Specifically, the authors adapted the two existing criteria: Hutson and colleagues (1998) and Lindsay and Lester (2004, 2008). Of particular note, a third of the fatalities met either of these criteria. These cases were significantly more likely to be of longer duration and be unplanned police operations initiated by the decedent than those not meeting the criteria for suicide by police. Mental or chronic physical illness, past suicide attempts, having experienced a recent stressor, alcohol intoxication, planning the incident in order to get the police to come to the scene, threatening officers with a weapon, refusing to drop the weapon, and advancing at officers were all significantly more likely to occur in the suicide by police group than the rest of the incidents. Police also used different tactical options with this group: They were more likely to attempt negotiation, tactical disengagement, and cordon and containment than in the rest of the fatality incidents.

Kesic and colleagues extended the examination of the link between mental disorders and use of force in encounters with the police through examining incidents of nonfatal use of force (Kesic, Thomas, & Ogloff, in press). The study aimed to examine the rates, characteristics of use of force, and injuries for those whom the police had perceived and recorded as "apparently mentally disordered" in a random sample of 4,267 cases of use of force that occurred between 1995 and 2008.

This study found that around 1 in 14 use of force incidents were those where the person appeared to have a mental disorder (Kesic et al., in press). More than half of these were mental health-related calls. Behaviourally, the majority of those who were deemed apparently mentally disordered were deemed irrational/unstable; more than half behaved violently, and almost a third used violent/abusive language. Whereas they were significantly more likely to be deemed irrational/unstable, they were less likely to appear alcohol affected, to use abusive/violent language, and to avoid police apprehension than the rest of the sample.

Those citizens who appeared mentally disordered were found to most likely use or threaten to use weaponless contact and verbal force on the police (Kesic et al., in press). Although only a quarter used or threatened to use weapons on the police, they were found to be two times more likely to use this force type on the police than the rest of the sample. The police, on the other hand, were most likely to threaten or use weaponless contact, followed by threat or use of restraints on those who appeared mentally disordered. Despite the fact that the police threatened to use or used weapons in 44% of these cases, they were significantly more likely to use or threaten to use weapons, and oleoresin capsicum (pepper) spray specifically, on those who appeared mentally disordered, controlling for other significant variables, such as age, gender, citizen use of force, violent behaviour, and intoxication. Although almost a half of those who appeared mentally disordered during these encounters were injured and one in seven also injured the police, they were no more likely to injure the police or to be injured than the rest of the people. Furthermore, the severities of received injuries were minor for both parties.

Therefore, these recent studies by Kesic and colleagues suggest that mental disorders are common in fatal force incidents with the police in Victoria. Similar to countries such as America and England, suicide by police appears to be a phenomenon common in fatal police shootings in Victoria as well. Additionally, people who appear mentally disordered at the time of the nonfatal force incident differed from the rest of the use of force cases on a number of indicators, including the types of force likely to be used on and by them.

Victorian Initiatives and the Way Forward

Mainly as a result of fatal force incidents involving people with mental illness and the most frequently reported claim that the police are not adequately trained to manage these incidents (Appelbaum, 2000), police forces have made (and continue to make) significant changes and improvements to the way in which they interact with people experiencing mental disorders.

The calls regarding better police training have been repeatedly made in Victoria (Brouwer, 2005; Pearson, 2009; Strong, 2009), and Victoria Police instituted the first comprehensive one-day training on dealing with citizens who have mental disorders in the first cycle of training in 2010. The training was delivered through a mix of classroom-based teaching and scenario-based experiential learning. It consisted of all operational Victoria Police receiving classroom-based teaching on what is mental illness, what are some of the most common types of mental illnesses, how to recognise signs of major mental illnesses, how to effectively engage and communicate with these and those people who are suicidal, hearing perspectives from the consumers of the mental health system, and what are the legal parameters of police obligations. The training emphasised slowing down their response to ensure that they conduct an appropriate risk assessment and management plan, and evaluating all available tactical options; providing clear and empathetic communication; adopting nonthreatening body language; and keeping a safe distance from the person. During scenario-based training, officers also practised how to manage an incident that involved a person experiencing active symptoms of psychosis.

In addition to these changes to training, Victoria Police announced that they have now implemented 82% of the 60 initiatives announced in their Mental Health Strategy (Mental Health Training Rise Among Members, 2010). Among these initiatives are optional training for police officers on mental health issues and the inclusion of a mental disorder person warning flag in the statewide LEAP database as of February 2010. The warning flag system works by adding specific fields to the contacts database so that when details of a person are requested by an officer, details pertaining to the person's mental health history, triggers and typical behaviours, effective communication strategies, known risks, and people to contact for support become available to assist the member in helping the person and resolving the situation (Mental Health Training Rise Among Members, 2010).

Although it is encouraging to observe that Victoria Police have begun to respond to repeated calls to improve their responses to people with mental disorders, it is important to note that this work must be continued and become a consistent consideration in their policy, training, and practise if it hopes to lead to lasting improvements. Namely, following the training changes of 2010, subsequent police training has emphasised firearms skills because of the recent introduction of semiautomatic firearms. Mental health training similar in content to the one received in 2010, delivered in an interactive online training format, started in June 2012 and is compulsory for all operational members. One of the major revisions to the new training is the introduction of examinations: Members must pass a test at the end of each deliverable module in order to proceed to the next module and to complete the training successfully.

It is important for Victoria Police to balance their training in firearms and other physical force techniques with training on nonphysical engagement: communication, verbal de-escalation, cordon and containment, and tactical disengagement. This not only would be in line with their philosophy and policy to only use the *minimum force*, but also will likely address the present concern regarding their forceful interacting and management of people who appear mentally ill. Although the police must receive regular training on an array of topics in order to maintain and improve their skill base, given the overrepresentation of mental disorders in use of force incidents, in police cells (Baksheev et al., 2010) and identified as one of the concerns for Victoria Police officers (Godfredson, Thomas, Ogloff, & Luebbers, 2010), this topic ought to be a consistent training requirement. Therefore, careful consideration of how to best integrate this training into the other important topics is necessary to increase its effectiveness and lead to lasting improvements.

In addition to receiving training in communication and de-escalation of people who appear to be experiencing a mental disorder, their overall management of critical incidents must be improved: Training on appropriate risk assessment and management, based on the information collated before attending the scene as well as the information available on the scene of these incidents, which is based on the principles of safety for all and minimum force, ought to be undertaken. These considerations should be reflected and consistently highlighted in their scenario-based training in order to increase their applicability and likelihood of use in routine practise. Although it is important to note that in some of these, regardless of police actions, fatal force is going to be the only option (Borum, 2000; Klinger, 2005), it is crucial to minimise the likelihood of this occurring through appropriate police training and practise changes.

Furthermore, including raising awareness about the prevalence and characteristics of mental disorders in incidents of fatal and nonfatal force with other mental health training might improve police perceptions of people with mental disorders and improve their confidence when dealing with this subgroup. The media represents the interface between Australian police and people with mental disorders as that where the use of force is the norm, and depicts those who experience mental illness in their encounters with the police as dangerous and a threat to police and the wider public (Kesic, Ducat, & Thomas, 2011). It is important that future police initiatives counter these popular public perceptions through raising awareness about these research findings among the police. It is hoped that such will minimise the belief that all mentally ill people are violent. Indeed, Godfredson and colleagues' (2010) survey of Victorian police officers revealed that "aggression/violence" was one of the top most common signs officers associated with mental illness, even more common than self-harm and psychotic symptoms. Therefore, it is crucial that these officers understand that persons who appear to have a mental disorder are not more likely to be violent or to injure them than those who do not appear to have a mental disorder, and therefore are unlikely to warrant a more forceful approach.

Perhaps most fundamentally, it is vitally important to consider the potentially deleterious impact of the traditional police communicative style when they engage in an encounter. Specifically, a forceful and authoritarian approach might actually escalate the incident when the person is in a mental health crisis and might be afraid and agitated (Borum, 2000; Fyfe, 2000). Keeping mental health on the regular training agenda is therefore essential to increase the likelihood that police officers will understand the complexities and facts regarding this interface, and use such to inform their decisions in future encounters with people who appear mentally ill.

However, just providing more training of police is not a panacea to problems in this, nor are police-only strategies going to be the only solution area (Borum, 2000; see Chapter 6 by Stuart Thomas for a discussion of broader systemic considerations at this interface). Quite apart from an effective diversionary scheme operating in the criminal justice system, adequate and well-resourced mental health services would be fundamental to facilitating the take up of these referrals in order to provide a seamless, alternative path for people experiencing mental disorders (Compton et al., 2010).

Lack of existing and effective partnerships between the mental health services and the police regarding the management of people in mental health crisis has been noted as one of the major problems to police effective management of these incidents internationally (Compton et al., 2010; Reuland, 2010) and in Australia (Brouwer, 2005; Pearson, 2009). Recently, Victoria's auditor general went even further to conclude that the joint responses of the mental health services, Department of Health, ambulance, and the police are not meeting the standards set out in the Mental Health Act (1986), where the needs, resources, and cultural and historical practises of these organisations sometimes come before the needs of mentally ill in crisis (Pearson, 2009).

Currently Victoria Police, in partnership with the Department of Health, is trialling a specialised response to dealing with people who are experiencing mental illness based on the mobile crisis team model, called the Police,

Ambulance, Clinical, Early Response (PACER) (Allen Consulting Group, 2012). In a nutshell, a response based on this model requires that a police officer and a mental health worker (e.g., nurse, social worker) respond together to calls involving people experiencing mental illness (Cotton & Coleman, 2010). The success of this specialised response is yet to be examined.

Additionally, a recently revised protocol between the Victoria Police and the Department of Health (2010) aims to further clarify roles and responsibilities of both sides in an attempt to improve the working relationship and their responses to people who experience mental disorders. This new protocol includes a number of improvements on the old protocol, including clarifying the roles regarding patient transfers and disclosure of client information. It also specifies that in high-risk encounters, such as siege and self-harm incidents, the police can notify the local mental health triage service and request telephone assistance regarding managing the incident and request any pertinent patient information (Department of Health, 2010).

It remains to be seen whether this type of assistance will be effective and enough to provide police with the necessary support in managing incidents where the person appears mentally ill and presents a threat to self or others. It is clear, however, that the mental health system requires more funding if it is going to be effective in (1) having enough staff and being able to assist police with the situation, whether on the scene or over the telephone, and (2) catering for the needs of these individuals following the incident with the police, such as providing them with timely, effective, and appropriate inpatient or outpatient mental health care.

Conclusions

Police are given vast legal powers, including the powers to use fatal and non-fatal force, in order to effectively perform their role of protecting and serving the community. This chapter reviewed the literature regarding the role that mental disorders play in these encounters, especially concentrating on the recent research from Victoria, Australia. Although fatal use of force was unavoidable in many incidents, the greater use of force on people presenting with apparent mental disorders is a notable and significant concern that suggests the need for a sustained collection of training reforms for police at this challenging interface. Fundamentally, it is considered crucial to not only provide police with a suit of options and additional supports when dealing with people experiencing mental disorders, but that also comprehensive broader systems' policy and practise initiatives, which would provide the backbone to interactions with this group, must be implemented to improve the experiences and outcomes at this interface.

References

Adang, O.M.J., Kaminski, R.J., Howell, M.Q., & Mensink, J. (2006). Assessing the performance of pepper spray in use-of-force encounters: The Dutch experience. *Policing: An International Journal of Police Strategies and Management, 29*, 282–305.

Appelbaum, K.L. (2000). Police encounters with persons with mental illness: Introduction. *Journal of the American Academy of Psychiatry and the Law, 28*, 325.

Baksheev, G.N., Thomas, S.D.M., & Ogloff, J.R.P. (2010). Psychiatric disorders and unmet needs in Australian police cells. *Australian and New Zealand Journal of Psychiatry, 44*, 1043–1051.

Best, D., Quigley, A., & Bailey, A. (2004). Police shootings as a way of self-harming: A review of the evidence for 'suicide by cop' in England and Wales between 1998 and 2001. *International Journal of the Sociology of Law, 32*, 349–361.

Borum, R. (2000). Improving high risk encounters between people with mental illness and the police. *Journal of the American Academy of Psychiatry and the Law, 28*, 332–337.

Brouwer, G.E. (2005). Review of fatal shootings by Victoria Police. Retrieved from Office of Police Integrity website: http://www.opi.vic.gov.au/index.php?i=88

Chappell, D. (2008). Policing and emotionally disturbed persons: Disseminating knowledge, removing stigma and enhancing performance. *Australian Journal of Forensic Science, 40*, 37–48.

Chappell, D. (2010). From sorcery to stun guns and suicide: The eclectic and global challenges of policing and the mentally ill. *Police Practice and Research: An International Journal, 11*, 289–300.

Clifford, K. (2010). The thin blue line of mental health in Australia. *Police Practice and Research: An International Journal, 11*, 355–370.

Coleman, T.G., & Cotton, D.H. (2010). Reducing risk and improving outcomes of police interactions with people with mental illness. *Journal of Police Crisis Negotiations, 10*, 39–57.

Compton, M.T., Broussard, B., Hankerson-Dyson, D., Krishan, S., Stewart, T., Oliva, J.R., & Watson, A.C. (2010). System- and policy-level challenges to full implementation of the crisis intervention team (CIT) model. *Journal of Police Crisis Negotiations, 10*, 72–85.

Dalton, V. (1998). Police shootings 1990–97. *Trends and Issues in Crime and Criminal Justice, 89*, 1–6.

Deane, M.W., Steadman, H.J., Borum, R., Veysey, B.M., & Morrissey, J.P. (1999). Emerging partnerships between mental health and law enforcement. *Psychiatric Services, 50*, 99–101.

De Leo, D., Bertolote, J., & Lester, D. (2002). Self-directed violence. In E.G. Krug, L.L. Dahlberg, J.A. Mercy, A.B. Zwi, & R. Lozano (Eds.), *World report on violence and health* (pp. 185–212). Retrieved from http://whqlibdoc.who.int/hq/2002/9241545615.pdf

Department of Health. (2010). *Department of Health and Victoria Police protocol for mental health*. Melbourne: Department of Health.

Fry, A.J., O'Riordan, D.P., & Geanellos, R. (2002). Social control agents or front-line carers for people with mental health problems: Police and mental health services in Sydney, Australia. *Health & Social Care in the Community, 10*, 277–286.

Fyfe, J.J. (2000). Policing the emotionally disturbed. *Journal of the American Academy of Psychiatry and the Law, 28*, 345–347.

Godfredson, J.W., Thomas, S.D.M., Ogloff, J.R.P., & Luebbers, S. (2011). Police perceptions of their encounters with individuals experiencing mental illnesses: A Victorian survey. *Australian and New Zealand Journal of Criminology, 44* 180–195.

Hartford, K., Heslop, L., Stitt, L., & Hoch, J.S. (2005). Design of an algorithm to identify persons with mental illness in a police administrative database. *International Journal of Law and Psychiatry, 28*, 1–11.

Hickman, M.J., Piquero, A.R., & Garner, J.H. (2008). Toward a national estimate of police use of nonlethal force. *Criminology & Public Policy, 7*, 563–604.

Homant, R.J., & Kennedy, D.B. (2000). Suicide by police: A proposed typology of law enforcement officer assisted suicide. *Policing: An International Journal of Police Strategies and Management, 23*, 339–355.

Hutson, H.R., Anglin, D., Yarabrough, J., Hardaway, K., Russell, M., Strote, J., Canter, M., & Blum, B. (1998). Suicide by cop. *Annals of Emergency Medicine, 32*, 665–669.

International Association of Chiefs of Police. (2001). *Police use of force in America 2001.* Alexandria, VA: Author.

Johnson, R.R. (2011). Suspect mental disorder and police use of force. *Criminal Justice and Behavior, 38*, 127–145.

Kaminski, R.J., DiGiovanni, C., & Downs, R. (2004). The use of force between the police and persons with impaired judgment. *Police Quarterly, 7*, 311–338.

Kerr, A.N., Morabito, M., & Watson, A.C. (2010). Police encounters, mental illness, and injury: An exploratory investigation. *Journal of Police Crisis Negotiations, 10*, 116–132.

Kesic, D., Ducat, L., & Thomas, S.D.M. (2011). Using force: Australian newspaper descriptions of contacts between the police and persons experiencing mental illness. *Australian Psychologist*, DOI: 10.1111/j.1742–9544.2011.00051.x.

Kesic, D., Thomas, S.D.M., & Ogloff, J.R.P. (2010). Mental illness among police fatalities in Victoria 1982–2007: Case linkage study. *Australian and New Zealand Journal of Psychiatry, 44*, 463–468.

Kesic, D., Thomas, S.D.M., & Ogloff, J.R.P. (2012). Analysis of fatal police shootings: Time, space and suicide by police. *Criminal Justice and Behavior*, DOI: 10.1177/0093854812440084.

Kesic, D., Thomas, S.D.M., & Ogloff, J.R.P. (In press). The use of nonfatal force on or by persons with apparent mental disorder in encounters with police. *Criminal Justice and Behavior.*

Klein, G.C. (2010). Negotiating the fate of people with mental illness: The police and the hospital emergency room. *Journal of Police Crisis Negotiations, 10*, 205–219.

Klinger, D.A. (2001). Suicidal intent in victim-precipitated homicide: Insights from the study of "suicide-by-cop." *Homicide Studies: An Interdisciplinary and International Journal, 5*, 206–226.

Klinger, D.A. (2005). Social theory and the street cop: The case of deadly force. *Police Foundation*, 1–15.

Knott, J.C., Pleban, A., Taylor, D., & Castle, D. (2007). Management of mental health patients attending Victorian emergency departments. *Royal Australian and New Zealand College of Psychiatrists, 41*, 759–767.

Lawton, B.A. (2007). Levels of nonlethal force: An examination of individual, situational and contextual factors. *Journal of Research in Crime and Delinquency, 44*, 163–184.

Lindsay, M., & Lester, D. (2004). *Suicide by cop: Committing suicide by provoking the police to shoot you*. Amityville, NY: Baywood Publishing Company, Inc.

Lindsay, M., & Lester, D. (2008). Criteria for suicide-by-cop incidents. *Psychological Reports, 102*, 603–605.

Lord, V.B. (2000). Law enforcement-assisted suicide. *Criminal Justice and Behavior, 27*, 401–419.

Lord, V.B., & Sloop, M.W. (2010). Suicide by cop: Police shootings as a method of self harming. *Journal of Criminal Justice, 38*, 889–895.

McCluskey, J.D., Mastrofski, S.D., & Parks, R.B. (1999). To acquiesce or rebel: Predicting citizen compliance with police requests. *Police Quarterly, 2*, 389–416.

McKenzie, I.K. (2006). Forcing the police to open fire: A cross-cultural/international examination of police-involved, victim-provoked shootings. *Journal of Police Crisis Negotiations, 6*, 5–25.

Mental health training rise among members. (2010, March). *The Gazette, 5*, 8.

Mohandie, K., Meloy, J., & Collins, P.I. (2009). Suicide by cop among officer-involved shooting cases. *Journal of Forensic Sciences, 54*, 456–462.

Mohandie, K., & Meloy, J.R. (2011). Suicide by cop among female subjects in officer-involved shooting cases. *Journal of Forensic Sciences, 56*, 664–668.

Moore, R. (2010). Current trends in policing and the mentally ill in Europe: A review of the literature. *Police Practice and Research: An International Journal, 11*, 330–341.

Morabito, M.S., Kerr, A.N., Watson, A., Draine, J., Ottati, V., & Angell, B. (2010). Crisis intervention team and people with mental illness: Exploring the factors that influence the use of force. *Crime and Delinquency, 20*, 1–21.

O'Brien, A.J., McKenna, B.G., Thom, K., Diesfeld, K., & Simpson, A.I. (2011). Use of tasers on people with mental illness. A New Zealand database study. *International Journal of Law and Psychiatry, 34*, 39–43.

Parent, R.B. (1996). Aspects of police use of deadly force in British Columbia: The phenomenon of victim-precipitated homicide (master's thesis). Retrieved from http://ir.lib.sfu.ca/bitstream/1892/8386/1/b18065880.pdf

Parent, R.B., & Verdun-Jones, S. (1998). Victim-precipitated homicide: Police use of deadly force in British Columbia. *Policing, 21*, 432–448.

Pearson, D.D.R. (2009). *Victorian auditor general's report: Responding to mental health crises in the community*. Melbourne: Victorian Auditor-General's Office.

Police Commissioners' Policy Advisory Group. (1992). *National guidelines: Police use of lethal force*. Payneham, SA, Australia: National Police Research Unit.

Police Complaints Authority. (2003). Review of shootings by police in England and Wales from 1998–2001. London: Police Complaints Authority. Retrieved from http://www.statewatch.org/news/2005/jul/pca-firearms-report-2003.pdf

Reuland, M. (2010). Tailoring the police response to people with mental illness to community characteristics in the USA. *Police Practice and Research: An International Journal, 11*, 315–329.

Ruiz, J., & Miller, C. (2004). An exploratory study of Pennsylvania police officers' perceptions of dangerousness and their ability to manage persons with mental illness. *Police Quarterly, 7*, 359–371.

Sced, M. (2006, August). Mental illness in the community: The role of the police. *ACPR Issues, 1*–12.

Smith, B.L. (2004). Structural and organizational predictors of homicide by police. *Policing: An International Journal of Police Strategies and Management, 27*, 539–557.

Strong, M. (2009). Review of the use of force by and against Victorian police. Retrieved from Office of Police Integrity website: http://www.opi.vic.gov.au/index.php?i=118

Task Force Victor. (1994). *Police shootings: A question of balance.* Melbourne: Author.

Terrill, W. (2005). Police use of force: A transactional approach. *Justice Quarterly, 22*, 107–138.

Terrill, W., & Mastrofski, S.D. (2002). Situational and officer-based determinants of police coercion. *Justice Quarterly, 19*, 215–248.

The Allen Consulting Group. (2012). Police, ambulance, and clinical early response (PACER) evaluation: Final report. Retrieved from http://www.allenconsult.com.au/resources/acgpacerevaluation2012.pdf.

United Nations. (1979). Code of conduct for law enforcement officials. Retrieved from the Office of the High Commissioner for Human Rights website: http://www2.ohchr.org/english/law/pdf/codeofconduct.pdf

United Nations (1990). Basic principles on the use of force and firearms by law enforcement officials. Retrieved from the Office of the High Commissioner for Human Rights website: http://www2.ohchr.org/english/law/firearms.htm#wp1019644

White, M.D., & Ready, J. (2010). The impact of the taser on suspect resistance: Identifying predictors of effectiveness. *Crime and Delinquency, 56*, 70–102.

Wolfgang, M.E. (1959). Suicide by means of victim-precipitated homicide. *Journal of Clinical and Experimental Psychopathology, 20*, 335–349.

World Health Organisation. (2009). Preventing suicide: A resource for police, firefighters and other first line responders. Retrieved from http://whqlibdoc.who.int/publications/2009/9789241598439_eng.pdf

World Health Organisation. (2010). Suicide prevention (SUPRE). Retrieved July 20, 2010, from http://www.who.int/mental_health/prevention/suicide/suicideprevent/en/print.html

Suggested Reading

Crawford, C., & Burns, R. (1998). Predictors of the police use of force: The application of a continuum perspective in Phoenix. *Police Quarterly, 1*, 41–63.

Ho, J.D., Dawes, D.M., Johnson, M.A., Lundin, E.J., & Miner, J.R. (2007). Impact of conducted electrical weapons in a mentally ill population: A brief report. *American Journal of Emergency Medicine, 25*, 780–785.

Kennedy, D.B., Homant, R.J., & Thomas, H.R. (1998). Suicide by cop. *FBI Law Enforcement Bulletin, 67*, 21–27.

Lee, S. (2006). The characteristics of police presentations to an emergency department in a community hospital. *Australasian Emergency Nursing Journal, 9*, 65–72.

Lord, V.B. (2010). The role of mental health in police-reported suicides. *Journal of Police Crisis Negotiations, 10*, 191–204.

Richardson, E., & McSherry, B. (2010). Diversion down under—Programs for offenders with mental illnesses in Australia. *International Journal of Law and Psychiatry, 33*, 249–257.

Mental Health Crisis Interventions and the Politics of Police Use of Deadly Force

9

KATRINA CLIFFORD

Contents

Introduction

Several decades have passed since the process of deinstitutionalisation commenced across Australia, shifting the care, treatment, and accommodation of mentally ill individuals from psychiatric custodial institutions to community-based settings. Despite many years of "reform," a number of prominent national and state-based inquiries have shown that the process of returning these individuals to community living and community care has been afflicted by significant deficiencies. Principal among these is an ongoing deficit in the requisite mental health funding, programmes, supervision, and support services required to fulfil the very ambitions of deinstitutionalisation—namely, a reduced incidence of both mental illness and the number (and mistreatment) of mentally ill individuals in society (Wylie & Wilson, 1990; Rosenberg, Hickie, & Mendoza, 2009).

Figures from the Australian Bureau of Statistics (ABS) reveal that the prevalence of mental illness in Australia has not diminished significantly over the past 10 years, and may have increased with regards to psychiatric problems, such as mood and anxiety disorders (Australian Bureau of Statistics, 2007; Cresswell, 2009). Studies have also shown that, similar to other countries, including Canada and the United Kingdom, increasing numbers of people with mental illness are coming in contact with the criminal justice system, be it as offenders or victims. At present, major mental illnesses, such as schizophrenia and depression, are thought to be between three to five times more prevalent among Australian prisoner populations than in the general community (Ogloff, Davis, Rivers, & Ross, 2007; *Because Mental Health Matters*, 2009; see also Australian Institute of Health and Welfare, 2011). The outcome is a national mental health system that has variously been described as failing, ineffective, and in crisis, with most people experiencing chronic mental illness (an estimated 60 to 65%) still unable to access the care they need (Mental Health Council of Australia and the Brain and Mind Research Institute, 2005; Sced, 2006; Rosenberg et al., 2009; National Health and Hospitals Reform Commission, 2009).

While there is undeniably a tendency within the literature to focus on the shortcomings rather than the successes of deinstitutionalisation, the extent to which appropriate care can be provided in community settings for individuals experiencing mental illness remains a valid concern, and one that is highly sensitive to and dependent on a number of factors, not least of all, resource constraints and work practises (Queensland Health, 2005). In Australia, as well as internationally, there is compelling evidence to suggest that police resources have been left to shoulder the burden of the inadequacies of deinstitutionalisation reforms, assuming a disproportionate share of the responsibilities in relation to managing mental illness in the community. This is in spite of the more recent development of formal protocols, such as memoranda of understanding (MOUs), which seek to provide clear and agreed guidelines on the parameters of engagement between mental health and law enforcement agencies in mental health crisis situations where these services are involved (Carroll, 2005). True of many communications frameworks and formal protocols relating to the separation of roles and responsibilities, MOUs are obviously only as effective on paper as they are enforceable in practise. Frontline police officers continue to report noncompliance with MOUs by some mental health staff and hospitals, who are perceived to be "abdicating their responsibilities, more often than not due to lack of funding and availability of positions" (Police Federation of Australia, 2005, p. 3; see also Carroll, 2005). Frontline police have become increasingly frustrated with the expectation that they will "fill the gaps" of mental health crisis response (Police Federation of Australia, 2005; Sced, 2006).

While, admittedly, such responsibilities have traditionally been a part of police work (Bittner, 1967), police interactions with mentally ill individuals post-deinstitutionalisation have become ever more frequent, according to available police data. In 2003, for example, Queensland Police responded to some 17,000 callouts across the state relating to people with a mental illness, a 17% increase from 2001 (Office of the Public Advocate—Queensland, 2005). In comparison, in 2004, New South Wales (NSW) Police responded to around 18,000 calls involving individuals with a mental disorder (Donohue, Cashin, Laing, Newman, & Halsey, 2008). By 2009, this had increased to

34,000 mental health-related incidents (Donohue, 2010). Writes Donohue and colleagues (2008, p. 25): "As the prevalence of mental illness increases so too does police involvement in dealing with such cases."

Some commentators, including those representing sector interests, have drawn particular attention to the frequency with which frontline police officers have been expected to deal with persons presenting with the acute symptoms of mental disorders in the community (particularly those of a co-morbid nature) and the complexities this has generated, including the stretching or overburdening of police resources (see, for example, Wylie & Wilson, 1990; Springvale Monash Legal Service, Inc., 2005; Sced, 2006; Police Federation of Australia, 2005; Carroll, 2005). This is a trend most readily measured by the millions of dollars spent in officer-hours each year on police involvement in mental health crisis interventions, and the management of hospital admissions and assessments, as well as the often unnecessary incarceration of mentally disordered and disabled individuals (Wylie & Wilson, 1990). As Teplin and Pruett (1992) point out, police officers are now typically the first, and often the only, responders to mental health crises, generally by virtue of the 24/7 nature of their work, and often as a consequence of community stereotypes, which view mentally ill individuals—particularly those exhibiting the disturbing signs of psychiatric crisis—as criminal and dangerous (see also Sced, 2006; Carroll, 2005). In many respects, police officers have become "streetcorner psychiatrists" (Teplin & Pruett, 1992).

Some operational police in Australia have expressed concerns over what they perceive to be a lack of necessary knowledge, skills, and resources to assess and respond appropriately to individuals with mental illness (Donohue et al., 2008; Fry, O'Riordan, & Geanellos, 2002). While frontline police should not be expected to undertake clinical diagnostic assessments, the Office of the Public Advocate—Queensland (2005, p. 13) has previously suggested that it is at least "imperative that they are familiar with, and learn to recognise, the likely symptoms and behaviours of a person who is experiencing acute mental illness" or a mental health crisis, given the increasing interactions of police with mentally ill individuals, and the serious consequences that can result. The (often unacknowledged) circumstances of an acute psychosis, where a mentally ill individual may be impaired in terms of his or her capacity to comprehend the severity of his or her situation and the need for police involvement, or the consequences of his or her actions (Patch & Arrigo, 1999), adds to this imperative.

In response, public discussion has increasingly turned to debate over practical factors, such as the introduction of less lethal weaponry (e.g., tasers) and the need for improved interagency coordination and communications. This has been matched by an identifiable trend toward the introduction of specialised mental health training programmes for frontline police officers in police jurisdictions across Australia. Such initiatives include the NSW

Police Force Mental Health Intervention Team (MHIT) programme, which is discussed in more detail in Chapter 4. Police initiatives such as these have sought to enhance the mental health literacy of frontline police officers and their professional practises of risk assessment, management, and communications with mental health consumers, their family members or carers, and other emergency responders, including mental health representatives and hospital staff. In short, they have been designed to facilitate a least restrictive approach to mental health crisis intervention by enhancing police awareness about mental illness, and alternative ways to address it by engaging with services in the community (Herrington & Clifford, 2012). Despite these objectives, there continues to be an overrepresentation of mentally ill individuals in the fatalities that have resulted from police use of force incidents, particularly police-involved shootings. This has led to questions about whether the positive impacts of mental health-related policing initiatives (some of which, like the NSW Police Force MHIT, have been independently evaluated) have yet to be realised in practise. Or is it that the circumstances that delineate these police-involved mental health crisis interventions from the other everyday encounters between frontline police officers and mentally ill individuals are so unique that no manner of least restrictive measures can neutralise the possibility of a fatal outcome?

In answer to these and other related questions about police use of deadly force, researchers in the field of policing studies have extensively theorised about the predictive determinants of police shooting behaviour and the influence of police culture and protocols on the outcomes of police-involved mental health crisis interventions. Within the literature, however, the degree to which the discretionary decision making of police officers is influenced by police attitudes toward mental illness, public expectations of police officers as frontline mental health responders, and the potential conflicts between these and the strict protocols of contemporary policing practises, has been insufficiently addressed. More significantly, the available literature—some of which relies on limited and imperfect statistical datasets—has paid minimal regard to the personal trauma narratives of those impacted by fatal police-involved shootings of mentally ill individuals. This is despite the fact that many of these trauma narratives offer unmediated evidence of recurrent themes and systemic deficiencies that might be better addressed in the critical (and human) response to mental health crisis incidents. It is especially rare, among the available literature, to locate detailed studies of the personal impacts of fatal mental health crisis interventions on police officers or their attempts to negotiate the "emotional labour" of their trauma work within the standard operating procedures (SOPs) and regulatory controls of contemporary policing practises. This is an area under current study by the author. This chapter draws on preliminary aspects of this research, which more broadly seeks to examine the ways in which fatal police-involved shootings of mentally ill individuals in crisis are represented and interpreted by and between news media and people traumatised by these critical incidents. This research has included personal communications, focus groups, and one-on-one semistructured interviews with individuals from key stakeholder groups, including police officers, bereaved family members, coroners, mental health advocates, and news media professionals responsible for the reporting of these critical incidents.

Fatal Mental Health Crisis Interventions in Australia

At present, encounters between police and mentally ill individuals generally result as a consequence of arrests for misdemeanours or petty crimes or, more crucially, when individuals have been detained for their own safety or the safety of others in response to critical situations variously referred to as some form of crisis (see, for example, Senate Select Committee on Mental Health, 2006; Sced, 2006; Commonwealth Department of Health and Family Services, 1998; Wooldridge, 2000; Springvale Monash Legal Services, Inc., 2005). A number of these individuals will come to police attention repeatedly as frequent presenters (Victoria Police, 2008). In most instances, the interactions police have with people with a mental illness are resolved safely and without incident (Office of the Public Advocate—Queensland, 2005). However, in a small number of cases, these encounters may involve levels of hostility that serve to heighten the resistance of a mentally ill individual toward attempts at negotiation by police officers, creating a situation that is beyond the point of de-escalation (Kerr et al., 2010). Notwithstanding stigmatising stereotypes that correlate mental illness with an inherent propensity for violence, the disturbed behaviour of individuals experiencing irrational thoughts and delusional beliefs associated with acute psychosis (which is frequently accompanied by some form of paranoia about police) can precipitate high-risk situations that require police use of force (Coleman & Cotton, 2010). These events may result in severe injury to or the death of the individual in psychiatric crisis—often, in the case of the latter, by police-involved shooting. These critical incidents, also referred to as fatal mental health crisis interventions, are invariably complex. They are typically distinguished from other interactions between mentally ill individuals and police "by virtue of a number of elements, such as the presence of or potential for violence or self-harm, the presence of firearms or other weapons, and the degree of distress experienced by the individual" (Office of the Public Advocate—Queensland, 2005, p. 15). Fatal mental health crisis interventions generate considerable controversy in news media and among the general public (see Clifford, 2012). In particular, when responses to mental health crisis incidents are mishandled or end in the use of deadly force by police, "our responses appear to be more complex"; the incident has the potential to arouse "serious concerns and passions" (Doob, cited in Chappell & Graham, 1985, p. v).

In Australia, fatal outcomes to police-involved mental health crisis interventions are relatively uncommon. What is troubling, however, is the prevalence of these critical incidents as a proportion of the total number of fatal police-involved shootings recorded. An examination of coronial findings and associated news media coverage of a number of fatal police-involved shootings over the past decade supports the proposition that, in Australia, mentally ill individuals are significantly (and, in many cases, increasingly) overrepresented among these fatalities (see also Kesic, Thomas, & Ogloff, 2010). Existing datasets, albeit limited in supply in the Australian context, also support this (see Godfredson, Ogloff, Thomas, & Luebbers, 2010). These trends are consistent with international research, which has found that individuals with a mental illness are four times more likely to be killed by the police (Cordner, 2006).

According to Dalton's (1998) seminal research report on police-involved shootings, between January 1, 1990 and June 30, 1997, Australian police fatally shot 41 people, with at least one-third of those identified as suffering from a diagnosed mental illness (requiring psychiatric treatment) or depression prior to police-involved crisis intervention. The peak during this period was 1994, during which time Victoria Police shot and killed nine people. At least four of those persons had a known psychiatric history (Dalton, 1998). In the first nine months of 1994 alone, there were twice as many fatal police-involved shootings in Victoria as in the previous six years in NSW (McCulloch, 2001). During the period covered by Dalton's (1998) report, eight persons were killed in total as a consequence of gunshot wounds inflicted by NSW Police. At least three of these had a known psychiatric history or had experienced depression prior to police-involved crisis intervention (Dalton, 1998).

In light of the untenable number of shooting deaths by Victoria Police throughout the 1990s, Project Beacon was established in September 1994, under the guise of ushering in the Victoria Police "Safety First Philosophy." The core principle underpinning the project was that the success of police operations, particularly those involving mentally ill individuals in crisis, would be consistent with and "primarily judged on the extent to which the use of force is avoided or minimised" (Brouwer, 2005). A review of the project's progress, conducted in 1995, speculated as to the reasons why Victorian police officers had fatally shot so many mentally ill individuals in crisis when deinstitutionalisation in other Australian states had not led to "the same dramatic increase in police shootings" (Victoria Police, 1995, p. 1). Misunderstandings by members of police as to "what the community expects of them," a heightened sense of vulnerability among police, and intensive firearms training (leading to police officers being more adept at their use of firearms) were implicated as contributing factors (Victoria Police, 1995, p. 1).

Overall, Project Beacon was considered a success in redressing some of the deficiencies of police training with regard to equipping operational police officers with techniques in nonphysical resolution of crisis incidents, and raising awareness of the "particular difficulties for police in dealing with people presenting with symptoms of mental illness or disorder" (Brouwer, 2005). Since 2005, however, there have been at least another eight Victoria Police reviews relevant to the use of force, some of which have published findings inconsistent with these earlier assessments (Office of Police Integrity Victoria, 2009). Despite recognising the improvements heralded by the introduction of Project Beacon, the Victorian Office of Police Integrity's *Review of Fatal Shootings by Victoria Police* concluded that "there remain aspects of policy and practice where Victoria Police performance against the 'Safety First Philosophy' requires improvement," particularly with regards to an identified increase in the proportion of mentally ill individuals shot by Victoria Police since the implementation of Project Beacon (Brouwer, 2005, p. 2). A subsequent report titled *Review of the Use of Force by and against Victorian Police* was critical of Victoria Police operational safety tactics (OST) training. The report noted that since June 2006, OST training had not focussed on mental health issues or on "making sure police have the crucial skills to identify and take appropriate action when someone may have a mental health problem" (Office of Police Integrity Victoria, 2009, p. 14). Recommendations were made in both cases for the development of strategies to redress the identified deficiencies in the mental health literacy of police officers, and to reintegrate tactical communications techniques, especially in relation to interactions with mentally ill individuals, into existing police training programmes (Brouwer, 2005; Office of Police Integrity Victoria, 2009).

In contrast to the overtly negative view of Victoria Police's (mis)handling of individuals suffering from mental illness, especially throughout the 1990s, an overall positive sentiment has typically been noted with regards to the operational approach of the NSW Police Force (Senate Select Committee on Mental Health, 2006). It could be argued that this is, in part, attributable to the "lower number of fatalities arising from high profile incidents between police and individuals suffering from a mental illness in NSW, as compared with Victoria" (Springvale Monash Legal Service, Inc., 2005, p. 23). This is not to say, however, that NSW Police officers have not endured their own share of negative public attention and high-profile scrutiny over the use of deadly force in interactions with mentally ill individuals in crisis. Most notably, in June 1997, 35-year-old Frenchman Roni Levi was fatally shot by police on Bondi Beach, Sydney, after allegedly lunging at attending police officers with a knife. At the time, Levi was suffering borderline delusional thought processes and had earlier disappeared from St. Vincent's Hospital, where he had voluntarily admitted himself the night before. Iconic images of the incident, captured by a professional photographer who happened to be on the beach that morning, reached international news audiences, and continue to resonate as culturally emblematic signifiers of these types of critical incidents. As is frequently the case with fatal mental health crisis interventions, the shooting was the subject of a highly publicised coronial inquiry, which was terminated on March 6, 1998, after the matter was referred by the coroner to the director of public prosecutions (DPP). In June of the same year, the DPP determined that there was no reasonable prospect of a conviction against either of the constables responsible for the discharge of firearms, and no prosecutions were brought against the officers in relation to the fatal police-involved shooting of Levi (NSW Police Integrity Commission, 2001; Chappell, 2008). The incident by no means did the NSW Police Force any favours, as allegations of police misconduct spilled over with suggestions that either one or both of the officers responsible for the fatal discharge of firearms had been affected by drugs or alcohol at the time of the shooting (for more on the death of Roni Levi and these claims, see Goodsir, 2001; Miller, J., 2000; and NSW Police Integrity Commission, 2001).

This is, of course, not the first (or sadly the last) critical incident in which allegations of police misconduct or operational deficiencies have been raised in relation to the fatal police-involved shooting of a person in psychiatric crisis. There are, indeed, a number of prominent fatal mental health crisis interventions in Australia that have captured public attention and attracted significant news media coverage over the past decade (see Clifford, 2010). Among these are the more recent deaths of Elijah Holcombe and Adam Salter, who both warrant mention in the context of this chapter for the criticisms expressed by the coroner in each case toward the actions of involved police officers. In the case of Salter's death, the police intervention was labelled "an utter failure" (Mitchell, 2011, p. 38) after it was revealed that one of the police officers in attendance had issued the warning "Taser, taser, taser" before discharging her firearm at Salter, who was, at the time, repeatedly stabbing himself in the chest in the kitchen of his father's house in the Sydney suburb of Lakemba in November 2009. At the time of writing, the critical incident was still the subject of a NSW Police Integrity Commission investigation into possible police misconduct.

The coronial inquest into Elijah Holcombe's death from a single bullet to the chest, fired by a plainclothed police officer on June 2, 2009, after a foot chase through the central business district of the northern NSW town of Armidale, was suspended before even half of the 71 listed witnesses could give their statements (Kennedy, 2010). The matter was referred to the DPP for the consideration of criminal charges against a "known person" whom the NSW state coroner suggested, "a jury, properly instructed, would convict … of an indictable offence" (Jerram, cited in Kennedy, 2010). Local police had earlier transported Holcombe to Armidale Hospital for psychiatric assessment after he was reported missing by his parents. He had reportedly not taken his medication for a mental illness, which was characterised by extreme fear and paranoia of police, for two days before his death (Walters, 2009). Holcombe was armed with a bread knife, taken from a local coffee shop, when he was shot in Cinders Lane hours after discharging himself from the hospital before a medical officer had been able to assess his condition. Police had been asked to return Holcombe to the hospital where nursing staff were concerned for his welfare. In late August 2012, the DPP confirmed that no charges would be laid against the police officer responsible for fatally shooting Elijah Holcombe (Olding & Davies, 2012).

Interpretations of Risk and Vulnerability

Beyond the statistics, the personal trauma narratives of those impacted by such critical incidents reveal that fatal mental health crisis interventions can have "devastating and long-term consequences—not only for the person's family and loved ones, but also for the police officer[s] involved and for community attitudes and perceptions" (Office of the Public Advocate—Queensland, 2005, p. 1). Previous research has shown that "vicarious experiences of policing have a substantial impact on perceptions of and confidence in police" (Herrington, Clifford, Lawrence, Ryle, & Pope, 2009, p. 35). In particular, news depictions of controversial police use of force against individuals in psychiatric crisis have important implications for how the public views police culture and mental illness more generally, and whether these incidents are considered typical or aberrations of contemporary policing practise (Hazelton, 1997). This, in turn, has significant implications for not only public trust in frontline police officers, but also the perceived legitimacy of police and the public's general willingness to cooperate and collaborate with them (Herrington et al., 2009; Myhill & Beak, 2008; Novak, 2009; Tyler, 1989). Such depictions may also have some bearing on the tenor of future interactions between police officers and mental health consumers. The impact and influence of news media reports of high-profile incidents involving police use of force, particularly where such force is lethal, is therefore a legitimate concern and ongoing consideration for police agencies—particularly since it is often through news media coverage that the public's knowledge of these critical incidents is constructed.

While the emotional impacts on family and friends of the deceased may be more immediately apparent to those who bear witness to such tragedies (researchers included), the trauma experienced by the police officers responsible for the discharge of firearms can be equally ruinous to the lives of these individuals. Many police officers "never recover from such circumstances and themselves suffer severe psychological problems after such incidents—often for the rest of their lives" (Carroll, 2005, p. 22). The personal testimonies and lived experiences of frontline police, where available, strongly support this—although, in keeping with official police protocols related to critical incidents, in the aftermath of a fatal mental health crisis intervention, these narratives are not able to be publicly shared by the individual police officers involved. Often, it requires others to articulate the trauma associated with such critical incidents. In 2008, for example, Rod Porter, a former detective inspector with Victoria Police, wrote an editorial for the Australian newspaper, the *Herald Sun*, in response to the fatal police-involved shooting of a 15-year-old Melbourne boy, Tyler Cassidy. Speaking from personal experience, having previously killed someone in the line of duty, Porter recalled that, at the time, preserving his own life was the priority. He wrote: "You have to act in what you think is the most appropriate way. But once that happens … you start to question yourself.… The fact I was involved in the taking of a life will stay with me until I die" (Porter, 2008).

The cumulative impacts of involvement in a fatal mental health crisis intervention on police officers *already routinely exposed to the negative effects of trauma work* are also evidenced in other police officer testimonies of this kind. These impacts are most readily identifiable in the references to fatal mental health crisis interventions as a "tipping point" in a police officer's decision to discontinue his or her service with the police force. As one police officer who had been involved in a fatal mental health crisis intervention told me, people tend to call the police when there is a problem of some kind, "so you're dealing with people's misery all the time … all of that can just chip away, and chip away, and chip away." More publicly, sentiments similar to these have been expressed by those such as Lenore Schiller, a former NSW police negotiator, who was involved in a siege on a property near Tumut, in the southwest region of NSW, in February 2001. The police operation concluded with the fatal police-involved shooting of Jim Hallinan, a local resident who, at the time, was delusional and experiencing the symptoms of acute psychosis associated with a preexisting mental disorder, which was known to police. Reflecting on the circumstances of the critical incident in an episode for the ABC TV programme *Australian Story*, Schiller (cited in "The Guns of Adjungbilly—Part 2") revealed:

> It just sent me into a complete state of anxiety.… Many years of policing and seeing horrific things, being at horrific events had all come to a head … this was just the one that tipped me, where my mind just apparently closed down and said, "That's it, no more."

There has been much made of the "special dangers" that are associated with the role of frontline police officers as the "vulnerable thin blue line between order and chaos" in society (Lawrence, 2000, p. 30; see also Kleinig, 2000). Frontline police officers are continually reminded of these risks by way of the mandatory requirements of police instruction, which advise that individual officers assess and manage the levels of risk they encounter as part of their everyday policing experiences in accordance with predefined operational protocols. This hypervigilance toward perceived levels of occupational risk may explain why some frontline police officers have demonstrated a tendency to overestimate the risks inherent to what might be considered by others as relatively routine police operations. In the broader area of field operations, the increasing frequency of interactions between frontline police officers and mentally ill individuals continues to be cited within policing circles as one of the single largest risks to police officer safety. For obvious reasons, such claims do not sit comfortably with mental health advocates and mental health consumers and their families and carers. For many of these individuals, police assumptions of dangerousness in relation to mentally ill individuals are often incommensurate with their own perceptions of risk and vulnerability, particularly as these relate to the hazards inherent to police involvement in mental health crisis interventions. All the same, there are real risks related to the interactions between police and mentally ill citizens in crisis, and these cannot be disregarded.

If the individual in crisis is both in a highly irrational state of mind and in possession of an edged weapon or firearm, the risk intrinsic to the situation will obviously increase relative to a mental health crisis incident where these factors are negligible or absent (Kaminski, DiGiovanni, & Downs, 2004). Risk, in this respect, is registered on a number of levels, not just in relation to the possible risk of harm (either to self or others) posed by the individual in crisis, but also in relation to the actual risks to which the person in psychiatric crisis is exposed as a consequence of the escalation of the volatility of the event, and the individual's disturbed or psychotic behaviour and the need for police presence. As Kerr, Morabito, and Watson (2010) explain, during a police-involved mental health crisis intervention, a mentally ill individual may be more vulnerable to injury because police officers may "misinterpret their behavior and demeanor," given that mental illness "can exacerbate a hostile demeanor or the appearance of resistance, depending on how the symptoms are manifested" (p. 119). Mentally ill individuals in crisis are also more likely to have an impaired sense of judgement and comprehension, and their mental disturbance may be exacerbated by the visible presence of police uniforms or police firearms. In these situations, mentally ill individuals in crisis are often unable to reflexively assess the level of threat they themselves are perceived to present to a police officer as a consequence of their carriage of knives or a firearm (which are often taken up for self-harm or self-protection during the onset of an acute psychosis) and the probable outcome of a failure to discard these "weapons." As Cordner (2006) explains, individuals experiencing an acute mental health crisis can appear to be ignoring a police officer when really they might not be able to understand the officer's instructions.

From Principles of Policing to Policing Practises

In all jurisdictions across Australia, "police are given wide-ranging power to intervene in the lives of the mentally ill and mentally disordered by virtue of the respective Mental Health Acts" (Police Federation of Australia, 2005, p. 4). Under these legislative statutes, police are commonly and legally authorised to use "reasonable" force or "reasonably necessary" use of force or restraints to assist with the apprehension and transportation of mentally ill or mentally disordered individuals to or from a mental health facility or other health facility. What is determined as reasonable, however, is commonly found to be indistinct in many mental health acts. "Thus," writes Pinto (2004), "as with other law enforcement decisions, the police must exercise discretion in choosing the best way to handle emergency situations involving the mentally ill" (p. 11). While national guidelines have previously established clear parameters for its application, the use of deadly force still ultimately remains *the discretion of the police officers involved.* This is supported by the body of scholarly research related to this issue, which confirms that police discretion plays an important role in managing crisis or arrest situations, particularly those involving mentally ill individuals (see, for example, Freeman & Roesch, 1989; Godfredson et al., 2010; Green, 1997; Kalinich & Senese, 1987; Lamb, Weinberger, & DeCuir Jr., 2002; Sellers, Sullivan, Veysey, & Shane, 2005).

The greatest amount of discretion in police-involved mental health crisis interventions is obviously available to police officers in situations where they have initiated contact with a mentally ill individual (Lamb et al., 2002). "In such situations," writes Lamb et al. (2002), "there is considerable potential for the disposition to be influenced by police officers' personal attitudes or beliefs" (p. 1267). Previous studies have shown that police officers, not unlike the broader public of which they are representative, often hold the illusionary belief that the risk of violence is much higher when mental illness is present (see Bolton, 2000; Kimhi et al., 1998; Lipson, Turner, & Kasper, 2010; Monahan & Steadman, 1994; Monahan et al., 2001; Ruiz & Miller, 2004). Research has also shown that police expectations that the acute symptoms associated with an individual's mental illness are under the individual's control, or that an individual with mental illness is inherently dangerous, can lead to police officer reactions ranging from avoidance to withholding help to the endorsement of coercive treatment (see Corrigan, Markowitz, Watson, Rowan, & Kubiak, 2003).

Situated knowledge, or rather, personal experience, can also play a fundamental and persuasive role in the development of these interpretive frameworks (see Angermeyer & Dietrich, 2006; Francis, Pirkis, Dunt, Blood, & Davis, 2002; Philo, 1996; van 't Veer, Kraan, Drosseart, & Modde, 2006; Wesley Mission, 2007). Personal experience of mental health problems—be it through one's own direct experience as a mental health consumer or as a carer to family or friends—can potentially predispose individuals involved in a mental health crisis intervention toward being "more informed and sensitive towards mental health issues than those without an appreciation of the actual reality of these experiences" (Morris, 2006, p. 7). Personal experience has also been shown to have a strong association with the adoption of "help-centred outcomes," as opposed to more restrictive options for dealing with mentally ill individuals in crisis (Godfredson, Thomas, Ogloff, & Luebbers, 2011). So too, specialised mental health training of frontline police officers has been shown to have a positive impact on police-involved mental health contacts (Herrington et al., 2009). These dynamics can produce differing strategic decisions about risk management and the responses of "experts" (Blood, 2002). It is the conflict between these subjective and technical (or more objective) definitions of risk—and the most appropriate and ethical police options for the management of this risk—that remains central to the enduring tensions identified between stakeholder interpretations of fatal mental health crisis interventions, particularly in the immediate aftermath of such traumatic events.

The Risk Logic of Deadly Offence

This inherent struggle to define the ways in which critical incidents, such as fatal mental health crisis interventions, are viewed and interpreted can be characterised in two ways. Primarily, it reflects a conflict between institutional (official) discourse, on the one hand, and lay (nonofficial) discourse, on the other. More specifically, the conflicts between institutional and lay discourse identifiable in the aftermath of such critical incidents may be traced to fundamental differences in the interpretive frameworks adopted by key stakeholders. Police organisations, for example, tend to evaluate the reasonableness of police use of deadly force according to the technical assessments and management of risks specified within the formal protocols and SOPs of contemporary policing. In contrast, the critical perspectives of family and friends of the deceased may be more readily guided by subjective measures that are often influenced by emotive responses to the death of a loved one. On occasion, this may lead to a situation where the risks inherent to a police-involved mental health crisis intervention, but particularly those presented by a mentally ill individual experiencing acute psychosis, may be under-estimated or unacknowledged by those closest to them. Bereaved family members often find it difficult to understand and reconcile, for example, the necessity for police officers to discharge their firearms when they have, for years, dealt with their mentally ill relative—who may have often become florid, deranged, and not rationally responsive, potentially violent—without having to resort to such extreme measures of force.

In Australia, the contentious issue of the use of lethal or deadly force against mentally ill individuals is quite often portrayed in media commentary and public debate as being indicative of or revealing much about a police officer's "commitment to the upholding of the civil liberties of the citizens they are required to protect" (Chappell, 2008, p. 40). This is particularly obvious where use of deadly force involving firearms is repeatedly framed as the by-product of a calculated "shoot to kill" policy or "shoot first" culture within the police force (see, for example, Brown, 2009; Kerbaj, 2007). In this context, the discretionary decision by police officers to discharge their fire-arm is framed as entirely incommensurate with both the reality and level of risk posed by a mentally ill individual in crisis who is, more often than not, armed with only an edged weapon, rather than a firearm. The difficulties often expressed by the public in reconciling the need for police use of deadly force against a person in possession of what is perceived to be a less lethal weapon, such as a knife, are well recognised by police officers themselves, albeit rarely contextualised within news media coverage.

It is not uncommon for family and friends of the deceased and other mental health advocates, after a fatal mental health crisis intervention, to hold fast to the notion that police officers could have availed themselves of other less lethal tactical measures in place of the decision to shoot. Quite often, this includes the argument that where it was necessary to shoot, police officers should have aimed for the individual's leg or arm, rather than the torso, and thereby, the outcome of shooting to kill. These perceptions are often vehemently maintained, regardless of whether the circumstances of the critical incident reasonably or even operationally would have enabled other-wise. The following comments from Melinda Dundas, the widow of Roni Levi, are representative of this recurrent news framing:

> The whole notion of a policy which says … when you use a firearm you've got to shoot to kill is really inhumane…. Roni was shot four times for God's sake … had he been shot once in the leg or the arm it would've been sufficient to hospitalise him, let alone four times. (Dundas, cited in McDermott, 2009)

These claims, as they relate to interpretations of the level of threat posed by an individual in psychiatric crisis and the appropriateness of police actions in response, are frequently informed by what is often framed in public discourse as the heavy-handedness of police officers and a systemic tendency among frontline police to routinely resort to unjustifiable displays of coercive force (over less excessive measures) in their everyday policing and as part of police culture more broadly. This is the notion that all police officers are "trigger-happy cops" (see Kaba, cited in Stephey, 2007). In some cases, the need for police use of firearms is also framed by lay discourse as a measure of the incompetence and negligence of frontline police officers to effectively respond to mental health crisis situations. But there are, at any given time, numerous mitigating factors that can influence a police officer's decision to use coercive force.

Mental health crisis interventions that result in violence or the use of deadly force by police typically escalate to such a point through a chain of events and perceptions (Lawrence, 2000), although this does not necessitate a corresponding escalation in the chain of tactical options available to police, regardless of public perceptions that often suggest the contrary. A senior police officer interviewed for the author's research acknowledged that it is commonly expected that frontline police officers will incrementally escalate their use of tactical options in response to a mental health crisis situation, starting with capsicum spray and then moving onto the use of a taser and finally the discharge of firearms as a "last resort." However, he was quick to point out that "it doesn't work that way." There is, he explained, "no staggered response" in field operations. Rather, police officers are educated to use "whatever tactical option is relevant under the circumstances and that's a judgement call, based on the circumstances you find yourself presented with," but one that usually starts with communication as "the first point of call."

Much less talked about (perhaps due to the sensitivity of the issue) is the idea that, in some instances, police discretion is informed by the necessity to shoot, that there are occasions where police officers have no other option but to use deadly force. In some cases, police may have a *legal and moral duty* to discharge their firearms in the protection of innocent lives, and may be found legally liable in situations where their failure to use deadly force results in the death of innocent citizens (Miller, S., 2000). In these scenarios, formal discretionary guidelines are of small relevance, because "by any reasonable standard, the officers involved have only one choice" (Fyfe, 1988, p. 185). This situation is obviously complicated by the phenomenon of suicide by cop or circumstances where the individual is not a fleeing felon, but a mentally ill person in psychiatric distress who likely does not have the capacity to control his or her behaviour or comprehend the implications of his or her failure to do so. The matter is further frustrated by the fact that, as Heath and O'Hair (2009) point out, issues of risk and crisis *are* "inherently matters of choice" (p. 22). The discourse related to police use of deadly force in these circumstances is therefore necessarily complex.

Bearing in mind that the specialist weapons training provided to front-line police officers instructs them to aim for centre body mass in the discharge of firearms, the likelihood of lethal force as the outcome of a decision to shoot a mentally ill individual in crisis is not implausible. In other words, if a police officer shoots "according to the rule book," it must be reasonably assumed that his or her actions require that he or she "shoots to kill," although this is not usually how an individual police officer will perceive his or her actions at the time. Nor is it a case that death is always the motive or intent when a police officer determines to discharge his or her firearm. The intentionality of a fatal police-involved shooting is, however, only ever debatable after the event, at which point it is regularly demonstrated that police officers, as Van Maanen (1980) contends, do not often regard shooting and killing as tightly coupled. Instead, fatal police-involved shootings are "more attuned to the fearful particulars of one's own safety than to a logic of deadly offense" (Van Maanen, 1980, p. 149). As one police participant in the author's research explained, "people see firearms and death; that's all they see.... We are trained to shoot centre body mass, which likely is going to result in somebody's death, but we don't shoot to kill people. We shoot to stop [them]."

Conclusion

In providing some context to critical incidents of this kind, it is important to recognise that the majority of police officers in the course of their everyday duties "do a difficult and stressful job in a professional and humane manner," for which they should be commended (Chappell, 2008, p. 39). As Godfredson and colleagues (2010) point out, this is not often reflected in the statistics cited in the critical literature on policing, particularly with regards to the "myriad police encounters that result in mental health dispositions or other less formal outcomes" (p. 1). These might include circumstances where a mental health crisis is resolved by other means of community intervention, such as police involvement of family members or through the use of de-escalation techniques that ultimately result in a scenario where the individual does not need to be scheduled or hospitalised or detained by police. Nevertheless, it is unsurprising that there continues to be significant interest in cases of police use of deadly force and in "ensuring that when force is used, this occurs in a way that is reasonable and proportionate" (NSW Ombudsman, 2008, p. 1). There are various reasons as to why public concerns about police use of force in mental health crisis interventions remain notable—among which, it could be argued, is the influence of news media coverage, which not all police officers believe always fairly represents them. Writes Lawrence (2000):

> Police often view the media with suspicion and express frustration and bitterness over what they see as the media's willingness to sensationalize the use of force without making the public aware of the difficulties and dangers faced by police officers. (p. 49)

The perpetuation (and, worse still, acceptance) of negative identity constructions, such as the presumption that all mentally ill individuals are inherently violent or that all police officers are trigger-happy cops, has significant real-world implications. As the *Final Report of the Mental Health Crisis Intervention Ad Hoc Advisory Group* suggests, one of the main reasons for "poor relationships between police and mental health consumers" is the combination of fear and stigma—of which police and mental health consumers are not immune, and news media coverage of fatal mental health crisis interventions and mental health issues more generally can be a contributing factor, given its tendency toward perpetuating "inappropriate stereotypes" (Commonwealth Department of Health and Family Services, 1998, p. 7). The personal narratives of those with lived experience of these encounters and the traumatic impacts of involvement in a fatal mental health crisis intervention therefore serve to not only complicate and counter such misrepresentations, but to also contextualise the complexities associated with these critical incidents. Moreover, they serve as timely reminders of the more acutely detrimental effects of deficient deinstitutionalisation reforms and the systemic failures that continue to proliferate from this. This includes the resulting and increasing (sometimes overwhelming) burdens placed upon those, such as police services, who are called (albeit reluctantly) to act as the frontline response to mental health crises in the community, often without the requisite knowledge, understanding, training, or resources to effectively do so. As Borum (2000) observes in an article on improving high-risk encounters between frontline police officers and mentally ill individuals: "It is unquestionably a tragedy when an encounter between a police officer and a person who has come to police attention solely because of symptoms of a mental illness ends in a fatal shooting" (p. 36). In these circumstances, there are no winners, and the traumatic impacts of such events can be profound and prolonged for the family and friends of the deceased as well as the individual police officers involved in the critical incident.

Attempts by police agencies across Australian jurisdictions to meet these challenges through improved preventive measures, such as interagency coordination, communication, and collaboration, and specialised mental health training for frontline police officers, are therefore to be commended. However, the continued overrepresentation of mentally ill individuals among the fatalities of police-involved shootings in the community warrants further in-depth analysis, if only to provide a deeper understanding of the contextual factors that typically contribute to such critical incidents and to more effectively inform the broader development of training and other preemptive mental health crisis intervention models across Australia (Kesic et al., 2010). To this end, the lessons derived from the Project Beacon experience offer some invaluable insights for successive mental health-related policing initiatives, such as the NSW Police Force MHIT and other crisis intervention team-oriented training programmes. Among these is the importance of maintaining the same vigilance and momentum that typically characterises the introductory phases of new programmes such as these. As Project Beacon has proven, with time, it is easy for police agencies to become either distracted from or complacent toward their original motivations and intentions for developing reforms that rethink the professional practises and risk conceptions of frontline police officers (Office of Police Integrity Victoria, 2009). To lose this focus may be to succumb to former negative habits, as more recent reviews of the resurgence in police use of force in Victoria have demonstrated. It is necessary, therefore, for shifts in the attitude and approach toward police interactions with mentally ill individuals in crisis to be embedded within the ethos and cultural structures of police agencies. Such reforms must be promoted as professional ideals that are championed throughout the police hierarchy—from senior management through to frontline police officers. The realisation of these shifts in professional practise is obviously predicated on a number of defining factors, not least of all resourcing and legislative constraints, the compatibility between this style of training and existing police protocols, and policy development, interagency cooperation, and the cultivation of valid and reliable performance measures that are not necessarily reliant on statistical correlatives and body counts.

There is an argument to suggest, however, that the adoption of these recommended measures should not be for politicians and bureaucrats alone to decide. They should also take account of the lived experiences of mental health consumers and their families/carers, as well as those of frontline police officers, particularly where these stakeholders have personal testimonies to offer in relation to the tensions between the subjective and objective experiences of mental health crisis interventions and risk interpretations. As Palmer (1995) has previously suggested, many of the major inquiries into contemporary policing practises and mental illness proceed on the assumption that "internal changes will right the wrongs," with no space given to raising "how the community might enter into open debate about the forms and practises of policing within the boundaries or principles of a liberal democracy" (p. 55). This requires that police agencies become more expansive and collaborative in their development of risk communications and response models, moving beyond the traditional conceptions of interagency relationships with mental health services to also consult with mental health advocates and mental health consumers/carers (as has been evident in the development of the

NSW Police Force MHIT and other "vulnerable people policing" models—see Bartkowiak-Théron & Crehan (2010)). This is not to suggest that recent developments in contemporary policing practises and improved interagency coordination should be dismissed or condemned, especially where positive outcomes have already been evidenced from the introduction of these initiatives. However, there is clearly room for continuous improvement. To a large extent, this requires a rethinking of the boundaries of risk communications as it relates to mental health crises in the community, and the stronger incorporation of lived experience in the public discourse surrounding these events. Sustainable risk communications, by definition, can never realistically be restricted to the autonomy of interagency relationships between police and mental health services. It would seem counterintuitive, therefore, to continue to exclude the voices of mental health consumers and their families/carers in this discourse, particularly when many of the triumphs of recent policing initiatives (such as specialised mental health training and preferred strategies of mental health crisis intervention) have been based on the development of risk communications models that have either been immediately shaped by these stakeholders or have at least engaged more actively with them.

As important, increasing police competence as a result of the commitment to training officers to recognise and respond more effectively to mental health issues in the community should not be viewed as an "alternative to filling service gaps within the health and disability support service systems" (Victoria Police, 2008, p. 21). Nor should it expand policing roles and involvement to include a wholesale adoption of the responsibilities of other service sectors, or come at the expense of developing partnerships with many of these (mental) health care providers, including consideration of the need for training of these same individuals in the roles, responsibilities, and functions of police (Sced, 2006; Victoria Police, 2008). Most of all, however, improvements in police training with regard to mental health literacy and more effective responses to mentally disordered individuals (be they in crisis or at the early onset of the illness) should never be seen as a means of addressing the problems deeply entrenched within Australia's mental health system (Sced, 2006).

References

Angermeyer, M.C., & Dietrich, S. (2006). Public beliefs about and attitudes towards people with mental illness: A review of population studies. *Acta Psychiatrica Scandinavica, 113*(3), 163–179.

Australian Bureau of Statistics. (2007). *National survey of mental health and wellbeing: Summary of results, 2007* (Cat. 4326.0). Canberra, ACT: Australian Bureau of Statistics.

Australian Institute of Health and Welfare. (2011). *The health of Australia's prisoners 2010* (Cat. PHE 149). Canberra, ACT: Australian Institute of Health and Welfare.

Bartkowiak-Théron, I., & A.C. Crehan. (2010). A new movement in community policing? From community policing to vulnerable people policing. In J. Putt (Ed.), *Community policing in Australia* (pp. 16–23). Canberra, ACT: Australian Institute of Criminology.

Because mental health matters: Victorian Mental Health Reform Strategy 2009–2019. (2009). Melbourne: Mental Health and Drugs Division, Department of Human Services.

Bittner, E. (1967). Police discretion in emergency apprehension of mentally ill persons. *Social Problems, 14,* 278–292.

Blood, R.W. (2002, October 2–3). Communication research in everyday contexts: Informing the Australian government's public health strategy on mass media reporting and portrayal of suicide and mental illness. Paper presented at the Communications Research Forum 2002. Canberra, Australia: DCITA.

Bolton, M.J. (2000). The influence of individual characteristics of police officers and police organizations on perceptions of persons with mental illness. PhD diss., Virginia Commonwealth University.

Borum, R. (2000). Improving high risk encounters between people with mental illness and police. *Journal of the American Academy of Psychiatry and Law, 28*(3), 332–337.

Brouwer, G.E. (2005). *Review of fatal police shootings by Victoria Police* [Report of the director, police integrity]. Melbourne: Office of Police Integrity Victoria.

Brown, R. (2009, July 16). Long wait on police shooting inquests. *PM with Mark Colvin* (Radio broadcast, transcript). Sydney: ABC Local Radio. Retrieved August 21, 2009, from http://www.abc.net.au/pm/content/2008/s2628113.htm

Carroll, M. (2005, December). Mental-health system overburdening police. *Police Journal,* 18–22.

Chappell, D. (2008). Policing and emotionally disturbed persons: Disseminating knowledge, removing stigma and enhancing performance. *Australian Journal of Forensic Services, 40*(1), 37–48.

Chappell, D., & Graham, L.P. (1985). *Police use of deadly force: Canadian perspectives.* Toronto, Canada: Centre of Criminology, University of Toronto.

Clifford, K. (2010). The thin blue line of mental health in Australia. *Police Practice and Research, 11*(4), 355–370.

Clifford, K. (2012). The vulnerable thin blue line: Representations of police use of force in the media. In I. Bartkowiak-Théron & N. Asquith (Eds.), *Policing Vulnerability* (pp. 101–114). Annandale, NSW: Federation Press.

Coleman, T.G., & Cotton, D.H. (2010). Reducing risk and improving outcomes of police interactions with people with mental illness. *Journal of Police Crisis Negotiations, 10*(1), 39–57.

Commonwealth Department of Health and Family Services. (1998). *Final report of the Mental Health Crisis Intervention Ad Hoc Advisory Group: An examination of mental health crisis intervention practices and policies regarding the fatal use of firearms by police against people with mental illness* (Whiteford Report). Canberra, ACT: Commonwealth of Australia.

Cordner, G. (2006). *People with mental illness: Problem-oriented guides for police problem-specific guides series.* Washington, DC: U.S. Department of Justice, Office of Community Oriented Policing Services.

Corrigan, P.W., Markowitz, F.E., Watson, A.C., Rowan, D., & Kubiak, M.A. (2003). An attribution model of public discrimination towards persons with mental illness. *Journal of Health and Social Behavior, 44*(2), 162–179.

Cresswell, A. (2009, March 26). Half suffer mental illness at some point. *The Australian.* Retrieved May 6, 2009, from http://www.theaustralian.news.com.au/business/story/0,,25243308-5018014,00.html

Dalton, V. (1998). Police shootings 1990–1997. In *Trends and issues in crime and criminal justice* (No. 89). Canberra, ACT: Australian Institute of Criminology.

Donohue, D. (2010). Corporate spokespersons message. In *NSW Police Force: Mental health.* Retrieved October 10, 2011, from http://www.police.nsw.gov.au/community_issues/mental_health

Donohue, D., Cashin, A., Laing, R., Newman, C., & Halsey, R. (2008, May). Mental health intervention. *Police News,* 24–25. Retrieved September 16, 2008, from http://www.pansw.org.au/PolNews/Police_News_May24–28.pdf

Francis, C., Pirkis, J., Dunt, D., Blood, R.W., & Davis, C. (2002). *Improving mental health literacy: A review of the literature.* Canberra, ACT: Centre for Health Program Evaluation.

Freeman, R.J., & Roesch, R. (1989). Mental disorder and the criminal justice system: A review. *International Journal of Law and Psychiatry, 12,* 105–115.

Fry, A.J., O'Riordan, D.P., & Geanellos, R. (2002). Social control agents or front-line carers for people with mental health problems: Police and mental health services in Sydney, Australia. *Health and Social Care in the Community, 10*(4), 277–286.

Fyfe, J.J. (1988). Police use of deadly force: Research and reform. *Justice Quarterly, 5*(2), 165–205.

Godfredson, J.W., Ogloff, J.R.P., Thomas, S.D.M., & Luebbers, S. (2010). Police discretion and encounters with people experiencing mental illness: The significant factors. *Criminal Justice and Behavior, 4,* 1–14.

Godfredson, J.W., Thomas, S.D.M., Ogloff, J.R.P., & Luebbers, S. (2011). Police perceptions of their encounters with individuals experiencing mental illness: A Victorian survey. *Australian and New Zealand Journal of Criminology, 44*(2), 180–195.

Goodsir, D. (2001). *Death at Bondi: Cops, cocaine, corruption and the killing of Roni Levi.* Sydney: Pan Macmillan Australia.

Green, T.M. (1997). Police as frontline mental health workers: The decision to arrest or refer to mental health agencies. *International Journal of Law and Psychiatry, 20,* 469–486.

The Guns of Adjungbilly—Part 2. (2005, September 19). *Australian story* (Television broadcast, transcript). Sydney: ABC TV. Retrieved August 18, 2010, from http://www.abc.net.au/austory/content/2005/s1464579.htm

Hazelton, M. (1997). Reporting mental health: A discourse analysis of mental health-related news in two Australian newspapers. *Australian and New Zealand Journal of Mental Health Nursing, 6*(2), 73–89.

Heath, R.L., & O'Hair, H.D. (2009). The significance of crisis and risk communication. In R.L. Heath & H.D. O'Hair (Eds.), *Handbook of risk and crisis communication* (pp. 5–30). New York: Routledge.

Herrington, V., & Clifford, K. (2012). Policing mental illness: Examining the police role in addressing mental ill-health. In I. Bartkowiak-Théron & N. Asquith (Eds.), *Policing Vulnerability* (pp. 117–131). Annandale, NSW: Federation Press.

Herrington, V., Clifford, K., Lawrence, P.F., Ryle, S., & Pope, R. (2009). *The NSW Police Force Mental Health Intervention Team: Final evaluation report*. Sydney: Charles Sturt University Centre for Inland Health and Australian Graduate School of Policing. Retrieved May 27, 2010, from http://www.police.nsw.gov.au/__data/ assets/pdf_file/0006/174246/MHIT_Evaluation_Final_Report_241209.pdf

Kalinich, D.B., & Senese, J.D. (1987). Police discretion and the mentally disordered in Chicago: A reconsideration. *Police Studies, 10*, 185–191.

Kaminski, R.J., DiGiovanni, C., & Downs, R. (2004). The use of force between the police and persons with impaired judgment. *Police Quarterly, 7*(3), 311–338.

Kennedy, L. (2010, November 14). Elijah was paranoid that police were chasing him. Then they did. *Sydney Morning Herald*. Retrieved October 17, 2011, from http:// www.smh.com.au/nsw/elijah-was-paranoid-that-police-were-chasing-him- then-they-did-20101114-17siy.html#ixzz1bpdUSem5

Kerbaj, R. (2007, February 22). Police defend fatal shooting of axe wielder. *The Australian*, 7.

Kerr, A.N., Morabito, M., & Watson, A.C. (2010). Police encounters, mental illness, and injury: An exploratory investigation. *Journal of Police Crisis Negotiations, 10*(1), 116–132.

Kesic, D., Thomas, S.D.M., & Ogloff, J.R.P. (2010). Mental illness among police fatalities in Victoria 1982–2007: Case linkage study. *Australian and New Zealand Journal of Psychiatry, 44*, 463–468.

Kimhi, R., Barak, Y., Gutman, J., Melamed, Y., Zohar, M., & Barak, I. (1998). Police attitudes toward mental illness and psychiatric patients in Israel. *Journal of the American Academy of Psychiatry and the Law, 4*, 625–630.

Kleinig, J. (2000). Police violence and the loyal code of silence. In T. Coady, S. James, S. Miller, & M. O'Keefe (Ed.), *Violence and police culture* (pp. 219–234). Carlton South, Victoria: Melbourne University Press.

Lamb, H.R., Weinberger, L.E., & DeCuir Jr., W.J. (2002). The police and mental health. *Psychiatric Services, 53*(10), 1266–1271.

Lawrence, R.G. (2000). *The politics of force: Media and the construction of police brutality*. Berkeley and Los Angeles, CA: University of California Press.

Lipson, G.S., Turner, J.T., and Kasper, R. (2010). A strategic approach to police interactions involving persons with mental illness. *Journal of Police Crisis Negotiations, 10*(1), 30–38.

McCulloch, J. (2001). *Blue army: Paramilitary policing in Australia*. Melbourne: Melbourne University Press.

McDermott, Q. (2009, October 26). *Lethal force* (Television broadcast, transcript). Four Corners. Sydney: ABC TV. Retrieved August 16, 2010, from http://www. abc.net.au/4corners/content/2009/s2722195.htm

Mental Health Council of Australia and the Brain and Mind Research Institute. (2005). *Not for service: Experiences of injustice and despair in mental health care in Australia*. Canberra, ACT: Mental Health Council of Australia.

Miller, J. (2000). *Shoot and demonise: The death of Roni Levi*. South Yarra, Victoria: Hardie Grant Books.

Miller, S. (2000). Shootings by police in Victoria: The ethical issues. In T. Coady, S. James, S. Miller, & M. O'Keefe (Eds.), *Violence and police culture* (pp. 205–218). Carlton South, Victoria: Melbourne University Press.

Mitchell, S. (2011, October 14). *Coronial findings: Inquest into the death of Adam Quddus Salter* (File 3333/09). Glebe, Australia: NSW State Coroner's Court. Retrieved December 6, 2011, from http://www.coroners.lawlink.nsw.gov.au/coroners/findings.html

Monahan, J., & Steadman, H. (1994). *Violence and mental disorder: Developments in risk assessment*. Chicago: University of Chicago Press.

Monahan, J., Steadman, H.J., Silver, E., Appelbaum, P.S., Robbins, P.C., Mulvey, E.P., Roth, L.H., Grisso, T., & Banks, S. (2001). *Rethinking risk assessment: The MacArthur study of mental disorder and violence*. Oxford: Oxford University Press.

Morris, G. (2006). *Mental health issues and the media: An introduction for health professionals*. London: Routledge.

Myhill, A., & Beak, K. (2008). *Public confidence in police*. London: National Policing Improvement Agency.

National Health and Hospitals Reform Commission. (2009). *A healthier future for all Australians—Interim report December 2008*. Canberra, ACT: Commonwealth of Australia.

Novak, K.J. (2009). Reasonable officers, public perceptions, and policy challenges. *Criminology and Public Policy, 8*(1), 153–161.

NSW Ombudsman. (2008). *The use of taser weapons by New South Wales Police Force: A special report to Parliament under Section 31 of the Ombudsman Act 1974*. Sydney: NSW Ombudsman.

NSW Police Integrity Commission. (2001). *Report to Parliament: Operation Saigon*. Sydney: NSW Police Integrity Commission.

Office of Police Integrity Victoria. (2009). *Review of the use of force by and against Victorian Police* (PP 165, Session 2006–09) Melbourne: Office of Police Integrity Victoria.

Office of the Public Advocate—Queensland. (2005). *Preserving life and dignity in distress: Responding to critical mental health incidents*. Brisbane, Queensland: Department of Justice and Attorney-General.

Ogloff, J.R.P., Davis, M.R., Rivers, G., & Ross, S. (2007). *The identification of mental disorders in the criminal justice system* (Paper from the *Trends and issues in crime and criminal justice* series, no. 334). Canberra, Australia: Australian Institute of Criminology.

Olding, R., & Davies, L. (2012, August 29). Officer who shot mentally ill man won't be charged. *Sydney Morning Herald*. Retrieved September 21, 2012, from http://www.smh.com.au/nsw/officer-who-shot-mentally-ill-man-wont-be-charged-20120829-250t7.html

Palmer, D. (1995). Excessive force. Beyond police shootings: Use of force and governing the Victorian Police force. *Alternative Law Journal, 20*(2), 53–56.

Patch, P.C., & Arrigo, B.A. (1999). Police officer attitudes and use of discretion in situations involving the mentally ill: The need to narrow the focus. *International Journal of Law and Psychiatry, 22*, 23–35.

Philo, G. (Ed.). (1996). *Media and mental distress*. London: Longman.

Pinto, S.M. (2004). Police response to mentally ill persons in crisis. PhD diss., Chicago School of Professional Psychology.

Police Federation of Australia. (2005, May 10). Submission to Senate Select Committee on Mental Health. Canberra, ACT: Police Federation of Australia.

Porter, R. (2008, December 13). The trauma of killing someone never goes. *Herald Sun*. Retrieved December 15, 2008, from http://www.news.com.au/heraldsun/story/0,,24792275-2862,00.html

Queensland Health. (2005). *Achieving balance: Report of the Queensland review of fatal mental health sentinel events. A review of systemic issues within Queensland Mental Health Services 2002–2003.* Brisbane, Queensland: Queensland Government. Retrieved February 7, 2009, from http://www.health.qld.gov.au/mentalhealth/docs/deidentified_report.pdf

Rosenberg, S., Hickie, I., & Mendoza, J. (2009). National mental health reform: Less talk, more action. *Medical Journal of Australia, 190*(4), 193–195.

Ruiz, J., & Miller, C. (2004). An exploratory study of Pennsylvania police officers' perceptions of dangerousness and their ability to manage persons with mental illness. *Police Quarterly, 7*, 359–371.

Sced, M. (2006). *Mental illness in the community: The role of police* (ACPR Issues 3). Retrieved October 9, 2006, from http://www.acpr.gov.au/pdf/Iss_3%20Mental.pdf

Sellers, C.L., Sullivan, C.J., Veysey, B.M., & Shane, J.M. (2005). Responding to persons with mental illnesses: Police perspectives on specialized and traditional practices. *Behavioural Sciences and the Law, 23*, 647–657.

Senate Select Committee on Mental Health. (2006). *A national approach to mental health—From crisis to community* (First report). Canberra, ACT: Commonwealth of Australia.

Springvale Monash Legal Service, Inc. (2005). *Police training and mental illness—A time for change.* Retrieved August 4, 2006, from http://www.smls.com.au

Stephey, M.J. (2007, August 8). De-criminalizing mental illness. *Time Magazine*. Retrieved February 1, 2010, from http://www.time.com/time/health/article/0,8599,1651002,00.html

Teplin, L.A., & Pruett, N.S. (1992). Police as streetcorner psychiatrist: Managing the mentally ill. *International Journal of Law and Psychiatry, 15*, 139–156.

Tyler, T. (1989). The psychology of procedural justice: A test of the group value model. *Journal of Personality and Social Psychology, 57*(5), 830–838.

Van Maanen, J. (1980). Beyond account: The personal impact of police shootings. *Annals of the American Academy of Political and Social Science, 452*, 145–156.

van't Veer, J.T.B., Kraan, H.F., Drosseart, S.H.C., & Modde, J.M. (2006). Determinants that shape public attitudes towards the mentally ill. *Social Psychiatry and Psychiatric Epidemiology, 41*(4), 310–317.

Victoria Police. (1995). *Project Beacon: Overview of progress.* No publication details given. Accessed May 21, 2008, via JV Barry Library at the Australian Institute of Criminology.

Victoria Police. (2008). *Victoria Police submission on the Green Paper: Because mental health matters.* Retrieved May 6, 2009, from http://www.health.vic.gov.au/mentalhealth/mhactreview/submissions/sub6.pdf

Walters, A. (2009, June 4). Elijah Holcombe shot dead by police in Armidale. *Daily Telegraph*. Retrieved December 5, 2011, from http://www.dailytelegraph.com.au/news/sydney-nsw/elijah-holcombe-shot-dead-by-police-in-armidale/story-e6freuzi-1225720594831

Wesley Mission. (2007). Living with mental illness: Attitudes, experiences and challenges. Retrieved May 8, 2008, from http://www.wesleymission.org.au/News/research/Mental_Health

Wooldridge, M. (2000). *Towards a national approach to information sharing in mental health crisis situations*. Expert Advisory Committee on Information Sharing in Mental Health Crisis Situations Report, National Mental Health Strategy. Canberra, ACT: Mental Health and Special Programs Branch, Commonwealth Department of Health and Aged Care.

Wylie, J.R., & Wilson, C. (1990). *Deinstitutionalisation of the mentally disabled and its impact on police services* (Report Series 93). Payneham, South Australia: National Police Research Unit.

Mental Health Frequent Presenters

10

Key Concerns, Case Management Approaches, and Policy and Programme Considerations for Emergency Services

GINA ANDREWS
EILEEN BALDRY

Contents

Mental health frequent presenters (MHFPs) are mentally ill or disordered consumers with multiple needs who frequently present to emergency services in mental health crisis. They often fail to have their complex health, social, and economic needs recognised or met, relapse quickly, and then present repeatedly to emergency services in the midst of mental health crises (Initiative Watch, 2005). Each mental health crisis experienced equates to a longer recovery period (Hudson, 2007; Hickie, 2008). Emergency services (police, ambulance, and emergency departments) invest substantial resources to manage and stabilise a mental health consumer in crisis. No one benefits in this cyclical crisis band-aid mode of addressing MHFPs' multiple concerns.

The purpose of this chapter is to identify the commonalities of MHFP as a population group (with particular attention given to the characteristics of MHFP to police), scope existing international and Australian mental health programmes and their responses to MHFP, and discuss potential changes to or new policies and programmes that could result in improved outcomes for all concerned. The context of the discussion will be Australian jurisdictions, with descriptions and brief analyses of some approaches undertaken in the United States. The rationale for including U.S. research in discussion is that some states in the United States seem relatively progressed on research, programme response, and evaluations for frequent presenters.

This chapter is divided into three sections. The first section explores key definitions of mental health frequent presenters, and specifically mental health frequent presenters to police, including the identification of salient population characteristics. The next section is a literature review of interagency case management and case coordination approaches for mental health frequent presenters. Finally, the last section contains concluding observations regarding future case management programmes and policy considerations for mental health frequent presenters.

Defining a Mental Health Frequent Presenter (MHFP) and Mental Health Frequent Presenters to Police

Definitions of *frequent use* of emergency and mental health services vary widely in the literature. There is no commonly accepted definition of a mental health frequent user or presenter. Dimensions considered in defining a frequent user include frequency (i.e., how many times a person presented and was admitted to an emergency department), what services were used by the individual (e.g., police, ambulance, emergency departments), and characteristics of the consumer (age, gender, ethnicity, socioeconomic, and health factors) (Andrews, 2012). Informally, representatives of emergency services agree that MHFPs are those persons who regularly present to emergency services with mental health problems in acute need of attention, but not always for their mental disorder. Definitions of frequent use surveyed in the academic literature range from as few as 3 visits up to 12 or more visits annually, as well as definitions incorporating consumption of a disproportionate amount of resources (Andrews, 2012, p. 10).

There is a paucity of government data available on this topic in Australia. Data held by agencies on MHFPs is neither readily accessible nor clearly defined. Thus, it has been difficult to develop a full picture of the scope of frequent presenting in Australia, of the range and frequency of services being used, or to make comparisons and integrate the results of the available studies. Further, the dearth of Australian academic research on the issue alone confirms the need for more robust data and scoping of the issue.

Despite the data difficulties, Australian and overseas studies reveal some important MHFP consumer trends and issues. Available studies confirm that a relatively small percentage of frequent presenters are responsible for a disproportionately large use of emergency services. Typically, most studies identified MHFP as the group that accounts for 15% to 25% of all emergency department (ED) presentations (Baldry, Dowse, & Clarence, 2012; Bernstein, 2006; Victorian DHS, 2005; Hunt et al., 2006; Fischer & Stevens, 1999; Chaput & Lebel, 2007; Fuda & Immekus, 2005, 2006; Lincoln & White, 2006; Mehl-Madrona, 1998).

It is apparent from analysis of international and Australian MHFP research that there are some common characteristics among the MHFP population (regardless of definitional anomalies). Consistently MHFPs:

- Consume disproportionately more emergency service resources, even when adjusting for the more frequent actual presentations at EDs, than infrequent presenters, for example, a significantly higher use of ambulance and police transports to EDs
- Are more likely to require intensive health treatment
- Typically have had early onset of mental health problems
- Are more likely to suffer from treatment-resistant severe mental disorders such as personality disorder or mental illnesses such as a psychotic disorder or schizophrenia
- Experience co-morbidity
- Are more likely to have come into contact with police (either apprehended by the police for their mental illness/disorder or come under police attention as a criminal or victim of crime matters) than nonfrequent presenters (Andrews, 2012, p. 12; Baldry et al.; Bernstein, 2006).

The frequency data survey by Baldry et al. in "Mental Health Frequent Presenters to NSW Police Force in 2005" made some research inroads with its quantitative data analysis of NSW Police Force Computerised Operating Policing System (COPS) data (Baldry et al., 2012). The study aimed to identify and describe cohorts of MHFPs specific to police who are dealt with due to a mental health-related condition three or more times in a given year. The research identifies the population characteristics of mental health frequent presenters to police via a frequency data analysis.

Key findings, noted below, from Baldry et al.'s NSW Police 2012 MHFP study are salient to this chapter's discussion:

- Overall, males were more often frequent presenters; however, females were overrepresented as MHFPs as frequency of presentation increased.
- Age is an important variable for mental health frequent presenting, with younger people more likely to be associated with higher rates of mental health frequent presenting. There is a trend of older MHFPs having lower levels of overall contact with police across all contact types.
- Australian aboriginal persons are disproportionately overrepresented in the police sample in spite of variable recording practises. For example, aboriginal female MHFPs were overwhelmingly represented longitudinally, having an average of 19 contacts with police under the Mental Health Act 2007 (NSW) for the period 2001–2009. This is in contrast to aboriginal male MHFPs having an average of 14 events, and the wider nonaboriginal population having an average of 11 events with police under the Mental Health Act 2007 (NSW) for the same period. These findings demonstrate that aboriginal persons, and in particular aboriginal women, are a specific subpopulation among MHFPs to the NSW Police Force—requiring a more culturally appropriate tailored programme response.
- NSW Police Force referrals to health facilities are associated with an individual's increased contacts and prolonged duration of contact with mental health services.
- While MHFPs to the NSW Police Force constituted less than 7% of all the individuals who have had matters dealt with by the NSW Police Force under the Mental Health Act 2007 (NSW), they were responsible for 23% of all mental health events in 2005.
- The disproportionate burden on the NSW Police Force of MHFPs extends beyond the Mental Health Act events. Out of the 1,010 individual MHFPs identified to police in Baldry et al.'s 2005 study:
  - Eighty percent of this cohort was also known to police as persons of interest (POIs). A POI is an individual in whom police have an interest as the consequence of a police-verified event or incident

(NSW Police Force, 2009, p. 31). As POIs, MHFPs are typically identified as being responsible for low-level criminal offences (e.g., low-level assault).

- Sixty percent of this cohort was likely to come under police notice as a victim of crime in that same year. NSWPF's definition of victim of crime is based on s. 5 of the Victims Rights Act 1996 (NSW), whereby a victim of crime is defined as a person who suffers harm as a direct result of an act committed, or apparently committed, by another person in the course of a criminal offence, and that the person suffers harm as a result of the offence (NSW Police Force, 2009, p. 23; Baldry et al., 2012).

Baldry et al.'s study confirmed the long-held anecdotal NSW Police Force view that MHFPs are interacting at a high and disproportionate rate with police on a range of event types (i.e., beyond police provisions in the Mental Health Act 2007) and with other agencies. Further, Baldry et al.'s findings echo and complement the international research findings noted earlier.

In the next section, six case examples of mental health frequent presenters to police are showcased. These case examples were extracted from the NSW Police Force Computerised Operating Policing System (COPS) in 2011 and selected on the basis that they reflect distinct subpopulation group characteristics of mental health frequent presenters to the NSW Police Force. The case examples are based on Andrews's thesis on MHFPs to police (Andrews, 2012, pp. 171–177).

Case examples have been de-identified, with salient population characteristics kept to enable a description of MHFPs to police subpopulation groups. Before proceeding, the following contextual information should be noted when reading the case examples that are sourced from NSWPF COPS database:

1. COPS records do not go back beyond the mid–late 1980s.
2. COPS records do not exist in the event that the person had contact with the criminal justice system as a juvenile.
3. A New South Wales Police Force "incident" recorded in the COPS database is a single criminal or noncriminal episode committed by a person or group of persons. In contrast, a COPS "event" consists of one or more criminal/noncriminal incidents, which are related to the same unique occurrence (i.e., course of conduct) and committed by the same person or group of persons (NSW Police Force, 2009, p. 5).
4. The Mental Health Act incident category only came into effect in 2001. In a number of the cases that follow, COPS records show police intervening in attempted suicides and the like at an earlier juncture. If the Mental Health Act incident category had existed in the COPS database

earlier, it might have been used in some of these instances. As a result, "first Mental Health Act record" is not necessarily the first contact with police in a situation where a person was exhibiting mental health issues.

5. Police enterprise data warehouse (EDW) records started only in 2000. The incidents shown for each case are only those over the past decade.

6. Person of interest (POI) can potentially include *all* crime categories (i.e., it may include assault and missing persons categories, etc.), and the reader should not mistakenly double-count it as additional total COPS incidents (Andrews, 2012, p. 171).

Mental Health Frequent Presenters to NSW Police Force: Subpopulation Case Examples

---

Case Study 1: Male With a History of Crime (including violence)

Description	Summary of COPS Recorded Incidents
<ul><li>Male, born 1968.</li><li>Aboriginal. COPS records show first contact was in his early 30s. COPS database also includes many warnings about his violent behaviour and threats to kill.</li><li>Unemployed.</li></ul>	<ul><li>First Mental Health Act record is 2001.</li><li>First COPS record was from 1994 (robbery and shoplifting).</li><li>190 COPS incidents in total; highlights include:<ul><li>POI = 61 incidents</li><li>Mental Health Act (MHA) = 52 incidents</li><li>Move-on orders = 36 incidents</li><li>Search orders = 29 incidents</li><li>Suicide/self-harm = 1 incident</li></ul></li></ul>

Case Study 2: Treatment-Resistant Male

Description	Summary of COPS Recorded Incidents
<ul><li>Male, born 1970.</li><li>Caucasian.</li><li>Unemployed.</li></ul>	<ul><li>First Mental Health Act record is from 2001.</li><li>First COPS record as offender was for stealing in 1990. He was listed as a missing person a number of times from 1988 and 2001.</li><li>261 COPS incidents in total; highlights include:<ul><li>POI = 213 incidents (include missing person incidents)</li><li>Mental Health Act (MHA) = 23 incidents</li><li>Missing person (MP) = 78 incidents</li></ul></li></ul>

Case Study 3: A Juvenile Female With a History of High-Level Interactions With the Police Under the Mental Health Act, and a Victim History of Sexual Assault

Description	Summary of COPS Recorded Incidents
<ul><li>Female, born 1993.</li><li>Caucasian.</li><li>Attending high school.</li></ul>	<ul><li>First Mental Health Act record is from 2006.</li><li>First COPS record as victim of sexual assault in 2006.</li><li>45 COPS incidents in total; highlights include:<ul><li>POI = 1 incidents (for use of a knife as a weapon)</li><li>Mental Health Act (MHA) = 40 incidents</li><li>Victim of sexual assault (incest) = 4 incidents</li></ul></li></ul>

Mental Health Frequent Presenters to NSW Police Force: Subpopulation Case Examples (continued)

Case Study 4: Female Diagnosed With a Personality Disorder	
Description	Summary of COPS Recorded Incidents

• Female, born 1970.
• Caucasian.
• Unemployed.
	• First Mental Health Act record is from 2001.
	• First record as an offender was in 1988 (various stealing and fraud offences); note that any possible juvenile offences from earlier than this are not recorded.
	• 151 COPS incidents in total; highlights include:
	  • POI = 51 incidents
	  • Mental Health Act (MHA) = 41 incidents
	  • Missing person (MP) = 4 incidents
	  • Suicide/self-harm = 13 incidents

Case Study 5: Mentally Ill Male With a History of Violence	
Description	Summary of COPS Recorded Incidents

• Male, born 1969.
• Caucasian
• Hep C and HIV positive.
• Unemployed.
	• First Mental Health Act record is from 2001.
	• First COPS record 1989—as an apprehended violence order defendant. Known drug detection.
	• 226 COPS incidents in total; highlights include:
	  • POI[a] = 150 incidents (includes AVO incidents)
	  • Mental Health Act (MHA) – 57 incidents
	  • Apprehended violence order (AVO) = 34 incidents
	  • Breach of AVO = 25 incidents
	  • Missing person (MP) = 1 incident
	  • Suicide/self-harm = 4 incidents

Case Study 6: Aboriginal Female	
Description	Summary of COPS Recorded Incidents

• Female, born 1962.
• Aboriginal.
• COPS records also mention numerous scars from self-inflicted wounds.
• Unemployed.
	• First records on COPS are from 1989—victim of common assault and also arrested stealing from retail store.
	• First mental health-related event was in 1994 (inflicted self-harm by slicing her stomach with a knife). At the time she was living with a de facto.
	• 138 COPS incidents in total; highlights include:
	  • POI = 15 incidents
	  • Mental Health Act (MHA) = 51 incidents
	  • Suicide/self-harm = 30 incidents
	  • Occurrence only = 13 incidents

[a] In COPS, *person of interest* can potentially include all crime categories (i.e., it includes assault, missing persons, etc.), and the reader should not mistakenly double-count it as additional total COPS incidents.

The six police case examples reflect NSW Police Force experience with persons who are MHFPs. They demonstrate the depth and breadth of medical, human service, and criminal justice issues that MHFPs to police experience, and the history they bring to their encounters with police and other service providers. Of note are the high rates of self-harm and missing persons events interwoven with frequent presentations for mental health events. These suggest extreme distress and volatility in the persons' lives, begging the question of the suitability of the crisis style of management afforded them. These cases provide real contexts to consider some case management programmes running in various jurisdictions that may be suitable for persons who are MHFPs.

Programme Response—Suitable Interagency Case Management Examples

Literature on mental health frequent presentations demonstrates that this population group is likely to come into contact with a range of government and nongovernment agencies at a higher rate than others, and that supporting them and addressing their needs requires interagency involvement.

This section provides an overview of interagency programmes that provide case management for mental health frequent presenters. The selected examples utilise robust programme design, and in some cases yielded identifiable programme results and data. Before discussing these programmes, we briefly identify the characteristics of health case management, as this is integral to programme responses for MHFP.

Case Management: What It Is and What Are Its Benefits?

In contemporary terms, case management implies a set of strategies that enable the consumer to engage with appropriate services, treatments, and stakeholders, with the aim of optimising the consumer's ongoing recovery (Andrews, 2012, p. 16).

A diverse range of case management models or approaches have been developed over the past 30 years (Andrews, 2012, pp. 16–17; Kelch Associates, 2003; Onyett, 1992; Mueser, Bond, Drake, & Resnik, 1998). Key case management models that have generated the most discussion and application in recent decades are:

1. Assertive community treatment (ACT) model
2. Intensive case management (ICM) model
3. Clinical case management model
4. The brokerage model
5. The recovery approach

While each of these models is different, they all have been developed for persons with severe mental illness (Andrews, 2012, pp. 16–17; Mueser et al., 1998). Analysis of each of these models finds there is no ideal case management model. However, each model has its benefits and deficits, and some models appear on the evidence to be better suited to MHFPs.

The benefits of each case management model vary greatly. A mixed medical and psychosocial case management model, such as the ACT or ICM, provides the opportunity to "glue fragmented services together into a continuous and coherent whole through locating responsibility for assessment and co-ordination with one person or agency" (Onyett, 1992, p. 21). There is strong evidence that shows that typically, ACT or ICM case management models, when delivered to frequent presenters, may yield positive outcomes for all stakeholders (Andrews, 2012, pp. 24–26; Berstein, 2006, p. 19; Mueser et al., 1998, p. 37; Phillips et al., 2001, p. 771; Onyett, 1992, p. 23).

Before examining the characteristics and outcomes of a number of case management programmes, we provide a note of caution. Policies and programmes from other states and contexts should not be transplanted uncritically to a new policy setting. For example, the health and criminal justice systems and settings in the United States, nationally and at state and local government levels, are significantly different from those in Australia. We note such differences where relevant.

Case Management for Mental Health Frequent Presenters: Programme Examples

Californian Frequent Users of Health Services Initiative

This initiative was a five-year (2002–2007) project that aimed to decrease avoidable emergency department (ED) visits and hospital stays through an ACT style case management model. It promoted a responsive system of care that addressed frequent user needs, improved consumer outcomes, and decreased unnecessary use of emergency rooms and avoidable hospital stays and medical crises. The initiative provided a strong evidence base of good practise for frequent presenters' case management.

Research preceding the *initiative* established that costly and ineffective use of EDs is often the result of medical crises that could often be prevented with ongoing, coordinated, and multidisciplinary care, provided in more appropriate settings. Under the initiative, mental health frequent presenters were identified as the project target population based on the following definition:

> [Frequent users are] often chronically ill, under- or uninsured individuals who repeatedly use emergency rooms and hospitals for medical crises that could be prevented with more appropriate ongoing care. They often have multiple psycho-social risk factors, such as mental illness, alcohol or substance

use disorders, and homelessness, and they lack social supports, which affects their ability to get continuous, coordinated care. (Initiative Watch, 2005, p. 1)

We note that the United States does not have a universal basic health care system like Medicare in Australia, so given the description above that a defining feature of the sample is its lack of private insurance, the persons frequently presenting to Californian EDs may not have the same profile or needs as MHFP in Australia. It is NSW Police Force experience, however, that MHFPs to police are also typically low income and socially excluded, and more likely to be 100% reliant on state health care provision (Andrews, 2012). The relevant principles of case management from the initiative that could be applied to Australia include multidisciplinary care, data sharing between agencies, and implementation of evidence-based best practises and engagement of patients in the most appropriate setting.

The initiative's results were promising, noting *declines* across the following services:

- ED re-presentations (including a reduction in the overall number of clients who visit the ED and in the number of visits per client).
- Hospital inpatient days (including a reduction in the number of clients with hospitalisations, their total number of inpatient days, and associated costs).
- Psychiatric emergency room visits and inpatient days.
- Jail bookings and days (Initiative Watch, 2005, p. 4). We note that jails in the United States are the local county level of incarceration, for remand and short-term incarceration. As Australia does not have an equivalent level of prison, and as California has such a massively higher rate of imprisonment than most states in Australia (over 700 per 100,000 compared with ~140 per 100,000 population), it is not clear whether there would be a comparable measure in NSW.

In summary, the Californian initiative's project evaluation found that the initiative had a positive impact on the presentation rates and costs associated with mental health frequent user's utilisation of emergency services and the consumer's quality of life outcomes. The key successful factor here appears to be the coordinated and integrated care and support ensured by a case manager liaising with relevant services.

San Diego: Intensive Case Management of Mental Health Consumers

This 1995 study evaluated the effects of an intensive case management model for frequent mental health consumers of a San Diego County mental health system:

- Use of inpatient and outpatient psychiatric care
- Cost of care

In the study, 90 MHFP clients of hospital inpatient services were randomly assigned to an intensive case management group, a traditional case management group, or a control group that received no particular services.

Outcome variables measured over two years included the number of units used by clients, costs of inpatient care in county and private facilities, and various types of outpatient care, including day treatment and use of an emergency psychiatric unit. Clients who received intensive case management had fewer inpatient days and reduced overall costs for mental health services throughout the trial (Quinlivan, Hough, Beach, Hofsetter, & Kenworthy, 1995).

Similar to the Californian initiative results, this project's results confirm that robust outreach and intensive case management can reduce MHFP hospitalisations. Interestingly, the San Diego study also found that mental health consumers employed as case management aides can play an integral role in the delivery of mental health services (Quinlivan et al., 1995).

Notable Australian Jurisdiction Interagency Case Management Models

In the past five years in Australia there have been a number of relevant interagency initiatives, two of which specifically target MHFPs. We will discuss these in detail now.

The Commonwealth's Personal Helpers and Mentors Program (PHaMs) is an initiative of the Council of Australian Governments (COAG) *National Action Plan* (COAG, 2006). PHaMs is administered by the Commonwealth's Department of Families, Housing, Community Services and Indigenous Affairs (FaHCSIA). PHaMs aims to assist consumers who have a severe functional limitation from a mental illness to better manage their daily activities and to access a range of appropriate services/supports when they need them. PHaMs target people who fit the profile of a MHFP. PHaMs aims to address the holistic situation of the consumer and seeks to remedy his or her situation from a health, socioeconomic perspective through a brokered style intensive case management model. PHaMs commenced in May 2007 with 140 case management staff placed in 28 metropolitan, rural, remote, and regional demonstration sites across Australia (eight in NSW).

The Personal Helper and Mentors Program role has three key functions to help persons over the age of 16 with severe mental illness live independently in the community:

1. *Direct involvement*: Helpers assess a consumer's needs, develop an individual recovery plan, and link with clinical case management, advocacy, peer support, and personal development. Helpers support a client's relationships and assist with mediation and the client's ability to manage his or her daily activities.

2. *Referrals to relevant services*: Helpers refer clients to housing support, employment, education, rehabilitation, living skills programmes, clinical and health services, and so on.

3. *Monitoring and reporting*: Helpers monitor participant referrals, progress against individual recovery plans, and reporting (FaHCSIA, 2012).

Programme evaluations for Personal Helpers and Mentors (PHaMs), while not rigorous, have been positive, but not without criticism. Some have suggested that the programme is not implemented, resourced, or evaluated equitably. In 2008 a Commonwealth Senate Committee noted that there had been no independent evaluation of the PHaM and recommended that the Commonwealth's FaHCSIA Department develop and publish an evaluation framework for the PHaM. The committee asked that the framework pay particular attention to who is accessing the programme and to consumer outcomes. The committee further recommended that all evaluations of the programme be made public (Senate Standing Committee on Community Affairs, 2008). We have been unable to find rigorous independent evaluation of PHaMs since the Senate Committee's 2008 comments.

The Victorian government's Multiple and Complex Needs Initiative (MACNI) is also worthy of discussion, as it is a progressive ICM style model that could be applied specifically to MHFPs to police. MACNI is run by the Victorian state government's Department of Human Services (DHS). MACNI provides an ICM and brokered case management to its clients, with a wide range of interactions with clients.

MACNI offers an effective and coordinated approach to enable participants to achieve stability in health, housing, social connection, and safety, and then be mainstreamed back into regular services at the conclusion of the intervention (Victorian DHS, 2012a). A point of difference between MACNI and other programmes explored is that it is underpinned by legislation, the Human Services (Complex Needs) Act 2009 (Vic). This legislation ensures interagency accountability, collaboration, and service delivery on behalf of MACNI clients (Victorian DHS, 2012b). Under s. 7 of the act, an eligible person is defined as a person who:

[a] has attained 16 years of age; and
[b] appears to satisfy 2 or more of the following criteria:
   • has a mental disorder within the meaning of the Mental Health Act 1986;
   • has an acquired brain injury;
   • has an intellectual impairment;
   • is an alcoholic or drug-dependent person within the meaning of the Alcoholics and Drug-dependent Persons Act 1986; and

[c] has exhibited violent or dangerous behaviour that caused serious harm to himself or herself or some other person or is exhibiting behaviour which is reasonably likely to place himself or herself or some other person at risk of serious harm; and

[d] is in need of intensive supervision and support and would derive benefit from receiving co-ordinated services in accordance with a care plan under this Act.

Participation in MACNI is voluntary. It targets a very small cross section of persons who pose a high risk to themselves and the community. In this respect, the model is pertinent to MHFPs to police. MACNI is underpinned with a strong evidence base. It was successfully trialled, and the trial was generally positively evaluated by KPMG (Victorian DHS, 2012a).

However, a concern with MACNI is that it is resource-intensive and costly (in personnel and budget terms), services are time-capped at 3 years, and it manages only approximately 45 persons at any one time—tailored to clients at the extreme end of the risk continuum. Further, with specific relevance to MHFPs to police, recidivism among MACNI participants was not assessed as part of the KPMG evaluation. This is a sizeable evidence gap.

Two other interagency case management programmes of note in Australia that target vulnerable clients with complex needs, including mentally ill persons, are noted briefly below:

- In NSW: *Integrated Services Project (ISP) for Clients with Challenging Behaviours* run by Ageing, Disability and Home Care NSW. The ISP intensively case manages a small number of people with complex needs who present often to human and criminal justice services but who have not received helpful or appropriate support. It has been positively evaluated with a main finding being that the majority of clients participating in the programme "experienced improvements in a number of key outcome areas over the course of their involvement with the project" (McDermott, Bruce, Fisher, & Gleeson, 2010).
- In Victoria: *Victorian Police, Ambulance and Clinical Early Response (PACER) trial.* The PACER pilot operated in the southern region of Melbourne from 2007 until late 2011. PACER was a joint crisis response from police and mental health clinicians to people experiencing a behavioural disturbance in the community. In 2011, Allen Consulting Group was commissioned by the Department of Health to evaluate the effectiveness and efficiency of the PACER pilot in managing and resolving mental health crises in the community (Victorian Department of Health, 2012). Evaluation findings were positive (Allen Consulting Group, 2012). From a police

perspective, evaluation results were assessed as positive, including the timely redeployment of police vehicles to other callouts (Allen Consulting Group, 2012; Victorian Police, 2010). The Victorian Police and the Victorian Department of Health have publicly stated that post the evaluation, they will continue to work together to improve responses to people experiencing a crisis in the community (Victorian Department of Health, 2012). Today, it is unknown if the PACER trial will be implemented. Rather, PACER-associated efficiencies are sought via strengthening existing emergency services triage practises (Victorian Department of Health, 2012).

Analysis of discussed international and Australian programmes confirms the following themes among the case management models:

- There is a need for structural change in the way agencies and services are organised rather than the provision of small-scale "boutique" programmes or trials that target specific MHFP population groups or MHFPs in specific geographic areas. MHFPs are likely to receive mainstream crisis attention in an emergency but are not receiving early or ongoing holistic social and health support and services that would assist in preventing them becoming MHFPs or at least reduce their frequent presenting.
- Appropriate administrative support structures are needed for MHFPs. Examples of administrative supports needed include supportive legislation, regulation and interagency service agreements, memoranda of understanding, and operational policy protocols between and among agencies. Such administrative agreements will ensure a cooperative, permeable, and integrated service approach.
- Strong governance structures are needed to ensure good practise, accountability, and equity (e.g., advisory panels or oversight steering committees).
- Consumer consent for case management, and interagency information exchange, needs to be addressed with both the person's human rights and well-being and the services' capacities in mind.
- Independent and robust programme evaluation is often lacking. Without independent evaluation there is no opportunity to learn from the programme—its successes and mistakes—regarding what is cost-effective, what works, and what is ineffective. Rigorous programme evaluation should be integral to a programme being developed and implemented because without it, evidence-based policy improvement and future programme design is extremely difficult.

MHFP Case Management—Future Programme and Policy Considerations

The evidence supports the hypothesis that MHFPs to police have higher levels of multiple health and welfare needs and use multiple services and service resources at a disproportionately higher rate than those who do not present frequently. So it is important to consider, as well as structural changes, what interventions may lead to the best outcomes for the persons and agencies involved. Three of the programmes explored in the second section of this chapter, the frequent presenters of ED in the California initiative, the San Diego intensive case management of mental health consumers, and the Victorian MACNI, demonstrate the benefits of interagency MHFP case management. This section identifies some of the programme and policy considerations to enable successful case management for frequent presenters. However, the advantages of case management are not automatic. There are potential costs to both the MHFP and investing agencies. Gains can only be achieved through careful consideration of the context, that is, the programme and policy environment (Onyett, 1992, p. 22).

MHFP Programme Considerations

The challenge for case managers in supporting MHFPs is to design programmes that will respond adequately to their diverse and often complex medical, psychosocial, and social disadvantage needs. Common mental health case management principles, identified in these programme examples above, are informed by Onyett (1992) and Rapp and Wintersteen (1989, as cited in Onyett, 1992, pp. 93–102) and can be applied to persons who are MHFPs:

1. Focus on consumers' strengths rather than pathology.
   Case managers should focus on consumer's strengths and skills rather than inabilities (Onyett, 1992, p. 95).
2. A close and professional case manager-consumer relationship is essential.
   The most influential aspect of the case management process is the quality of the personal commitment that the case managers develop toward their clients (Intagliata, 1982, p. 660, cited in Onyett, 1992, p. 96).
3. Consumer consent to case management.
   Integral to the success of interagency case management is consumers' consent. Consent to case management ensures informed consumers' awareness and involvement, as well as potentially alleviating

interagency information exchange issues. Supporting MHFPs who do not consent to case management and continue to cycle in and out of the hospital, prison, and homelessness falls to emergency services as demonstrated above, so it is most beneficial to carefully explain and assist MHFPs to see the positive aspects for themselves in consenting to case management.

4. Interventions are based on the principle of user self-determination.
   Self-determination maximises the power of consumers and carers in decision making and taking control over their lives (Onyett, 1992, pp. 93–102).
5. Prioritising assertive outreach as a mode of early intervention.
   Evidence shows that early intervention works when it comes to managing persons with acute mental health problems (Onyett, 1992, p. 97).
6. People with severe mental health problems can learn and grow.
   There is considerable literature on the positive outcome of recovery-focussed interventions with people who have long-term and severe mental illness, even those who have been damaged through institutional care (Liberman et al., 2008; Tarrier, 1986, as cited in Onyett, 1992, p. 98).
7. Case management resources lie beyond traditional mental health services.
   Stakeholders and the wider community, local communities, nongovernment organisations, and families all play a role in this approach.

These principles are core to a case management design that will deliver positive outcomes for MHFPs and agencies alike. These principles aim to overcome some of the barriers that mental health frequent presenters face in their interactions with the health and justice system, and provide insights into how barriers to care might be preempted (Kushnal, 2003, p. 23).

MHFP Case Management: Policy Considerations

This section identifies policy considerations that may inform future MHFP policy design.

1. *Respecting the human rights of persons with disability.* Australia is a signatory to the United Nations Convention on Human Rights and the Convention on the Rights of Persons with Disabilities (NSW Consumer Advisory Group, 2011). These conventions require that persons be treated with equal respect irrespective of race, gender, age, and disability. An underlying drive in these conventions is to ensure that systemic changes are necessary to ensure that persons with disability are treated equitably.

2. *Government agreed definition of MHFP.* As discussed in the first
   section, the definition of *frequent user* varies. It is important to
   agree upon a shared interagency definition that reflects consumers
   with mental health disorders and the most complex needs who are
   repeatedly presenting to emergency services in mental health crisis.
   However, the definition has to be flexible enough to capture people
   who are otherwise excluded by siloing policy and programme criteria. Accordingly, a definition of MHFP must not rely solely on an
   individual's quantity of presentations, but should take into account
   the range of issues experienced by persons with mental health disorders or illness.
3. *Whole-of-government policy.* There is little whole-of-government
   policy on MHFP. The result is limited programmes that respond to
   the compounding and complex needs of MHFPs. Few programmes
   engage across agency boundaries and provide integrated service support. Due to the policy void there is little statewide accountability
   to encourage or require cross-agency cooperation and planning for
   this client group (Kelch Associates, 2003). MHFPs' needs must be
   integrated into government policy to ensure appropriate interagency
   management of MHFPs. Such policy needs to have clear, attainable
   objectives incorporated to ensure the agency's accountability.
4. *Fragmented care delivery.* Divisions between human and justice services, and even within individual human services, such as within
   health (for example, between medical health, mental health, and drug
   and alcohol services), limit the ability of agencies to address the needs
   of MHFPs in a coordinated manner (FUHSI, 2005, pp. 2–3). Despite
   the years of rhetoric regarding joined-up whole-of-government services, integration and coordination have not been achieved (Kelch
   Associates, 2003, p. 6). Given the multiple and complex needs of MH
   frequent presenters, meeting their needs effectively requires a range
   of simultaneous health, human, and justice service interventions.
5. *Adequate training and staffing levels.* Government agencies, researchers, and professionals have consistently documented a shortage of staff
   and appropriately trained mental health staff. Staff members often lack
   the training and ability to respond to the diversity and interagency
   needs of MHFPs. Snoyman's study of the NSW criminal justice system demonstrated the profound lack of knowledge about and understanding of MHFP, of the nature of mental disorders in combination
   with other disorders and impairments, among staff in police, courts,
   health, and corrective services (Snoyman, 2010). These factors are compounded by the reality that, in some rural and urban communities,
   there are facility and staffing shortages as well as the inability to serve
   specialised populations, including those with co-occurring disorders.

6. *Appropriate budget and flexible funding systems.* Funding levels need to enable programme longevity and continuity of case coordination. Furthermore, programmes need to have inbuilt flexible funding streams to enable case managers access to a range of services that may fall outside the scope of traditional health care (Kelch Associates, 2003, p. 8; FUHSI, 2005, pp. 2–3). An example of such a system is a brokered funding approach whereby funding for an individual can be used flexibly for a range of services suitable to the consumer's needs. Research indicates that individualised approaches to budgets bring additional benefits to disabled persons, "especially in terms of choice and control" (Siska & Beadle-Brown, 2011, p. 125; Andrews, 2012, p. 152). Decisions to implement individual budgets should be informed by consumer interest and capacity to consent.

7. *Good communication among service providers* is vital for a number of reasons. Poor communication and resistance to sharing information often result in consumers' needs not being adequately met, the duplication of service provision, or misuse of resources. The Australian Commonwealth states and territories lack information sharing between departments on the services provided, their interagency clients, and the results of the services delivered.

8. *Privacy and information exchange considerations.* One challenge common to agencies is an understanding of the parameters of privacy law and information sharing about MHFPs. This is an issue noted by a number of jurisdictions and stakeholders (Andrews, 2012, p. 153; Kelch Associates, 2003, p. 7). Despite the existence of documents such as the NSW Emergency Mental Health Memorandum of Understanding and policy directives that articulate privacy law and the parameters for interagency information exchange, lack of clarity and understanding persists. This often results in police and health officers' caution in exchanging information, and has an adverse impact on consumers' case management, as officers err on the side of not sharing information in order to avoid potential breaches of privacy law (Andrews, 2012, p. 153). Ultimately, this confusion results in a lack of policy and programme response to MHFPs. Clear direction from government is required to achieve whole-of-government policy and legislation regarding information exchange parameters involving MHFPs.

9. *Quality data and interagency data integration* (Kelch Associates, 2003). The lack of common data management approaches as well as poor or nonexistent integration of agencies' programmes and services' data complicates the process of sharing information and collection and analysis of meaningful data. The challenges experienced by Baldry et al. (2012) in their quantitative study of MHFPs attest to

the depth of this problem. Matters of capacity and quality of agency data are equally concerning (Andrews, 2012; FUHSI, 2005, pp. 2–3). Poor data gathering results from both a lack of optimal data sharing between programmes and agencies and the collection of incomplete or inadequate data (Kelch Associates, 2003, pp. 6–8).

The benefits for government of accruing quality data on MHFPs include:

- The potential to develop clear client profiles (clinical, forensic, psychosocial, etc.) of people with mental illness and disorder and other compounding disability and disadvantage in order to better tailor future programmes and policies
- The capacity for governments to use this information to develop evidence-based policies and case management programmes
- Improve resource allocation by federal and state/territory governments (based on evidence) to providers of services to MHFPs

10. *The possible role of Australian Medicare rebates.* There may be a role for Australian Medicare in funding MHFP case management. MHFP interagency case management could be aligned to Medicare mental health initiatives and be bulk billed. This could result in health system savings.

11. *Negative stereotypes.* Most MHFPs suffer from multiple challenges, including chronic health problems, homelessness, justice system involvement, mental illness or substance abuse, and behavioural issues, any of which might subject them to social stereotyping and isolation. Such stereotypes can result in policy and programme makers putting MHFP into the "too hard basket" due to their complex service delivery needs. Educational challenges exist in both the policy and the public arena to increase understanding, and in turn support for improved care and services for MHFP.

Conclusion

Research demonstrates that MHFPs represent a relatively small number of people whose use of emergency services, including police, is disproportionately high, and their crisis-led use of services results in poor outcomes. MHFPs to police utilisation patterns are due to compounding factors, including disability, low socioeconomic status, drug and alcohol dependency, and criminal behaviour (as both victim and perpetrator).

Programme evaluations from the United States and some Australian programmes demonstrate that case management for MHFPs can have a positive effect for service providers and the consumer. These include a reduction in the number of presentations to emergency services as a result of the stabilisation of their condition and circumstances. To achieve positive outcomes, interagency case management strategies must be flexible, individualised, and comprehensive in addressing the often complex health conditions and related socioeconomic needs of each consumer.

In the Australian context, it is essential that MHFP services be integrated into whole-of-government policy. Currently, there is a MHFP policy void, despite the highly disproportionate resources they consume. There is an urgent need for applied MHFP research leading to policy responses and strategic programmes for MHFPs. Quantitative research such as Baldry et al.'s (2012) and Andrews (2012) research into MHFPs to the NSW Police Force and available international research provide profiles of and information on the population characteristics and problems at hand for MHFPs to emergency services. But there are yawning knowledge gaps in Australia about what specific populations of MHFPs (e.g., aboriginal MHFPs) require, what are acceptable and appropriate support and services, and most importantly, how to prevent persons becoming MHFPs in the first place, as well as avert them continuing as frequent presenters. Such research is needed to develop informed policies and tailored MHFP case management programme responses.

References

Allen Consulting Group. (2012). *Police ambulance and clinical early response: Final evaluation.* Report to the Department of Health, Victoria. Retrieved September 22, 2012, from http://docs.health.vic.gov.au/docs/doc/57EE551A9F8F3263CA 257A0600065B14/$FILE/PACER_Eval_18April2012_FinalFinal.pdf

Andrews, G. (2012). Mental health frequent presenters to police: Who are they and what can we do? University of Sydney Master's of Administration Law and Policy thesis 2011, NSW Police Force website: www.police.nsw.gov.au/ communityissues/mental health

Australian Government Department of Families, Housing, Community Services and Indigenous Affairs. (2012). Personal helpers and mentors. Retrieved September 17, 2012, from http://www.fahcsia.gov.au/our-responsibilities/communities-and-vulnerable-people/programs-services/personal-helpers-and-mentors

Baldry, E., Dowse, L., & Clarence, M. 2012. Mental health frequent presenters to NSW Police Force in 2005: Police data. Retrieved September 17, 2012, from http:// www.police.nsw.gov.au/__data/assets/pdf_file/0019/238222/Mental_Health_ Frequent_Presenters_to_NSW_Police_Force_.pdf

Bernstein, S.L. (2006). Frequent emergency department visitors: The end of inappropriateness. *Annals of Emergency Medicine, 48*(1), 18.

Chaput, Y.J.A., & Lebel, M.J. (2007). Demographic and clinical profiles of patients who make multiple visits to psychiatric emergency services. *Psychiatric Services, 58*(3), 335.

Council of Australian Governments (COAG). (2006). *National Action Plan on Mental Health 2006–2011.* Commonwealth Government.

Fisher, S., & Stevens, R. (1999). Subgroups of frequent users of an inpatient and mental health program at a community hospital in Canada. *Psychiatric Services*, 50(2), 244–247.

Frequent Users of Health Services Initiative (FUHSI). (2005). Policy brief: Frequent users of health services: Barriers to care.

Fuda, K.K., & Immekus, R. (2005). A statewide study of frequent users of emergency departments of Massachusetts. Paper presented at the Academic Health Annual Meeting, Boston, MA.

Fuda, K.K., & Immekus, R. (2006). Frequent users of Massachusetts emergency departments: A statewide analysis. *Annals of Emergency Medicine*, 48(1), 16.e1.

Hickie, I. (2008). *A new model for delivering selected mental health services in Australia.* Brain and Mind Institute University of Sydney.

Hudson, Beaver, Interview with, Deputy Director Mental Health Services, St. Vincent's Hospital NSW. (2007, May 29).

Human Services (Complex Needs) Act 2009 (Vic).

Hunt, K., et al. (2006). Characteristics of frequent users of emergency departments. *Annals of Emergency Medicine*, 48(1), 1.

Initiative Watch. (2005). Frequent service users of health services initiative 1. Summer.

Kelch Associates. (2003). Policy scan: Legislation environment: Final working draft (p. 6). Frequent Service Users of Health Services Initiative.

Kushnal, M. (2003). Policy scan: Care provision challenges: Final working draft. University of California.

Liberman, R., Drake, R.E., Sederer, L.I., Belger, A., Keefe, R., Perkins, D., & Stroup, S. (2008, May 1). Science and recovery in schizophrenia. *Psychiatric Services*, 59(5). Retrieved September 22, 2012, from http://ps.psychiatryonline.org/article.aspx?articleID=99354

Lincoln, A., & White, A. (2006). A re-examination of frequent users of psychiatric emergency room services. Paper presented at Annual Meeting of the American Sociological Association 2006. Retrieved September 22, 2012, from http://citation.allacademic.com//meta/p_mla_apa_research_citation/1/0/4/3/6/pages104360/p104360-2.php

McDermott, S., Bruce, J., Fisher, K.R., & Gleeson, R. (2010). *Evaluation of the Integrated Services Project for Clients With Challenging Behaviour (PDF)* (SPRC Report 5/10). Prepared for Ageing, Disability and Home Care, Department of Human Services NSW, University of NSW.

Mehl-Madrona, L. (1998). Frequent users of rural primary care: Comparisons with randomly selected users. *Journal of American Board of Family Practice*, 11(2), 105.

Mental Health Act 2007 (NSW).

Mueser, K., Bond, G., Drake, R., & Resnik, S. (1998). Models of community care for severe mental illness: A review of research on case management. *Schizophrenia Bulletin*, 24(1), 37.

NSW Consumer Advisory Group. (2011). Human rights. Retrieved September 2011 from http://www.nswcag.org.au/page/human_rights.html

NSW Police Force. (2009). NSW Police Force crime recording standards (Unpublished).

Onyett, S. (1992). *Case management in mental health* (1st ed.). New York: Chapman & Hall.

Phillips, S., et al. (2001). Moving assertive community treatment into standard practice. *Psychiatric Services, 52*(6), 771.

Quinlivan, R., Hough, A., Beach, C., Hofsetter, R., & Kenworthy, K. (1995). Mental health case management services. *Psychiatric Services, 46*, 365–371.

Senate Standing Committee on Community Affairs. (2008). Towards recovery: Mental health services in Australia. Commonwealth of Australia. Retrieved September 20, 2012, from http://www.aph.gov.au/senate/committee/clac_ctte/mental_health/report/c05.htm

Siska, J., & Beadle-Brown, J. (2011). Developments in deinstitutionalisation and community living in the Czech Republic. *Journal of Policy and Practice in Intellectual Disabilities, 8*(2), 125.

Snoyman, P. (2010). Staff in the criminal justice system's understanding of people with and without disability who offend. Doctorate of philosophy, University of NSW. Retrieved September 21, 2012, from http://primoa.library.unsw.edu.au/primo_library/libweb/tiles/lrs/unsworks/datastream.jsp?pid=UNSWorks8332

Victorian Department of Health. (2012). *Police, ambulance and clinical early response evaluation report.* Retrieved September 22, 2012, from http://docs.health.vic.gov.au/docs/doc/Police-Ambulance-and-Clinical-Early-Response-(PACER)-Evaluation-Report

Victorian Department of Human Services. (2005). Mental health presentations to the emergency department.

Victorian Department of Human Services. (2012a). Multiple and Complex Needs Initiative. Retrieved September 15, 2012, from http://www.dhs.vic.gov.au/about-the-department/plans,-programs-and-projects/projects-and-initiatives/cross-departmental-projects-and-initiatives/multiple-and-complex-needs-initiative

Victorian Department of Human Services. (2012b). *MACNI development—KPMG evaluation reports.* Retrieved September 15, 2012, from http://www.dhs.vic.gov.au/about-the-department/documents-and-resources/reports-publications/macni-development-kpmg-evaluation-reports

Victorian Police. (2010). Annual report. Retrieved September 20, 2011, from http://www.vicpolannualreport.net.au/default.aspx?iid=40339&startpage=page0000043

Compounding Mental and Cognitive Disability and Disadvantage

Police as Care Managers

11

EILEEN BALDRY
LEANNE DOWSE

Contents

Introduction

The presence of highly disadvantaged people with multiple mental and cognitive impairments and problematic alcohol and drug (AOD) use in criminal justice systems is not a new phenomenon. But international and national evidence points to increasing widespread overrepresentation of these individuals in police work, the courts, and juvenile and adult prisoner populations, as both victims and offenders. The rate of contact with police of people with what recently has been termed complex needs (Carney, 2006; Draine et al., 2002) has increased over the past two decades (Hayes, Shackell, Mottram, & Lancaster, 2007). We discuss the term *complex needs* further below, but here we note the specific vulnerability of individuals in this group to a range of harms, involvement in the criminal justice system, and social disadvantages. They are more likely than people with only one impairment or none to have earlier contact with police, be victims as well as offenders, be a client of juvenile justice, have more police contacts, have more police and prison custody episodes (Baldry, Dowse, & Clarence, 2012; Dowse, Baldry, & Snoyman,

2009; New South Wales Law Reform Commission (NSWLRC), 2012, p. 63), and be refused bail and imprisoned (Lyall, Holland, & Styles, 1995).

Other chapters in this book examine closely the work of police with people with mental impairment and the various approaches to and outcomes of those interactions. This chapter adds to these discussions the experiences of and interactions with those with cognitive as well as mental impairment, along with AOD and social disadvantages. The majority of people with cognitive impairment enmeshed in the criminal justice system also have a mental impairment or problematic AOD use (Baldry, 2010; Baldry et al., 2012, p. 5; NSWLRC, 2012, p. 65). We draw on a linked and merged dataset of 2,731 people whose diagnoses are known, and who have been in prison in New South Wales (NSW), to explore police interactions with those with complex needs. These diagnoses were determined for this group of prisoners in NSW by Justice Health and staff of the Statewide Disability Service in Corrections NSW, using the Composite International Diagnostic Interview (CIDI), which yields both DSM-IV and ICD-10 diagnoses, and by the administration of the *Wechsler Adult Intelligence Scale* (WAIS). Mental impairment among this cohort refers to psychosis, anxiety disorder, affective disorder, personality disorder, or neurasthenia (Butler & Allnut, 2003). People with cognitive impairment include individuals with intellectual disability (ID) (IQ < 70), borderline intellectual disability (BID) (IQ > 70 and < 80), and acquired brain injury (ABI) who, as well as possibly experiencing physical, sensory, psychological, and communication difficulties, also experience disability related to cognitive function (as defined in the NSW Corrective Services Statewide Disability Dataset).

More research has been done and there is more information on police work with people with mental impairment than with individuals with cognitive impairment. There is even less known about police work with people with multiple impairments. Police carry the major burden of attending to psychiatrically disturbed people behaving in an antisocial or offending manner, and they must make the determination whether to take such persons to a psychiatric unit, arrest them, or do nothing (Fry et al., 2002; Lamb, Weinberger, & Gross, 2004). Police often find such individuals may not be accepted into the mental health system due to lack of space, the person being deemed not ill enough, or able to be handled by the criminal justice system, or importantly for our discussion, that they have other diagnoses that preclude them from admission to a psychiatric service (New South Wales Legislative Council Select Committee on Mental Health, 2002: NSWLRC, 2012; Lamb, Wenberger, & DeCuir Jr., 2002). Differentiating the manifestations of mental health or psychiatric disabilities from those associated with cognitive impairment is a challenge for many practitioners outside specialist medical or disability fields. Police training tends to be largely focussed on the recognition of mental or psychiatric disabilities and generally does not extend to the development of capacity to discern that a person has a cognitive impairment, never mind both a mental and a cognitive impairment. It is difficult enough for the untrained to identify any one of these impairments, while the combined effects of the presence of more than one can be easily misinterpreted and misunderstood. As we reveal, many police, informed by their experience of frontline work, *suspect* that a person may have a number of problems, but their capacity to recognise, ascertain, and respond to people with impairments is limited by the absence, within policing practise, of a coherent framework for dealing with this group and by lack of information or assistance from support services.

Some recent studies have examined police encounters with people with intellectual disability (Henshaw & Thomas, 2012), perceptions of police identification of and responses to such people (Spivak & Thomas, 2012), and issues of police discretion as it applies to encounters with people experiencing mental illness (Godfredson, Ogloff, Thomas, & Luebbers, 2010). Henshaw and Thomas (2012) investigated the experiences and perceptions of operational members of Victoria Police in relation to their contacts with people with intellectual disability, finding that police surveyed believed that they come into contact with people with intellectual disability on a regular basis. In the absence of agreed approaches to recognising intellectual disability and differentiating ID from mental illness, participants identified the most common challenges in their policing work with this group as communication, and gaining access to assistance and cooperation from other service providers (Henshaw & Thomas, 2012, p. 620). Beyond the perceptions of frontline police, Spivak and Thomas (2012) found that independent third-person volunteers generally regarded police as competent at identifying those with cognitive deficits and seeking appropriate supports for the person with ID in the interview context. Research exploring police discretion in dealing with people experiencing mental illness, however, indicated that there was a range of intervening factors, which could impact negatively on police efficacy in dealing with such encounters, primarily the severity of symptoms presented and the officers' attitudes to people experiencing mental illness (Godfredson et al., 2010, p. 1392). Taken together, these findings suggest that while awareness of issues in and responses to cognitive impairment and mental illness in frontline policing may be growing in some jurisdictions, there is a lack of coordinated and evidence-based frameworks for addressing police responses to those who experience issues related to these impairments simultaneously and as part of an interlocking multiplicity of need.

Although there is evidence that police events attending to people with mental impairment in NSW represent a very small proportion of all police events, at 1.75% in 2009 (Herrington, 2009, p. 15), an earlier survey of 131 police officers in Sydney found the reported police *time* spent dealing with mentally disturbed people was an average of 10%, with responses ranging from 0% to

60% (NSWLRC, 2012). So although mental health-related events make up only a small proportion of events dealt with by police, the time dealing with them is disproportionate to their representation in number of events. There is no similar data on events with people with cognitive impairment or those with complex needs. Analysis of our data suggests that although people with complex needs represent a small proportion of people in the general population, they attract a significantly disproportionate large amount of police time and attention. Before moving to this evidence, we try to tease out the concept of complex needs.

Complex Needs

The challenge of adequately recognising and appropriately responding to individuals experiencing multiple and simultaneous mental, cognitive, and substance abuse problems is significant. The lack of agreed terminology in the field is evidence of underdeveloped conceptual and practise frameworks, which struggle to move beyond limited categorisations such as dual diagnosis or co-morbidity. These terms remain firmly rooted in a medicalised approach to characterising and understanding complex problems that are most commonly presented as a substance misuse problem coexisting with a serious mental health problem or a mental health problem coexisting with intellectual disability (Rankin & Regan, 2004, p. 9). These categorisations are limited in that they assume that an individual is defined by the presence of a primary medical diagnosis, that only two disorders or impairments can exist simultaneously, and that these attributes are in some way static within each individual and do not interact. More significantly, the underpinning assumption is that the presence of a particular characteristic, impairment, or dysfunction, or combinations of these, is attributed primarily to the individual. The individual is more often than not understood and portrayed as someone who should be able to control or manage or organise treatment for his or her "problem." Their problems are individualised (he or she is the person with complex needs), and any social and structural factors that have created and maintained the need or dysfunction are written out of an understanding of the person's immediate situation and out of a criminal justice response.

The term *complex needs*, although problematic and contested as an explanatory term that potentially ignores the systemic and institutional aspects of this phenomenon, as noted in the previous paragraph, does at least try to capture the simultaneousness of the experience of these many factors and aspects. For example, a person with a cognitive impairment experiences an anxiety attack or chronic depression at the same time as being homeless, stealing to buy alcohol, and being a victim of physical bullying, an intimidation to which they acquiesce as a result of their cognitive impairment. These experiences are multifaceted and compounding, are complex because they are difficult and convoluted, and form a complex in the sense of a web or set of circumstances that grows as it is fed by more abuse, teasing, anxiety, and disadvantage. As an overarching concept, the term *complex needs* at least provides a framework for understanding *multiple interlocking* (to which we would add compounding) experiences and factors that span health and social issues (Rankin & Regan, 2004, p. i).

Two conceptualisations of complex needs are broadly evident in the existing literature addressing this phenomenon, one that describes the population of individuals who could be thought of as complex and the other that looks at the composition and conglomeration of the needs of individuals in this group. Broadly, those with complex needs are seen as people who require fairly high levels of health, welfare, and other community-based services and include individuals who experience various combinations of mental illness, intellectual disability, acquired brain injury, physical disability, behavioural difficulties, homelessness, social isolation, family dysfunction, and have problematic drug or alcohol use (Hamilton, 2010). Those with complex needs are also frequently defined in the context of their relationship or otherwise to service systems. These systems, such as the child protection, health, housing, and criminal justice systems, struggle to work with and support effectively such individuals. The supports they need are usually based in services focussed on efficient, specialist service delivery, an approach inimical to messy, broad-based, multilayered support. In short, contemporary evolution of the service sector appears not to have responded well to those with multiple needs and disadvantages (Hamilton, 2010).

An important element in working with and supporting a person with complex needs is the recognition that it is not simply a matter of compiling a checklist of needs. It may be helpful to think of a three-dimensional web of factors, elements, and circumstances that interact simultaneously and across time. The interactions have a compounding effect (like interest on money in a bank account) in that the effect is not just the sum of the individual parts, but each aspect adds to and increases the potency of each of the other effects. The result of these interlocking and compounding elements is that the total is more than the sum of its parts (Rankin & Regan, 2004). There is both a breadth and depth of needs as each increases the other. For example, it is very likely that a person from a cultural and linguistically diverse (CALD) or indigenous background who has experienced severe trauma as a young person, is living in out-of-home care or precarious housing, and has cognitive impairment will experience these factors in a heightened negative manner and develop further impairment out of his or her interactions if there is no holistic intervention. We discuss examples of such compounding interactions in the case studies below.

Conceptualisations of risk and vulnerability and the interactions between them are key to understanding the notion of complex needs where the presence of one need tends to heighten or increase the risk of experiencing another need—this in turn heightens the vulnerability to experiencing further needs. Perversely assessing these factors and interactions as risks has taken a negative turn among service providers and the criminal justice system in that high needs has been transformed into high risk (needs and risk have been conflated; see Hannah-Moffat (2010) for this discussion), and high risk into dangerous, and dangerous into needing to be dealt with by the criminal justice system (in which the police force is the front line). Taken together we have developed these elements into a framework, captured in Figure 11.1, which attends to the dynamic interaction of individual, social, and systemic experience, highlighting the breadth, depth, and interconnectedness of the experience of complex need. Most critically, it repositions an atomised notion of additive individual dysfunction or disability toward a dynamic, interactive, and multidimensional concept, which is created and sustained by social arrangements and systems.

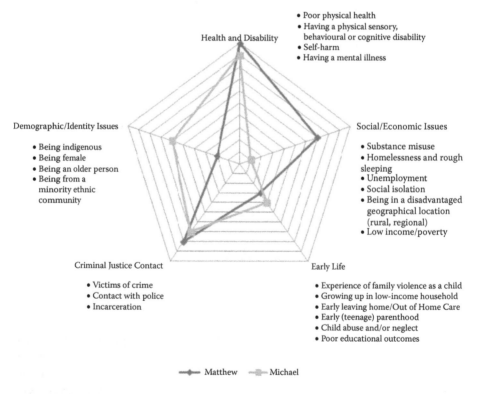

Figure 11.1 The complex needs a web, here capturing the breadth, depth, and interlocking nature of disadvantageous factors that coalesce to create complex needs. The dimensional complexity of the interactions created by the compounding of the factors is illustrated by mapping the case studies of Matthew and Michael.

Despite the problems with the term *complex needs*, we use it in this chapter as a term now in common use to describe a group of people (as discussed above) who experience the compounding effects of these many disadvantages and impairments.

Involvement in the Criminal Justice System

To explore the dimensions and elements of and interactions between people with complex needs and the police force, institutional life course events and interactions of a cohort of people who have been in prison, and whose impairment and other diagnoses and social disadvantages are known, were analysed. A large number ($N = 2,731$) of individual life course pathways into various forms of institutional control, including into prison, have been derived from linked and merged datasets from all the criminal justice and some human service agencies in New South Wales, Australia.* The cohort was derived from the NSW Inmate Health Survey 2001 (Butler & Milner, 2003) and updated with the 2009 survey (Indig et al., 2011) and from the NSW Corrective Services Statewide Disability Dataset. Both datasets were provided after ethics clearance to the project team to create the group of 2,731 people and their identification details. The project obtained ethics clearance from all the appropriate ethics bodies, including from Justice Health and the University of New South Wales (UNSW) ethics committee, and was able then to draw data and identifiers on the 2,731 people across the two datasets, merge them and link data of each of the individuals from other agencies, and merge them and then de-identify all the data. A Structured Query Language (SQL) server was used to manage and store the data. Data on the life involvement with each agency, of all the individuals, were obtained from NSW agencies: police, health, corrective services, juvenile justice, legal aid, the courts, social housing, disability services, and child services. The data were divided into those with more than one impairment or disorder (and these were further divided according to the main diagnoses, for example, those with mental and intellectual impairment, with borderline intellectual impairment and alcohol or other drug disorder, and so on), those with only one, and those with none, so that comparisons could be made between the complex needs groups and those without complex needs. The analyses of human service and

* ARC linkage grant at UNSW: People With Mental Health Disorders and Cognitive Disability in Then Criminal Justice System. Chief Investigators (CIs): Baldry, Dowse, and Webster; Partner Investigators (PIs): Simpson, Butler, and Eyland. Partner organisations: Justice Health NSW; Corrective Services NSW; NSW Police; Department of Housing NSW; NSW Department of Juvenile Justice; and NSW Council for Intellectual Disability. See http://www.mhdcd.unsw.edu.au/.

criminal justice life course histories highlight points of agency interactions, diversion, and support, and identify gaps in policy, protocols, and service delivery and areas of potential improvement for criminal justice and human service agencies. In particular, of relevance to this chapter, analyses of these histories reveal the high level and types of police interactions with people with complex needs.

We use mixed methods to explore these aspects, with aggregated data analysed via a number of key factors, as well as using case studies to flesh out and provide examples of the quantitative findings. As seen in Figure 11.1, we have created from both the literature and our data exploration a web of factors, elements, and dimensions that interact to create the complex needs just discussed and that appear to work in synergistically negative manners in an individual's life unless appropriate social intervention and support are provided.

We now focus on points and aspects of these contacts drawn from the data and case studies to develop our discussion regarding police interaction with people with complex needs. Most, but not all, of the case studies are of Indigenous Australians from regional or rural towns reflecting the study findings of the higher likelihood of Indigenous Australians having higher rates of mental and cognitive impairment, having complex needs, and being enmeshed in the criminal justice system. Some may have faetal alcohol spectrum syndrome disorder (FASSD), but this is rarely diagnosed once a person is past childhood, and as almost all those in the cohort with cognitive impairment were not diagnosed until reaching adult prison, this is difficult to determine.

Police First Contact

The first recorded contact with police for people with mental and cognitive impairment is a key event: The earlier the first recorded event, the more contact over life is likely. The first police event may be in response to the person committing an offence, being the victim of a crime, or being a child at risk. The average age at first police contact for people who have any form of cognitive impairment plus another disorder, that is, those with complex needs, in the cohort is significantly lower than for those with a single or no diagnosis. The average age for first recorded police contact for the cognitive complex groups is 15.5 years, whereas it is 20 years for those with no diagnosis and 21 for those with a mental disorder only (as mental disorder when not accompanied by other impairment or disorder often emerges after the mid to late teens).

Indigenous children and young people experience first police contact at a significantly lower age than the rest of the cohort, and there is much less difference across the different diagnostic groups for first police contact for Indigenous young people than non-Indigenous youth; in other words, indigenous young people, whether they have an impairment or not, are far more likely to have earlier police contact than any non-Indigenous young people, with the average age being between 14 and 15 years. Nevertheless, those groups of people with cognitive impairment and complex needs again have the lowest average ages at first police contact, of under 15 years.

Matthew's case illustrates this early contact.

Matthew, now in his early twenties, was diagnosed with "behaviour defiance syndrome" as a child and has been diagnosed subsequently with a borderline intellectual disability with an overall IQ of 70 and substance use disorder. He attended school on and off until year 8, but his school attendance was very poor and he effectively ceased to engage with school around the fourth class. Both Matthew's parents came from highly disadvantaged backgrounds and used alcohol to excess. He was surrounded from birth with drugs and alcohol. A number of times before the age of 12 police noted that Matthew was with one or the other of his parents, who were intoxicated, at a pub. Matthew lived between the streets and various relatives from very early in his life and had "no fixed address," a fact noted often by police and community services. At age 7 Matthew had his first police event and was also known to them for being a child at risk, with police recording sadistic and threatening behaviour. As he was under the age of 10, no formal action was taken. He started to go in and out of state care, eventually coming under permanent out-of-home care (OOHC). But all his foster care arrangements broke down quickly due to his behaviour. Between the ages of 7 and 11 Matthew had over 70 contacts with police as a person of interest (POI), often for minor thefts of money and retail items (usually food), and some for more serious matters. Matthew went on to have hundreds of contacts with police for both offending and being a child at risk, and many juvenile justice orders before the age of 18, and then hundreds more police events and many adult custody episodes to date, as an adult. He has not lived in an ordinary community space as a small child, youth, or adult but has been in marginal community/criminal justice spaces controlled by the criminal justice system, with police his frontline "carers." He did not receive disability support as a child or adult. All but the police washed their hands of him by the time he was 14, by which time he had become entrenched in this criminal justice management system.

Matthew may sound like an extreme case, but he is not, as there are many with complex needs in the study cohort who experience their first police event before the age of 10 and whose contact with the police persists as they get older. Eventually, police were left to manage the whole range of Matthew's childhood needs from his neglect, use of alcohol, homelessness, and poor school attendance, to his cognitive and mental impairments. Police case notes indicate they often contacted other services that may or may not have responded, but if they did, they did not take a holistic or long-term approach to his multiple needs.

First Police and Juvenile Justice Contact

Earlier average first police contact is not associated with earlier first juvenile justice involvement for the complex diagnosis group. All groups, except the mental disorder-only group (that was significantly older), had an average of 15 to 16 years at their first juvenile custody. There were significantly more police contacts prior to first juvenile custody for the complex needs groups, that is, those with mental disorder and intellectual disability and those with cognitive impairment and problematic AOD use, at an average of 15, compared with 10 for those with no diagnosis. Although there are some like Matthew who go on to juvenile justice orders and into custody very early, the evidence just presented suggests police and perhaps community advocacy groups worked to keep these groups out of custody for as long as possible. These attempts, though, did not result in these young people being diverted to disability or health services that should have provided the kind of care and support they needed as children. Rather, it appears that police spent more time managing and trying to get other service support and had more events with this group of young people before they moved into juvenile justice. Eddie's case (like Matthew's) shows the almost inevitable move into juvenile justice for young people with complex needs who are not supported by appropriate services and who are in frequent contact with the police for difficult and offending behaviour.

Eddie's first recorded contact with police for a property offence was when he was 11. Eddie has an intellectual disability, and a long history of problematic drug use beginning at the age of 6, including use of prescription drugs, amphetamines, alcohol, cannabis, heroin, methadone, and buprenorphine. Much of his contact with police is in relation to his drug use and property offences that escalated, as he got older, into violence. He regularly attempted self-harm from a young age. He did not attend school past the age of 12. By age 9, Eddie was experiencing frequent short periods in OOHC.

After his first police charge Eddie came to the attention of police, often with records noting he was uncontrollable and attention seeking and was living on the street. He was placed on a juvenile control order on bail at age 12, on the condition that he only left his mother's home address in the company of his mother or a responsible adult. But he constantly breached bail conditions, as he did not understand them and had no responsible adult to go out with him in any case. He began a series of juvenile detention episodes from age 13.

When he was out of juvenile detention he would attend the emergency department of the local hospital seeking assistance. Hospital staff often requested a police escort due to his history of violence and aggression and his threats to kill himself and family members, and he was often restrained and sedated. Eddie has been variously diagnosed with or noted as having adjustment disorders, disorders of adult personality and behaviour, a conduct disorder, somatoform disorder, mental and behavioural disorders due to use of cannabinoids, alcohol, and volatile solvents, acute and transient psychotic disorder, schizotypal disorder, and unsocialised and conduct disorder, with notes of his "loss of love relationship in childhood and other negative life events in childhood." Despite all these diagnoses, police notes state he was assessed as "being not mentally disturbed" when a teenager.

In Eddie's case the police tried numerous times to have him assessed as mentally disordered or at least in need of long-term care, but no social or human service intervention seemed able or willing to grapple with Eddie's complex needs, and he was left to the police and then juvenile justice to manage.

Police Custody

The complex needs groups have much higher rates of police custody episodes than the no-diagnosis and single-diagnosis groups in the cohort. There are frequent references in police notes to not having anywhere to take someone whom they recognize as vulnerable due to an impairment, and of keeping him or her in custody as a result. Concern for the public and the individual's safety appear to drive this. There are references by police to people they recognize as having "something wrong," a "mental illness," as "very unwell," as being homeless, or a child at risk being turned away from psychiatric units, hospitals, youth refuges, and child protection services because the person is not unwell enough, is known to the service and considered too high risk to take in as a client, or there is no service suitable for the multitude of problems faced by the person. Sometimes the police noted that it was Friday afternoon or the weekend and services said they could do nothing until Monday morning. Police notes often contain indications of the officers' sense of despair at the position they find themselves in, recognising that they are the only ones who cannot turn the person away. Casey is a young woman who has been managed by the police since she was 12 and has been held in police custody many times, as there was no where else to take her.

Casey, now 22, was diagnosed with a range of mental and cognitive conditions, including behavioural and emotional conditions emerging in childhood and adolescence: ADHD, conduct disorders, adjustment disorders, and personality disorder. These diagnoses were maintained as she entered adulthood with an additional diagnosis of bipolar affective disorder. Casey also has intellectual disability. She had a long history of self-harm, physical abuse, and trauma as a young person. She started problematic AOD use as a child and had very poor school attendance, ceasing any attendance at 13. Police began to note that Casey, aged 12, was walking the streets at night, threatening suicide, and was "highly agitated and suffering from a mental illness."

Police events with Casey were prolific. For example, when she was 13, she was the subject of 87 events, with almost half of those resulting in her being taken into police custody (35 times) overnight and charged on 56 different counts.

Police noted that on numerous occasions services failed to support Casey, with workers from a local mental health service no longer agreeing to have Casey released from police into their custody, and community services informing the police "they have nowhere to place the child" and refusing "to have her in their custody." No family member was able to have her, and "there is no other option available to police than to house the child." Sometimes she was scheduled under the Mental Health Act, but she was always released very quickly or not accepted at all at the hospital. Police noted their concern that "this child is in need of medical and mental treatment. She has been bounced around between police and the hospital at least three times in the past two weeks." They made multiple reports to community services as they held fears "that the young person may be physically, emotionally, or psychologically abused." She was homeless. Casey's bail conditions continued to require that she "reside in her family home and not be absent between the hours of 6 p.m. and 6 a.m.," creating a situation in which she breached her bail conditions and was again picked up by the police in an ongoing cycle of police acting as her manager.

Many of the people in the cohort had been held in police custody for one or two nights as both children and adults; this applied to Indigenous people in particular. This practise was not favoured by police in many instances, as evidenced in their notes about Casey, but they had become the carers and protectors of people like Casey. This use of police time and custody could be understood as a perverse outcome for both police and the person with an impairment.

Police Contact Over Time

For the complex needs groups with any form of cognitive impairment, first police contact for 80% of the group had been before age 20. This initiated continued police contact at a rate of over an average of four per year, over their lifetime. This early and continuing police contact was associated with higher ongoing rates of juvenile and adult prison custody than for those with no diagnosis or with a single diagnosis only. Ned's history is one of lifelong frequent interactions with police.

Ned, now 40, has an IQ of 65 and a history of mental illness, including diagnoses of personality and behaviour disorders, schizophrenia, and mental illness related to psychoactive substance use. He had a very disrupted childhood and did not receive any support at school for his disability. Ned stopped attending school when he was 13. At the same time, he was arrested by the police for the first time. Subsequently, he was arrested and charged many times before the age of 18, but there is no record that his cognitive impairment or mental disorders were recognised or addressed. As an adult, his offending behaviour has included domestic violence, property damage, and stealing, and he has gone in and out of police custody and prison numerous times. Police have often noted Ned's desperate state as a result of his addictions, his homelessness, his depression, and his frequent attempts at suicide. The police are his care managers, often picking him up and taking him to the hospital after a suicide attempt or when severely affected by amphetamines. He has been on a methadone programme a number of times with no ongoing success, and has often been in breach of various Apprehended Violence Orders (AVOs). Ned of course has very poor comprehension of the requirements of these sorts of orders due to his intellectual disability and little capacity to respond to programmes due to his various impairments.

Nowhere does it appear that his cognitive impairment was recognised by police, school education, or juvenile justice. Ned's life course exemplifies the management role police play in controlling someone with multiple diagnoses who, from birth, is deeply affected by dispossession, disadvantage, and trauma. In fact, he is so completely enmeshed in police control that he is often stopped and searched without there being good reason for suspicion other than he is known well to the police. A strong disability response to Ned earlier in life may have channelled him into a community support service rather than into police management.

It appears that once police effectively begin managing people with complex needs, usually at a fairly young age, the police (and subsequently juvenile justice and corrections) manage them by attending to crises, ferrying them from children's services, mental and other health services, disability services, and homeless shelters, as well as not infrequently keeping them in police custody for short spells. They become well known to the police, and this way of managing people with impairment is normalised for all parties. Human and social services leave this group of people's care and management to the police.

Discussion and Conclusion

It is apparent from both the aggregate data analysis and the case studies that the NSW Police Force is the frontline manager of people who have mental and cognitive impairment, who have had long histories of disadvantage and trauma, are seen as having challenging and risky behaviour, and at times as being dangerous. Despite often having been victims of abuse and other criminal acts as children and young people and having impairments and disorders, their primary identity develops quickly as *offender*. They move from being *at risk* as a child to being *a risk* as an older teenager and adult without the benefit of appropriate, integrated, supportive disability and other social services. Matthew, for example, began life without any of the usual care or support afforded to children in twenty-first-century Australia. He was neglected, did not go to school regularly, was not identified as having a disability, and so received no disability support—he was left to fend for himself on the streets. Although police realised he was a child at risk, they were unable to engage wraparound disability service supports and acted as emergency triage staff for him. His behaviour, unsurprisingly, became more aggressive as he became older, and he became a risk to others. The same pattern, with minor variation, is evident in each of the case studies.

The themes in regard to the experiences, support, and management of people with complex needs emerging from the findings are that this group, in comparison to those without complex needs, has had:

- Significantly earlier contact with police
- Higher rates of contact with police continuing through life
- Escalating and damaging contact with the criminal justice system
- High and damaging use of alcohol and other drugs
- Very poor support from human and social service agencies

People with complex needs who become enmeshed in the criminal justice system early in life are likely to continue that involvement, having frequent police events and cycling in and out of police and prison custody. They are also likely to be victims of crime as well as offenders. The case studies suggest that police have great difficulty knowing what to do or how to handle people in this group, especially when the people are young, as they try to engage human and social services, often to little effect, and are left to manage the many difficulties this group of people has. The evidence also shows that police frequently target people in this group for searches and regular surveillance, as they often behave in an unusual manner and are known to police. This often causes severe anxiety in people with mental and cognitive impairment and can result in resistance and behaviour that could be misinterpreted as offending, although of course sometimes is offending behaviour.

The prominence of cognitive impairment among those with complex needs who experience the greatest difficulties is obvious in the aggregated analysis. Those with intellectual disability, borderline intellectual disability, or acquired brain injury along with a mental disorder or substance abuse disorder are the most likely to experience the highest levels of difficulties throughout life, the least likely to be afforded appropriate support, and the most likely to be managed by police.

This fairly small group of individuals takes so much time and costs so much in regard to the number of police staff tied up in managing them. Alternative avenues of supporting and managing people with complex needs must be made available to the police and to families and communities when these individuals are young or when the impairments first become obvious. These programmes need to be available in the most disadvantaged suburbs and in rural and remote towns. There are some programmes in some jurisdictions in Australia, the Integrated Services Program in NSW, for example, that work in an appropriate and beneficial way with this group. But these programmes are not early prevention programmes, are extremely limited in the numbers they take in, are not available for children or young people, are available only in one or two centres, and find it very difficult to recruit skilled staff as there are very few people trained in this area. The challenge is for governments to ensure police are not the designated care managers for people with complex needs in the future.

References

Baldry, E. (2010). Women in transition: Prison to .... *Current Issues in Criminal Justice, 22*(2), 253–268.

Baldry, E., Dowse, L., & Clarence, M. (2012). *People with intellectual and other cognitive disability in the criminal justice system.* Report for NSW Family and Community Services Ageing, Disability and Home Care. Retrieved from http://www.adhc.nsw.gov.au/publications

Butler, T., & Allnut, S. (2003). *Mental health among NSW prisoners.* Sydney: Corrections Health Service.

Butler, T., & Milner L. (2003). *The 2001 New South Wales inmate health survey.* Sydney: Corrections Health Service.

Carney, T. (2006). Complex needs at the boundaries of mental health, justice and welfare: Gatekeeping issues in managing chronic alcoholism treatment? *Current Issues in Criminal Justice, 17*(3), 347–361.

Dowse, L., Baldry, E., & Snoyman, P. (2009). Disabling criminology: Conceptualizing the intersections of critical disability studies and critical criminology for people with mental health and cognitive disabilities in the criminal justice system. *Australian Journal of Human Rights, 15*(1), 29–46.

Draine, J., et al. (2002). Role of social disadvantage in crime, joblessness, and homelessness among persons with serious mental illness. *Psychiatric Services, 53*(5), 565–573.

Fry, A., O'Riordan, D., and Geanellos, R. (2002). Social control agents or front-line carers for people with mental health problems: Police and mental health services in Sydney, Australia. *Health and Social Care in the Community, 10*(4).

Godfredson, J., Ogloff, J., Thomas, S., & Luebbers, S. (2010). Police discretion and encounters with people experiencing mental illness. *Criminal Justice and Behaviour, 37*(12), 1392–1405.

Hamilton, M. (2010). People with complex needs and the criminal justice system. *Current Issues in Criminal Justice, 22*(2), 307–324.

Hannah-Moffat, K. (2010). Sacrosanct or flawed: Risk, accountability and gender-responsive penal politics. *Current Issues in Criminal Justice, 22*(2), 193–216.

Hayes, S., Shackell, P., Mottram, P., & Lancaster, R. (2007). The prevalence of intellectual disability in a major UK prison. *British Journal of Learning Disabilities, 35*(3), 162–167.

Henshaw, M., & Thomas, S. (2012). Police encounters with people with intellectual disability: Prevalence, characteristics and challenges. *Journal of Intellectual Disability Research, 56*(6), 620–631.

Herrington, V. (2009). *The impact of the NSW Police Force Mental Health Intervention Team: Final evaluation report.* Charles Sturt University.

Indig, D., et al. (2011). *2009 NSW inmate health survey: Key findings report.* Sydney: Justice Health NSW.

Lamb, H.R., Wenberger, L.E., & DeCuir Jr., W.J. (2002). The police and mental health. *Psychiatric Services, 53*(10), 1266–1271.

Lamb, H.R., Weinberger, L.E., & Gross, B.H. (2004). Mentally ill persons in the criminal justice system: Some perspectives. *Psychiatric Quarterly, 75*(2), 107–126.

Lyall, I., Holland, A.J., & Styles, P. (1995). Incidence of persons with a learning disability detained in police custody: A needs assessment for service development. *Medicine Science and Law, 35*(1), 61–71.

New South Wales Legislative Council Select Committee on Mental Health. (2002). Final report. Sydney: NSW Parliament.

NSWLRC. (2012). *People with cognitive and mental health impairment in the criminal justice system—Diversion.* Report 135. Sydney: NSW Law Reform Commission.

Rankin, J., & Regan, S. (2004). *Meeting complex needs: The future of social care.* London: Institute for Public Policy Research.

Spivak, B.L., & Thomas, S.D.M. (2012). Police contact with people with an intellectual disability: The independent third person perspective. Retrieved May 4, 2012, from http://onlinelibrary.wiley.com/doi/10.1111/j.1365-2788.2012.01571.x/abstract

Suggested Reading

Baldry, E., McDonnell, D., Maplestone, P., & Peeters, M. (2006). Ex-prisoners, accommodation and the state: Post-release in Australia. *ANZ Journal of Criminology, 39*(1), 20–33.

Legal Myth Busting and Frontline Mental Health Decision Making

12

SIMON BRONITT
JANE GATH

Contents

Introduction

An individual's mental health is vital to a person's ability to lead a satisfying and rewarding life. In recognition of this fact, the Australian government has introduced a number of initiatives, including the National Standards for Mental Health Services, to assist in the continuous improvement of the quality of mental health services being delivered across Australia. Underpinning these standards are a number of key principles consistent with national policy aimed at ensuring mental health treatment and support that imposes the least personal restriction on the rights and choices of mental health patients, clients, and consumers. The Queensland government has also developed and introduced a number of plans and programmes aimed at improving the delivery of mental health services in Queensland, including the Mental Health Intervention Project (MHIP) and the Queensland Mental Health Commission, which became operational on July 1, 2012. The prioritisation of providing mental health treatment within the community has led frontline police and ambulance officers to assume a more prominent first response role to mental health-related incidents. In this chapter, we examine some of the unintended effects of community-based mental health policies and programmes, including challenges that frontline police and ambulance officers face in complying with the key principles and legal requirements of mental health legislation.

Partnership Models: Coordinating Police, Ambulance, and Mental Health Responses

The introduction in Queensland of the Mental Health Intervention Project (MHIP) in 2005 has seen a number of positive outcomes in the management of mental health crisis situations in Queensland. MHIP, which is an agreement between Queensland Ambulance Service (QAS), Queensland Police Service (QPS), and Queensland Health (QH), has produced a memorandum of understanding (MOU) that aims to focus on the prevention and safe resolution of mental health crisis and improve the formal work practices and procedures both within and between the three frontline agencies. MHIP's aspiration to provide a more dignified approach to the management of people experiencing mental illness or disorder has led to over 7,000 police officers receiving training in de-escalation techniques.[1] It has also led to a policy that requires the QAS, rather than QPS, where practicable, to provide the first response to mental health-related incidents within the community.

Since these changes were introduced in 2005, however, there is evidence of emerging professional defensive practices, driven by uncertainty over legal rights and responsibilities and a fear of litigation. The impact of this professional defensive culture on people with mental health problems has been negative and discriminatory, increasing the likelihood of outcomes with marginal therapeutic benefit for patients. Under the 2005 agreement, the role of police was modified, with officers authorised to respond to mental health-related matters in the community *only* where the situation is deemed unsafe or as otherwise requested by QAS. While QAS is clearly an appropriate and humane alternative to using QPS, ambulance services are not generally equipped to manage mental health presentations, and their role involves transportation of persons presenting with mental health-related issues to an emergency department, often in the absence of identifiable clinical concerns or significant risk of harm to self or others. There appears to be no expectation within the MOU for mental health acute care teams to provide home-based assessment or treatment notwithstanding significant evidence, both internationally and nationally, that assertive mobile mental health crisis teams who provide crisis assessment and treatment within the community show increased levels of patient satisfaction, significantly reduced need for use of mental health acts, and decreased hospital admissions.[2]

Prioritisation of home-based crisis or semicrisis assessment and treatment to people with mental health problems conforms with the principles under mental health law that require the continued participation in community life and to the greatest extent practicable the provision of treatment in the community in which the person lives. In Queensland, the *Mental Health*

Act 2000 (Qld) underscores the importance of respecting liberty in exercising powers and functions under the Act. Section 9 of the Act provides:

Principles for exercising powers and performing functions

A power or function under this Act relating to a person who has a mental illness must be exercised or performed so that—

(a) the person's liberty and rights are adversely affected only if there is no less restrictive way to protect the person's health and safety or to protect others; and

(b) any adverse effect on the person's liberty and rights is the minimum necessary in the circumstances.[3]

Notwithstanding the legal and policy priority attached to the principles of autonomy and "least coercive" treatment for patients, there has been a systemic failure to adhere to these principles by frontline decision makers. As demonstrated above, people with mental health issues are being routinely denied their rights to autonomy, notwithstanding that, in many cases, they display little or no evidence of impaired capacity or lack ability to consent to treatment.

These concerns are not merely anecdotal. The Director of Mental Health in Queensland has recently reported an 18% increase in the number of emergency examination orders (EEOs) issued by police and ambulance officers in the last 12 months, with a 72% cumulative increase over the last five years.[4] There is no evidence that persons experiencing mental health issues in the community are presenting more frequently with greater risks to self or others to justify this increase. Indeed, in relation to persons placed under an EEO in the 2009–2010 period, 39% subsequently reviewed by a clinician required ongoing involuntary treatment under the *Mental Health Act 2000* (Qld). Put another way, over 50% of people presented to the emergency department under an EEO were either agreeable to treatment or were no longer believed to be suffering from a mental illness.[5]

The precautionary use of the EEO to detain people with mental health issues "just in case" flatly conflicts with the guiding principles of the *Mental Health Act 2000* (Qld), which seek to ensure that individuals with mental illness are afforded the same basic human rights and respect for their human worth and dignity as any other individuals, and also that their rights to consent to voluntary treatment are respected (*Mental Health Act 2000* (Qld), s. 9).

In fairness to frontline decision makers, there are various factors that contribute to the above position. These include the lack of mental health training, particularly in relation to the legal powers, and severe time pressures, which impair the ability of police and ambulance officers to make appropriate judgements. Also, there is a culture of professional defensive practise in relation to mental health clients, supported by the widely held but erroneous assumption that a person exhibiting any mental health problem or suicidal behaviour lacks legal capacity to consent to treatment. In response to paramedics voicing concerns regarding their ability to adequately assess mental health patients without adequate mental health education, Shaban conducted a study in Queensland in 2007 to determine how paramedics managed decision making when faced with mentally ill patients. The study found that Queensland ambulance officers did not view transporting patients to the hospital as providing good patient care; rather, it was viewed as a way of meeting their legal obligations as an employee.[6] A further study examining how ambulance officers make decisions regarding mentally ill patients identified a professional culture that was prepared to run the risk of committing an unlawful assault, battery, or imprisonment in transporting a person with mental health issues, rather than risk exposing themselves and their organisation to civil charges of professional negligence.[7]

Is this fear of the law of negligence among frontline decision makers well founded? It is widely reported that there is a "litigation crisis" in Australia's health care system, a view perpetuated by sensational media coverage of cases, as well as the lobbying efforts of unions, professional associations, and the insurance industry.[8] Indeed, the perceived crisis led to Justice Ipp being appointed to chair a review of the law of negligence in 2002. The Ipp Review's primary purpose was to address the public perception of escalating, "unsustainable public liability insurance premiums and damages awards for those injured through another's fault."[9] That review led to significant changes in the law, and limits on damages introduced across Australia.[10] As the Law Council of Australia pointed out in research it commissioned in 2006, there was no evidence that there was indeed a litigation explosion in the years before the Ipp Review.[11]

> There was no evidence of a sustained, significant increasing trend in claims prior to the Ipp inspired reforms. Likewise, however, that data indicates in most jurisdictions that there has been an appreciable (in some states dramatic) decline in litigation since the tort law reforms were enacted.

It would be fairer to say that this was an insurance rather than a litigation crisis, with increased premiums rather than damages awards placing unfair strains on the cost of medical services. Clearly then, *perceptions* of legal risk seem to be more influential than reality (based on litigation data). Surveys of professionals groups in Australia—whether from policing, paramedic, or health care professions—reveal that "fear of litigation" (and the negative professional impact of being sued) rates as a major concern.[12]

Contrary to widely held perceptions of the growing scope of negligence, the risk of liability faced by public sector professionals is not "writ large." Yet this perception clearly has bearing upon strategies taken by frontline professionals exercising mental health powers.

Legal Myth Busting and the Overriding Duty of Care to Prevent Self-Harm

The law of negligence, rather than expanding the scope of liability for police and ambulance officers, has a fairly circumscribed field of operation in relation to frontline mental health decision making. The leading Australian authority is the High Court decision of *Stuart & Anor v. Kirkland-Veenstra & Anor* (2009) HCA 15. The case addressed whether or not a duty of care is placed on the police to prevent suicide. In the early hours of August 22, 1999, two police officers observed Mr. Veenstra sitting in his vehicle in a car park on the Mornington Peninsula, with a vacuum hose leading from the exhaust pipe to the vehicle interior. The engine was not running and the bonnet was cold. Upon questioning, Mr. Veenstra persuaded the police he had been in the car for approximately two hours and had been thinking about doing something stupid, but he was an intelligent person and there were other options available to him other than suicide. He admitted to having marital problems. He declined their various offers of assistance. He removed the hose from the exhaust and the officers let him go. They checked the vehicle and found no alcohol, drugs, or medication. (The police were not aware that Mr. Veenstra was about to be charged with a number of fraud offences arising from his former employment.) The officers did not consider him to be mentally ill and did not detain him, stating he was "rational, cooperative and very responsible" with no apparent "disturbance of thought, perception or mood." They did, however, think he was "depressed," which Mr Stuart described as "unhappy," and asked if they could ring his doctor or a number of other support people and agencies, including the crisis assessment team. Mr. Veenstra declined their offers, stating he would visit his doctor later in the day. Mr. Veenstra killed himself by carbon monoxide poisoning in his own vehicle, near home, later the same day. His widow sued the police officers and the state of Victoria, alleging that the officers had breached their duty of care toward her husband and herself by failing to exercise their powers under Section 10 of the *Mental Health Act 1986*. At trial, the judge ruled that there was no duty of care and denied the claim. The widow appealed to the Court of Appeal, which, by majority, allowed the appeal. The officers were then granted special leave to appeal to the High Court.

Almost 10 years after the incident, on April 22, 2009, the High Court unanimously held there was no legal duty of care owed by the police officers on the grounds that the relevant statutory power (s. 10 of the *Mental Health Act*) had not been enlivened in the circumstances. Chief Justice French pointed out that the police officers had not formed the view that Mr. Veenstra was mentally ill, and therefore there was no statutory power to apprehend him. In their joint judgement, Gummow, Hayne, and Heydon JJ pointed out that personal autonomy is a paramount value protected by the common law, and the law of negligence, and that mere knowledge of a risk of harm and power to avert or minimise that harm does not, without more, give rise to a duty of care at common law.[13]

Crennan and Kiefel JJ similarly held that the common law generally does not impose a duty upon a person to take affirmative action to protect another from harm, and underscored the importance that individuals should take responsibility for their own actions. Thus, the statute supplied no relevant statutory power to which a common law duty of care could attach.[14]

As one legal summary of the case concluded:

> This is an important decision in putting a check on the widening of the scope of duty of care and gives police officers and similar workers, particularly in the area of mental health, some assurance that they will not be found liable for the self harm actions of persons who seemingly do not appear to be mentally ill....
>
> In each of the judgments it was pointed out that the Mental Health Act was not designed to prevent suicide; it was addressed to the protection of mentally ill persons. It would be wrong to assume that all persons who attempted suicide were mentally ill; the Mental Health Act contained no such assumption.[15]

Some commentators criticised the High Court, taking the view that the decision gives too much weight to autonomy interests, and insufficient weight to the welfare of vulnerable persons. As one clinician (a leading forensic psychiatrist) observed in a commentary on the High Court ruling, the decision "can be criticised as atomistic and predicated on excessive deference to the shibboleth of self-determination and 'personal autonomy' and the 'least restrictive option' principle enshrined in all mental health legislation."[16] Instead, the clinician calls for a wide interpretation of mental health powers:

> [These powers] should be widely interpreted to empower police, acting in good faith and with reasonable care, to err on the side of caution in exigent circumstances where a person appears to be in "crisis" and at risk. Such a benevolent intervention should not offend the sensibilities of any but the most rigid civil libertarian.[17]

With respect, this argument misunderstands the nature of the ruling. It also places no weight on the mandated principles that the legislature has stipulated must guide decision making. The High Court decision did not deny that police officers (or ambulance officers) have the *power* to intervene, where they believe on reasonable grounds the statutory conditions are satisfied; it simply refused to compel them to act in the absence of a belief that there were grounds to do so! To go further, and impose a duty to intervene, would extend negligence liability too far. The clinician's proposed precautionary rule of thumb for police to "err on the side of caution" offends not only the High Court's ruling, but also violates the clear statutory intent of the mental health legislation (and its guiding principles), which aims to protect human rights of the mentally ill, including that their liberty should be only infringed in cases of demonstrable necessity.

The current law of negligence, put simply, enables frontline decision makers (whether police or ambulance officers), within the limits of their own competence, to exercise their own professional judgement about whether the triggering statutory thresholds of mental illness or disorder have been met. The decision underscores that police and ambulance officers are not held to the clinical standard of care and do not share the same duties of mental health professionals. The decision is a reminder that in the absence of a statutory compulsion, there is no general duty to rescue another at common law, even in order to prevent another person's suicide. In making such assessments, the courts give consideration to public policy (either expressly or implicitly), as well as fundamental principles such as respect for personal autonomy and liberty. With respect, beneficence and good therapeutic intentions, as the above senior clinician proposed, should not, without sound reasons and express legislative authority, override the individual autonomy interests of the patient.

Conclusion

In the field of mental health, as in other areas, it is important to recognise that the legal norms (rules and principles) that support decision making are rarely clear-cut. Indeed, it may be more helpful for professionals to view law as a toolkit of norms for guiding and enabling conduct, rather than a simply as a rule book constraining and restricting conduct. This is not to imply a crude reductionism that rules are meaningless, capable of being distorted to achieve any particular policy, institutional, or personal outcome. Rather, it means that the rules must be understood by examining the guiding principles and underlying policy that motivate the relevant Act, and to develop policies and practises that both operationalise and align with those legal norms.[18]

There are many legal myths pervading our health system. While a perfect state of legal certainty is unattainable, the present system must strive for better understanding and compliance with the guiding principles and rules. Like the defence of superior orders in military trials, there is no overriding duty of care, as often claimed by frontline decision makers, that trumps patient rights. The High Court decision *Stuart & Anor v. Kirkland-Veenstra & Anor* (2009) HCA 15 exemplifies that.

Decision making by police and ambulance officers is beset by uncertainty. Uncertainty, whether factual, clinical, or legal, is pervasive. Clinical knowledge about mental disorders is constantly changing. Frontline decision making involves discretionary judgement—depending on the particular provision, the decision maker *may* exercise a particular power rather than *must*. Discretion needs to be recognised and valued more explicitly in policy and protocols, rather than be defensively policed out of existence. Leaving room for discretion does not necessarily equate with arbitrariness, inconsistency, or unlawfulness.

This Queensland case study reveals how a defensive professional culture can trump patient rights and the statutory principles that have been adopted (ostensibly) to uphold and maximise protection of those rights under the *Mental Health Act 2000* (Qld), including the presumption that persons with mental illness have the capacity to make, and should be encouraged to take part in, decisions about assessment and treatment, unless proven otherwise. The increasing numbers of EEOs issued by police and ambulance officers suggest a professional culture dictated by defensive rather than therapeutic imperatives for managing people with mental health problems. This trend in EEOs is at odds with the growing community awareness of the importance of patient autonomy and the legal precedents that underscore the fundamental importance of respecting patient autonomy and self-determination.

The inadequate resourcing of services in crisis or acute assessment and treatment invariably falls heavily on the shoulder of frontline agencies, such as police and ambulance officers. This has in turn led to people with mental health issues being denied their rights to autonomy. A form of professional practise is required that focusses more strongly on therapeutic needs, as well as approaching legal compliance in a more principled, rather than defensive, manner. Gratifyingly, in the Queensland context, a recent review of the EEO processes by QAS and QH has led to a policy directive that clarifies that ambulance officers must uphold the principle of least restrictive treatment and respecting the rights of those patients, who do not lack capacity, to voluntarily consent to treatment.[19] The restructuring and resourcing of acute care teams to focus *exclusively* on providing crisis or acute assessment and treatment service would be consistent with the principles in the *Mental Health Act 2000* (Qld), but would also likely improve patient outcomes. It would also have some collateral payoffs in terms of reducing the pressures on emergency departments. These teams working in partnership with police and ambulance services, to provide community-based crisis assessment, treatment, follow-up, and referral, would ensure the rights of mental health clients are respected, and they receive the treatment and care they deserve.

Disclaimer: The views expressed in this chapter should not be attributed to either Queensland Health or the Queensland Police Service. The authors alone are responsible for the views and errors. Professor Bronitt acknowledges the financial support of the Australian Research Council. We also thank Professor Chappell for soliciting this paper in the first place and patience in waiting for the final version, and Lisa Gilmore for her research assistance. The chapter is based on a conference paper delivered at the 31st International Academy of Law and Mental Health, Berlin, 2011.

References

Australian Medical Association Media Release. (2000a, November 2). AMA calls for government action on medical indemnity crisis. Retrieved from http://ama.com.au/node/826

Australian Medical Association Media Release. (2000b, December 8). Doctors sign up for widespread reforms to medical litigation. Retrieved from http://ama.com.au/node/696

Australian Medical Association Media Release. (2003, July 1). Medical indemnity like a three-legged dog—Glasson. Retrieved from http://ama.com.au/print/1272

Barker, V., Taylor, M., Kader I., Stewart K., & Le Fevre P. (2011, March). Impact of crisis resolution and home treatment services on user experience and admission to psychiatric hospital. *The Psychiatrist Online, 35,* 106–110. Retrieved from http://pb.rcpysch.org/content/35/3/106#BIBL

Commonwealth of Australia. (2002). Review of the law of negligence: Final report. Retrieved from http://revofneg.treasury.gov.au/content/review2.asp

Dixon, D. (1997). *Law in policing: Legal regulation and police practices.* Oxford: Oxford University Press.

Glover, G., Arts, G., & Babu, K.S. (2006). Crisis resolution/home treatment teams and psychiatric admission rates in England. *British Journal of Psychiatry, 189,* 441–445. Retrieved from http://bjp.rcpsych.org/content/189/5/441#BIBL

Jellet, S., Pope, N., & Voges, K. (1994). The stress of litigation: Fear of litigation as a stressor in Queensland Police officers. *Australian Police Journal, 48*(4), 163–167.

Lavan Legal Publications (law firm). (2009, April 30). Is there a duty of care to prevent suicide? *Pulse.* Retrieved from http://www.lavanlegal.com.au/index.php/publications/publicationdetail/there_a_duty_of_care_to_prevent_suicide

Law Council of Australia. (2005). *Higher insurer profits allow better benefits to the injured.* Retrieved from http://www.lawcouncil.asn.au/programs/national-policy/tort-law-reform/research.cfm

Law Council of Australia. (2006). *National trends in personal injury litigation: Before and after Ipp.* Retrieved from http://www.lawcouncil.asn.au/programs/national-policy/tort-law-reform/research.cfm

MacLennan, A., & Spencer, M. (2002). Projections of Australian obstetricians ceasing practice and the reasons. *Medical Journal of Australia, 176*(9), 425–428. Retrieved from http://www.mja.com.au/public/issues/176_09.html

Mental Health Act 2000 (Qld).

Police Too Scared to Make Arrests. (2003, July 12). *Illawarra Mercury*, p. 27.

Queensland Ambulance Service. (2012, January 19). *Medical director's circular no. 03/2012—Emergency examination orders.*

Queensland Department of Health. (2010). *Annual report of the director of Queensland Health 2009–10.* Retrieved from http://www.health.qld.gov.au/mentalhealth/pub/qld_pub.asp

Queensland Police Service. (2010). *Annual report of the Queensland Police Service 2009–2010.* Retrieved from http://www.police.qld.gov.au/services/reportsPublications/annualReport/20092010/performance/sds/Clientservice.htm

Scott, R. (2010). The duty of care owed by police to a person at risk of suicide. *Psychiatry, Psychology and Law, 17*(1), 1–24. Retrieved from http://dx.doi.org/10.1080/13218710903518871.

Shaban, R.Z. (2009). Paramedics and the mentally ill. In P. O'Meara & C. Grbich (Eds.), *Paramedics in Australia: Contemporary challenges of practice* (pp. 1–15). Sydney: Pearson.

Spigelman, J. (2006). Tort law reform: An overview. *Tort Law Review, 14*, 5–15.

Stuart & Anor v. Kirkland-Veenstra & Anor (2009) HCA 15.

Townsend, R., & Morgan, L. 2009. Protective jurisdiction, patient autonomy and paramedics: The challenges applying to the NSW Mental Health Act. *Journal of Emergency Primary Health Care, 7*(4), 1–8 (Article 990375). Retrieved from http://www.jephc.com/full_article.cfm?content_id=554

Endnotes

1. Queensland Police Service (2010).
2. Barker (2011, p. 108). Glover, Arts, and Babu (2006, p. 442).
3. Policy and ethical norms should play an important role in guiding and supplementing (rather than subverting and denying) discretion. In this respect it is worth recalling the relevant UN Mental Health Principles that provide valuable guidance as to how rights ought to apply to people with mental illness. Principle 7 emphasises the right to be treated and cared for as far as possible in the community; Principle 9 emphasises the importance of the least restrictive alternative in relation to treatment; Principle 15 states that voluntary treatment is to be the preferred form of hospital treatment of people with mental illness.
4. Queensland Department of Health (2010, p. 22).
5. Ibid., p. 25.
6. Townsend and Morgan (2009, p. 3).
7. Shaban (2009, p. 7).
8. In 2000 Australia's peak medical colleges and medical bodies lobbied all health ministers and attorneys general seeking urgent reforms to the medical litigation system (Australian Medical Association Media Release, 2000b, Article 696). The call for reform followed a crisis meeting where doctors voiced concerns about the soaring costs of medical insurance premiums and the costs of litigation. The federal president of the Australian Medical Association also met with the Commonwealth Attorney General in 2000, raising concerns about the increasing cost of insurance due to the fact that Australians were increasingly resorting

to litigation to solve grievances, with the courts increasingly awarding larger awards in damages (Australian Medical Association Media Release, 2000a, Article 826).

9. Commonwealth of Australia (2002, pp. 25–26).

10. Spigelman (2006). p. 11.

11. Law Council of Australia (2006). Another Law Council study funded showed that the Ipp reforms had increased insurers profitability (from 6–8% to over 20%) with no significant decline in premiums, concluding that the pendulum had swung too far and advocated that reform was needed to ensure the injured received a "fair go": Law Council of Australia (2005). Both reports are accessible online at www.lawcouncil.asn.au/programs/national-policy/tort-law-reform/research.cfm.

12. In 2001 an opinion survey of 1,116 obstetricians conducted by the Royal Australian and New Zealand College of Obstetricians and Gynecologists revealed a number of reasons why specialists were ceasing public and private practise. One of these reasons was fear or trauma of litigation, with 25% of public practice obstetricians citing this as the reason why they left their profession. Thirty-nine percent of private practice obstetricians cited fear or trauma of litigation as the reason why they left private practice (MacLennan & Spencer). A survey of 81 Queensland Police officers conducted in 1994 found that over 50% of respondents were worried about civil lawsuits as a result of their police work, with only 8% of respondents indicating their fears of litigation were irrational and excessive (Jellet, Pope, & Voges, 1994, p. 167). The NSW Police Association contends that it is the fear of being sued that stops some police from making arrests (Police Too Scared to Make Arrests, 2003). The Australian Medical Association continues to argue that it is the desire of doctors to work in environments that do not expose them to litigation (Australian Medical Association Media Release, 2003, Article 1272).

13. *Stuart & Anor v. Kirkland-Veenstra & Anor* (2009) HCA 15, 237 CLR 215 at p. 58 per French CJ, at p. 88 per Gummow, Hayne, and Heydon JJ.

14. *Stuart & Anor v. Kirkland-Veenstra & Anor* (2009) HCA 15, 237 CLR 215 at p. 127 per Crennan and Kiefel JJ.

15. Lavan Legal Publications (2009, p. 2).

16. See also a comprehensive analysis of the decision in Scott (2010).

17. Idem.

18. A point made in Dixon (1997).

19. Queensland Ambulance Service (2012).

Police Officer Mental Illness, Suicide, and the Effects of a Policing Organisation

13

STEPHEN BARRON

Contents

Introduction

Mental health is an important concern in many occupations, including the policing profession. The literature relating police stress and its effects, on both the individual officer and organisation, clearly reflects the importance of mental health and well-being. Yet this area has been beset with controversy for many years: Is it the nature of policing with its inherent problems and occupational risks, or is it the policing organisation that provides the stressful events that might affect the officer's mental health. The more extreme outcome of poor mental health policies and practises within a police organisation is suicide (Barron, 2010). These are the issues that form the gist of this chapter.

It is a prevailing and strongly held belief in policing circles that the psychological trauma experienced by some police officers is an important source of work-related stress, leading to mental health issues and problems. More recent research tends to suggest, however, that the single most important contributor to the mental health issues experienced by many police officers is their police organisation and principally problematic management practises,

(Barron, 2008a, 2010). Rather than address work-related stress and outcomes such as officer suicide on an individual officer level, a more effective intervention is at the organisational level. Such an intervention is required by both occupational health and safety (OHS) and antidiscrimination legislation and makes good business sense when well-being initiatives significantly improve the productivity of employees and decrease work-related absences and workers' compensation costs.

In what follows, attention is first directed to the general relationship between mental health and physical health, and research that has linked this relationship to the law enforcement working environment. A brief review is then made of the research literature regarding the links between mental illness and suicide as an entry point to a more substantial review and discussion of the occupational risks of suicide within the policing profession, and of mental health and stress-related issues. Particular attention is given to the risks involved when operational police officers suffering some form of depressive illness for which they are receiving medication continue to have access to firearms. The chapter concludes with some suggested ways forward in the promotion of organisational change in law enforcement agencies designed to reduce or eliminate the factors known to produce poor mental health outcomes for their employees.

Linking Mental Health With Physical Health

The relationship between mental health and physical health may be summarised by three points: First, mental health problems, particularly conditions such as depression and anxiety, often manifest themselves in physical symptoms for which there is no detectable underlying physical condition; this process is commonly referred to as somatisation (Parsons, 2004). As such, it is probable that a significant proportion of work-related absence and poor performance may be incorrectly ascribed to physical illness when the underlying features are either psychological or emotional. Second, there is considerable evidence that indicates that mental health issues are implicated in a range of physical ailments, such as heart disease, diabetes, cancer, and respiratory illnesses (Joseph et al., 2009). An example is the strong connection between depressive or mood disorders and coronary arterial disease. Further, underlying both mental and physical health is a wide range of lifestyle-related risk factors, such as alcohol abuse, poor diet, poor physical fitness, and smoking. There is also some evidence that prolonged stress has a negative effect on the immune system, increasing the vulnerability to a range of diseases (Parsons, 2004).

Finally, there is evidence that mental health issues have adverse effects on the prevalence and prognosis of other physical illnesses. Co-morbidity of psychological disorders and physical illnesses has implications on life expectancy, medication compliance, stigmatising of sufferers, nonreporting of health concerns (reducing early intervention), and a range of self-harming behaviours (alcohol and drug abuse, domestic violence, aggression, and other self-destructive behaviours) and suicide (Barron, 2010). While these relationships cause significant impacts in the general population, they are also featured in the range of and in the severity of a range of negative outcomes for law enforcement (police) officers.

A study completed by McCraty, Tomasino, Atkinson, and Sundram (1999) explored many of the physiological, behavioural, and psychological effects of stress on police officers as described by the literature. The study reviewed 65 police officers as they were subjected to a range of medical and psychological assessment techniques while being exposed to a number of different scenarios based upon their duties as police officers (building search, high-speed pursuit, attending a domestic violence incident). The rationale for the study was the presence of an extensive literature and research on police stress and its negative effects, on both the individual and society (McCraty et al., 1999). The negative effects included were the potential for errors, accidents, overreaction, and exposure of the police organisation to significant liability costs from officer misconduct, accidents, corruption, and complaints from the public.

Areas that were assessed, during the scenario exposures, included "physical health, emotional well-being, coping and interpersonal skills, work performance, workplace effectiveness and climate, family relationships, physiological and psychological recalibration following acute stress" (p. 1). The study referenced other literature where officers were twice as likely to develop cardiovascular disease as other occupational groups, and have a higher mortality rate from cancer as the general population. Similarly, police were found to have high levels of anxiety, anger, depression, alcohol use, and a suicide rate that was "nearly three times higher in police than in other municipal employees" (McCraty et al., p. 3), citing a study by Violanti, Vena, and Petralia (1998).

The tested group included patrol officers, with the majority having less than 15 years' experience (36 of the 65 study participants), 55 males and 10 females, with an average age of 39 years. While the programme was designed to support a range of coping and assessment strategies for the participants to manage their stress and return to a lower post-incident stress level—the baseline measures recorded prior to exposure and at the completion of the programme indicated that in almost every case, officers had moderate to high levels of arousal, heart rates, blood pressure, and stress levels.

The study demonstrated that even exposure to simulated scenarios of police work generated high levels of physiological and psychological stress. About 11% of the participants were found to be at high risk of cardiovascular disease, caused by structural changes in the cardiovascular system by repeated exposure to stress. A heart rate variability (HRV) analysis found that 27 officers tested fell "below the normal ranges for their age groups in several key measures of autonomic nervous system function and balance" (Violanti et al., p. 14).

The study stated that HRV is also a marker for the efficiency of the body's neural feedback mechanisms and is a reflection of our capacity to gather physiological and behavioural resources to the demands of our environment. A poor HRV rating may reflect a potential for slow adaptability and poor flexibility under stress. Though the body may adapt to a lower HRV rating, the consequences of a poor outcome are increased.

Parsons (2004) examined the health and safety risks of police officers from a large number of agencies in Canada, the United States, and Europe by reviewing the available literature on police occupational safety. Part of that review included areas such as work-related injuries and death, cardiovascular disease, fatigue, cancer, communicable diseases, back problems, psychosocial risks, and suicide. Overall, the research indicated that findings were comparable between countries, though there are considerable gaps in the research undertaken, with most research being in areas such as stress, homicide, and fatigue. The research completed on individual characteristics of police officers and their stress indicate that the stress often generates "general attitudinal behavioural characteristics" such as suspiciousness, rigidity, cynicism, and negative attitudes toward work (Parsons, 2004, p. 21).

Joseph et al. (2009) reported that "police work was associated with increased subclinical cardiovascular disease (CVD) compared to a similarly aged general population sample from the same geographical area" (Joseph et al., 2009, p. 706). Winwood, Tuckey, Peters, and Dollard (2009) indicated that the costs of poor mental health among police officers were the financial costs of compensation, sick leave, lost productivity, and the considerable emotional costs to the officer. They identified the duty of care of the organisation toward the officer as well as the "powerful economic argument to prevent, or at the very least limit, such injuries" (Winwood et al., p. 1057).

For police agencies and organisations, there is a clear business, legal, and ethical (including duty of care) case for strategies, policies, and interventions to address the mental health and well-being of police officers.

Mental Illness and Suicide—A Brief Overview of the Research

Police officers are drawn from the general community, and factors such as the presence or absence of mental illness in serving officers are usually determined by the effectiveness of recruit selection, screening, and training. In many cases, officers with a mental health issue may escape initial identification, while others with an underlying vulnerability or suffering from specific conditions within the policing environment may later develop mental health concerns.

Within the general community, increasing levels of sickness absence and increasing numbers of those on incapacity benefits have made health and well-being at work a major priority for many policy makers and governments in the developed world. Mental disorders are now the leading cause for sickness absence, accounting for about 40% of the total time lost to work-related sickness and absenteeism (Harvey, Henderson, Lelliot, & Hotopf, 2009). These authors also report that mental illnesses account for around 35% of all disability benefits. Major causes of these disabilities are anxiety, depression, physical symptoms, and musculoskeletal problems, which may also feature in undiagnosed mental disorders. In a study reported by the UK Health and Safety Executive (HSE), 20% of workers indicated that they felt "very" or "extremely" stressed at work, with percentages rising to 40% in some occupational groups (HSE, 2000).

In a 2007 report by the Sainsbury Centre for Mental Health (UK), the estimated cost of absenteeism was determined to be around £8.4 billion a year (US$13.14 billion). Further costs in terms of lost production were £15.1 billion (US$23.5 billion), and the costs associated with mental ill health were estimated at £2.4 billion (US$3.7 billion) each year. The report concluded that changing the management of mental health in the workplace, including prevention and early identification of problems, would enable employers to make savings of around 30% of these costs (£8 billion or US$12.5 billion) each year.

According to the Sainsbury report, the costs of mental ill health at work are reflected in increased sickness-related absence, reduced productivity at work, and staff turnover. Average workforce rates for mental ill health are around 23.4% of the adult population. The Sainsbury report indicated that similar findings were reported in the United States, Canada, and Australia, with the increased legal risks associated with not responding to work-related health issues, including mental health of employees, as required under health and safety legislation.

Within the general community, the determination of risk indicators or risk factors in suicide are used in assessment and treatment of persons who present with a range of mental illness, as well as those who communicate suicide intent via many different means. The use of the term *risk factor* is to indicate a nonrandom association between characteristics of completed suicides and the suicide as an outcome, with the added requirement that the factor(s) precede that outcome. The earliest studies of risk factors are found in retrospective analysis of completed suicides such as those undertaken by

Robins, Gassner, Kayes, Wilkinson, and Murphy (1959), and Shneidman and Farberow (1965). Though it is consistent in this and other research that persons who have been exposed to diseases, traumatic life events, abuse, stress, or other personal problems are at an increased risk of suicidal behaviour, only a small number of them commit suicide, despite having been exposed to the same risk factors.

Hawton and van Heeringen (2002) outlined many of the factors associated with suicide; they considered a range of both individual and environmental factors that research has indicated are related to suicide. Among the individual or demographic factors are age (where suicide is regarded as being more frequent among younger age groups), gender (where males are more likely to commit suicide than their female counterparts), and marital and parental status. Being married appears to act as a protective factor, reducing a number of risk factors in suicide, such as isolation and low support. There was also a linear decrease in suicide for females with increasing numbers of children. Other factors, such as race, ethnicity, and culture (suicide rates tend to mirror the rates of the country of origin; some cultures saw suicide as a traditional way of dealing with failure, shame, and distress or physical illness) and sexual orientation (gay, lesbian, and bisexual young persons have a higher risk of suicide than heterosexual comparison groups) also have been found to have an influence on suicide rates. Some occupational groups also feature more than others in terms of suicidal behaviour (included here are risk factors such as occupational stress and available means such as firearms (Hawton & van Heerington, 2002)).

Police Suicide—An Occupational Review

There have been a number of studies that have attempted to identify specific occupations that are featured in suicidal behaviours and ideation. Kposowa's (1999) study conducted a review, by occupation, of suicide outcomes. In a 2006 paper, the World Health Organisation considered a number of occupations with high suicide rates: physicians, some chemical workers, pharmacists, lawyers, teachers, counsellors, farmers, and "some police officers (such as those who are retired or suffering the effects of psychological trauma)" (WHO, 2006, p. 8).

Stack (2000) identified four factors that were important in the relationship between occupation and suicide: demographics, preexisting psychiatric morbidity, internal occupational stress, and access to lethal means. Some occupations appear to have an elevated rate of suicide, but when demographic variables such as sex, age, ethnicity, marital status, and level of education are controlled for, the occupational risk of suicide is no longer statistically different from that of other populations (Agerbo, Gunnell, Bonde, Mortenson, & Nordentoft, 2007). That is, suicides within occupations may be a product of the people who work in those occupations rather than the characteristics of the job itself. As mentioned, effective screening for mental illness is a suicide protective factor that distinguishes police work from other occupations. A number of authors (Hem, Berg, & Ekeberg, 2004; Loo, 2003; Violanti, 1996) have identified screening as a probable reason for relatively low suicide rates. The general literature suggests that police work is inherently stressful, and therefore warrants specific attention for any issue(s) related to the health, well-being, and safety of those who serve and protect. Most of the studies into police suicide, as an extreme end result outcome of policing, have tended to focus on two main areas: suicide rates of police officers and risk factors unique to police work and police organisational culture. Though the research into police suicide appears divided on the prevalence of suicide among serving police officers, more recent research indicates that police officers are more likely to die by their own hand than by generally perceived dangers of law enforcement.

Information regarding the numbers of police officers who commit suicide each year is generally difficult to obtain. In a 2010 study completed by Barron, there were 41 police officer suicides between 1990 and 2008 in the New South Wales Police Force, which is the largest policing agency in Australia, with more than 15,000 sworn police officers. Figures released by the National Coroner's Information System (NCIS) database in Australia reported that there were 47 police officer suicides in the period between July 2000 and August 2011 across all of the police forces within the country. In an article by O'Hara (2011), there were 141 suicides within law enforcement agencies across the United States in 2008, and 143 suicides in 2009. O'Hara reported that within the state of New Jersey, there were 9 suicides documented in 2008, 10 in 2009, and in 2010 the number had increased to 13. These figures do not accurately reflect those officers who attempt suicide or other self-harming behaviours, suffer from some psychiatric illness, or utilise long-term sick leave or make workers' compensation claims. Since the figures for police suicide are usually more able to be estimated, this area has tended to remain a focus of research into the mental health of those engaged in the occupation of law enforcement. In recent research the only significant risk factor in police officer suicide is the availability of lethal means, specifically a firearm.

The figures of reported police suicides do not reflect the actual number of suicides committed by police officers. The accurate figure is usually viewed as between 14% and 20% higher (Barron, 2007; Violanti, Vena, Marshall, & Petralia, 1996). Coronial legislation, systematic procedures, judicial discretion, and a reluctance to report police officer suicides to avoid stigmatising the deceased officer (or his or her family), as well as insurance concerns, are indicated as the more common reasons for this underreporting. Single-accident deaths and drug-related deaths remain the more problematic areas of suicide (or equivocal death) investigation.

Generally, the literature reports that the important contributors to police suicide are depression, relationship problems, financial problems, substance abuse, alcohol abuse, and access to firearms, as well as organisational issues such as corruption and management decisions. Other risk factors for police suicide include one or more diagnosable mental or substance abuse disorders, impulsivity, history of alcohol abuse, adverse life events, family history of suicide, physical and sexual abuse, a prior suicide attempt, and exposure to other suicidal events (contagion effect), similar for those found in general population studies of suicide.

Shift work and the resultant loss of family time and family disruption, ineffective communication, and lack of support from administration have been identified as contributing to the range of individual factors in suicide (Barron, 2010). Suicide by police officers is similar in almost every respect to suicide by those who are not police; the differences lie in the characteristics of those who seek employment and remain as police, in their psychological adaptation to the demands and stressors within the occupational and social environment, and the range of organisational and professional expectations of the police department. Shneidman (1994) indicated the importance of lethality of means as a factor in completed suicide; the ready availability of firearms in policing leaves officers in a constant state of potentially high lethality regarding suicide ideation, attempts, and completed suicide. Although suicide causation is multidimensional, availability of means remains an important factor and part of the explanation as to why the rate of suicide for police officers remains higher than for many occupational groups. The presence of occupational factors/stressors and availability of firearms account for many of the differences that exist in the literature for what is believed to be an elevated level of risk for suicide among this particular occupational group.

Violanti (2004) found that the suicide risks for police were similar to those found in the general population—depression, family dysfunction or conflict, personal stress, alcohol abuse, occupational work trauma, and the availability of firearms. This view has been held by other researchers who found similar common risk factors for suicide in general population studies and specific industrial groups (Hawton & Vislisel, 1999; Kposowa, 1999).

Previous studies (Friedman, 1968; Nelson & Smith, 1970; Heiman, 1975; Dash & Reiser, 1978; Aussant, 1984; Loo, 1986; Vena, Violanti, Marshall, & Fiedler, 1986; Curran, Findlay, & McGarry, 1988; Hill & Clawson, 1988; Josephson & Reiser, 1990; Wagner & Brzeczek, 1993; Cantor, Tyman, & O'Brien, 1994; Stack & Kelley, 1994; Violanti, 1996; Violanti et al., 1998) have all suggested that suicide rates for police are higher than those of the general population, though these increased rates often vary considerably. Kapusuta et al. (2010), in a study of suicides within the Federal Austrian Police Corps, concluded that rates were not higher than the age-adjusted levels within the general population; however, "given the healthy-worker effect, one would expect these rates to be lower than the general population" (p. 269).

Suicide studies involving police and nonpolice share considerable overlap in relation to the social stressors, psychological factors, biological factors, risk factors, and demographic characteristics. As Shneidman (1996) suggested, all suicides have common factors; the presence of more than one of these factors may constitute a suicidal crisis. The key is reaching a critical mass of predisposing factors, which as a suicide threshold would be different between individuals and within occupational groups. The influence of lifestyle and life events considerably impacts on the presence of this suicide threshold.

Ivanoff (1994) reported that the important contributors to police suicide are depression, relationship problems, financial problems, substance abuse, alcohol abuse, and access to firearms, as well as organisational issues such as corruption and management decisions. This is largely supported by the literature on suicide generally, apart from the availability of firearms. Other risk factors for police suicide include one or more diagnosable mental or substance abuse disorders, impulsivity, adverse life events, family history of suicide, physical and sexual abuse, a prior suicide attempt, and exposure to other suicidal events (contagion effect) (Herndon, 2001). Janik and Kravitz (1994), in a review of 134 officers who had reported for fitness for duty evaluations, found that only marital problems and work suspension were statistical predictors for suicide attempts. Lester (1993) found that alcohol use and interpersonal relationships appeared to play a significant function, while Violanti (1995) cited alcohol and mental illness as significant. He later added an overbearing police bureaucracy, shift work, social strain, and lack of control over work and personal lives as important factors in police suicide (Violanti et al., 1998).

Kimbrough (1999, cited in Herndon, 2001) added hopelessness, internal investigations, suicide ideation, a desire to punish someone, fear of retirement, and maladjustment to illness, injury, or psychiatric symptoms. Despite the range and commonalities in risk factors of police and others in suicide, it remains almost impossible to predict. Friedman (1968), in an early study of police suicide, found that marital discord (often a precipitating factor), psychological dysfunction, and consuming alcohol at the time of the suicide (or a history of heavy alcohol use) were significant factors in the decision to suicide. An additional feature was the reluctance of officers to seek assistance with their personal and other problems that might be the cause of their suicide ideation. Campbell (2001), in a study of the suicides among officers with the FBI, found that in addition to those already mentioned above, investigations, increase in paranoia, and indecisiveness were also factors. For

Campbell (2001), the communication of intent was a common feature among agents, who were often reluctant to pass on this information to managers. This issue is an important feature of the suicide prevention packages developed and delivered to U.S. military personnel.

Slosar (2001) described the importance of perfectionism in police suicide, or setting exceedingly high self-imposed standards, with both personal and social components. These persons are especially vulnerable to experiences of failure, poor adaptability to stress and negative events, and difficulty in establishing and sustaining interpersonal relationships, and more likely to attempt suicide. In an occupational environment where high standards are set, unrealistic expectations form part of a cycle of self-critical thought, which may lead to self-destructive behaviours, including suicide. Perfectionism may also be linked with anxiety, depression, and a prominent feature in obsessive compulsive disorder (OCD).

Seltzer, Croxton, and Bartholomew (2001) found that police suicides are unique in that the manner and cause of death is often determined in the presence and use of the officer's firearm. The other unique aspect of police officer suicide is the considerable amount of background and occupational material available. Since the late 1990s, police officer suicides in New South Wales have been regarded as "critical incidents," and as such, attract a significant amount of investigative resources and produce a large amount of documentation. The need to interview informants and witnesses post-death is minimised by the interviews conducted by the original investigators and coroner's death reviews. Factors such as alcohol abuse, legal and financial problems, relationship issues, changes in behaviour, communication of intent to others, performance issues, and other contributing factors are frequently documented.

Lennings (1995), who conducted a study into the risk factors of suicide and suicide ideation among police officers, found that a history of negative life events appeared to have a large impact on suicide ideation among the sampled officers. They appeared to use less problem-focussed coping skills than the sampled student participants and reported greater negative impact in using their avoidant coping skills. The presence of negative life events and depression implied an increased suicide risk. Loo (2003) undertook meta-analyses of studies examining suicide rates for police officers, and commented on the large variability found in some studies. While the access to firearms may partially explain this variability, there were other explanations, including cross-national and cross-cultural differences as well as cultural differences in the results found in international studies. Another possibility was the social, economic, and political context in which the suicides took place (Benner, 2001). For Loos (2003), the review of 28 studies of 101 different international sample suicide rates for officers resulted in markedly different rates depending on the reported statistics. Violanti (2004) found that the suicide risks for police were similar to those found in the general population: depression, family dysfunction or conflict, personal stress, alcohol abuse, occupational work trauma, and the availability of firearms.

Violanti (2001) reviewed the contribution of psychological autopsies in police suicide and suggested that unlike many other research designs, this methodology is able to estimate the presence and levels of high risk factors, but fails to sufficiently explain the individual and social factors that may be involved in police suicide. This insufficiency has implications in the efficacy of occupation-specific suicide prevention programmes and the clarification of police suicide precipitants. A result supported by research undertaken by Brent, Perper, Kolko, and Zelenak (1988) was where findings by psychological autopsy were found to be consistent across studies and population groups.

Many police suicides are characterised by active and lifetime diagnoses of major affective disorders, a presence of violence of aggression, experiencing more and severe life event stressors, a history of alcohol abuse, access to firearms, untrusting of health professionals, and more likely to have been exposed to traumatic and stressful occupational events (Violanti, 2001). Further, it was "understanding the nature and association [between suicide and immersion in work culture] that may provide insight into the aetiology of suicide and possible means for its prevention in the police and possibly other populations as well" (in Sheehan & Warren, 2001, p. 446).

In a 2007 study into police officer suicide within the New South Wales Police Force (Barron, 2010), reviewing 41 suicides by serving police officers, the significant identifying features of those suicides were:

1. Alcohol and drugs affected at time of death—53.5% of suicides
2. Suicides who were smokers at time of death—66%
3. Visits to medical practitioner within 12 months prior to death—68%
4. Those with a diagnosis of mental illness, including depression, at time of death—77%
5. Organisational referral (welfare/psych/medical/EAP)—51.5%
6. Presence of negative life event(s) within 12 months of death—63%
7. Relationship breakdown within 12 months of suicide—60% of suicides

With respect to operational stressors, work-related trauma only featured in 9.5% of those officers who committed suicide. Performance and work-related adjustment issues were present in 43% of the officers, almost one-third had problematic work relationships, and one-third were under internal investigation or subject to a workplace review. Organisational factors, including problematic management and leadership practises in policing, appear to be an increasing feature in police officers who develop work-related stress and psychiatric illnesses (Barron, 2008b).

The prevalence of psychiatric illness in this study reflects the prevalence of psychiatric illness in general populations of suicide. About 70% of the police officers were diagnosed or determined to have symptoms of mental health issues in the three months prior to death, with depression being the most prominent. There was also co-morbid alcohol abuse in about 30% of the officers.

The development of a risk profile for police officers who may, in some circumstances, commit suicide is a subtle part solution only to the problem of police officer suicide. From this study it is clear that a complex interaction between organisational stresses, work-related cumulative stress, poor adaptability to changing family and environmental factors, emotional avoidance as a protective strategy, and developing cognitive rigidity all play important parts in the problem of police officer suicide (Barron, 2008a).

It was apparent in the Barron (2007) study that a number of organisational factors may have featured in the development of the suicidal behaviour(s) leading to the decision to suicide. These factors appeared to include poor management practises, poor communication, an absence of training in the recognition and assessment of self-harming behaviours, inadequate supervision (including access to firearms), and a lack of continuity of care.

Many of the suicide risk factors for police officers in suicides by New South Wales police officers (Barron, 2007) appear consistent with those found in research conducted on general population samples, though the officers in the study were different from general population characteristics in significant ways. In contrast to suicide risk factors that exist in general population suicide studies, this group is employed, and the officers (at least upon recruitment and subsequent screening) do not display any overt psychopathology or mental illness, fall within an age group of 19 through 55 (excluding high population rates for the young and elderly), have available a range of in-house and outsourced support systems, including Employee Assistance Programs (EAPs), are usually closely supervised, and generally report a positive occupational outlook in culture surveys.

What was not clear in the Barron (2007) study is why other police officers with similar negative life events did not choose to commit suicide as a means of escaping their particular situation. Many of the officers in this study who committed suicide communicated clear and repeated intention to do so to family members, colleagues, and others. They were predominantly males, tended to demonstrate poor problem-solving skills, held a problematic social identity or occupational identity, had a recent history of conflicts and disputes with family members, colleagues, or others, demonstrated low connectedness with others and their occupation, tended to have poor family and social supports, increasingly isolated themselves from others, and had poor help-seeking behaviours.

Occupational stress, alcohol use and abuse, frustration and impulsivity, the presence of some mental health problem, and firearm accessibility all feature in the lives of the officers in this study who committed suicide

(Barron, 2008a). What is not clear is the extent to which each of these factors contributed to the decision to suicide (assuming that none of these officers died by accident in changing their intention too late). This study did indicate that many of these officers did not have supportive, positive, and productive personal relationships. Others who appeared to have such positive relationships with family, children, and peers had poor organisational relationships and were subject to management action in some form.

Police Occupational Stress and Mental Health

A long-held view in the literature is that cumulative stress as a consequence of the occupation of policing is a major contributor to many of the problems faced by police. This cumulative stress is manifested in lower cognitive and emotional functioning, difficulties in social, occupational areas, and increasing incidents of physical injury and disability. The growth of Employee Assistance Programs for police in the 1970s was recognition that many police found coping with the dangers and difficulties of the occupation damaging to their health and family (Raue, 1989). Early researchers documented and described the social isolation, normlessness, role conflict, powerlessness, suspiciousness, anomie, public mistrust, cynicism, and alienation that were features of policing (Klockars, 1980). Klockars' research suggested that police may engage in unethical, morally corrupt, and questionable behaviours that are seen as justification of dirty means.

The research is not clear about the psychological changes that may take place over many years of policing duties, but there is some indication that officers who spend too long in undercover work and being attached to special crime units investigating child abuse and homicide can experience an erosion of individual psychological defence systems to mediate stress (Campion, 2001). Violanti (1996) explained: "Acquisition and maintenance of the police role restricts cognitive flexibility and the use of other life roles by police officers, thus impairing their ability to deal with psychological distress" (p. 709), but this does not explain the relatively few suicides and attempted suicides as compared to the large number of officers who manage the same amount of occupational stress. The importance of individual characteristics, personality, domestic developmental background, adaptive reasoning, restricted affect, and so on, appears to be the significant key to understanding and predicting suicide—hence the present inability to predict suicide.

In a survey of police officers and their responses to police suicide by Campion (2001), 35% of officers strongly agreed that in their personal experience of police suicide, the officer "never should have been a police officer" (p. 428); a further 30% "agreed or somewhat agreed" to the same proposition. Other areas in this study that reviewed officers' attitudes to the reasons why police officers commit suicide are personal stress, alcohol abuse, mental problems other than depression, relationship conflicts off the job, depression off the job, and family problems (not job related), with the highest job-related reason of suicide as attendance at critical incidents (ranked 11 of 28 items).

Aamodt and Werlick (2001) in a study of police officer suicide found that in almost 24% of suicide cases, there appeared no obvious or discernable reason for that suicide. Explanations as to why United Kingdom and Canadian police suicide rates are much lower than those in the United States tend to focus on the different policing styles and the lack of connectedness with the officer and their home society in the United States, despite the methodological, measurement, and classification problems associated with such research.

Kasperczyk (2010) reported that there was a corporate responsibility for occupational stress prevention; this view is particularly relevant to police organisations. The view of the author was that "if occupational stress is understood as a transaction between the worker and the work environment then it has significant implications for corporate governance in the areas of organisational effectiveness, employee health, employee performance and risk management" (p. 52). Traditionally, stress has been conceptualised by business and public sector management as an individual problem rather than a corporate one. This is observable in many of the welfare policies and protocols established for police officers specifically. In managing police (and to a lesser extent, administrative staff), the emphasis of support policies (emotional health, stress debriefing, alcohol and drug counselling, etc.) has rested on the individual officer—where the officer was expected to self-refer or comply with policies designed by, or for, the police organisation. Since the experience of individual officer stress is seen as some personal characteristic of the officer, stress prevention strategies tend to address individual factors as being more prevalent than organisational factors. Both of these approaches are quite different in managing stress in the work environment.

Kasperczyk (2010) estimated that, in Australia, there has been a significant increase in mental stress compensation claims as a part of work-related injury, from 4,440 claims in 1997–1998 to 8,665 in 2004–2005—representing a 95% growth. This increase was against a decrease of 13% in the annual workers' compensation claims for all injuries over the same period. Though contributions to such an increase may be affected by the increased focus on workplace well-being and mental health, the increased number of claims for mental stress represents a significant and growing proportion of the overall national workers' compensation allocation. Kasperczyk (2010) reported similar significant increases across Europe and the UK. Additional costs to all industries are reflected in changes to unplanned absences, increased industrial accidents, lower morale, and lower productivity. Much of these costs are directly related to established causal links between psychosocial problems in the work environment and poor health and diseases, such as cardiovascular, coronary, blood pressure, and poor mental health outcomes.

One of the first corporations that took a strategic approach to workplace health, well-being, and safety of employees was Rolls-Royce in 2006. The research conducted into workplace stress prevention concluded that organisational-level interventions were more effective than individual-level interventions (Cooper, 2001). The view that organisational stress should be addressed by organisational responses is not unchallenged. Kinman and Jones (2005) suggested that though it was accepted that workplace stress was largely organisational by nature, the individual held the responsibility with managing that stress.

Collins and Gibbs (2003) concluded that for many occupations (including policing), the research was compelling that organisational issues created more stress for employees than operational duties related to those occupations (despite stress associated with policing duties and responsibilities). The focus of primary interventions for workplace stress is in improving the environment in which the individual operates, and consequently, they are likely to involve organisational change initiatives.

Mental Illness and the Occupation of Policing

> Our officers and staff are our most valuable asset. Their health, safety and well-being are critical to forces' ability to deliver the services which society needs and expects. Sickness has a major impact on efficiency in terms of absence, financial resources and the effect on the staff that are left to cover for those who are absent. It also impacts on a wider group, namely the families of the officers and staff, and the communities we serve. (Chief Constable, UK, 2009)

Many policing organisations express similar views regarding their most important asset: their people. These statements are usually located in annual reports, human resource documents, and policy documents relating to welfare, health, and well-being of employees, both sworn and nonsworn. The largest single budget item in any police agency is likely to be its salaries paid to the officers and administrative staff. The cost of recruitment, training, and professional development for many agencies is a significant investment in terms of public confidence in police, the popular media, political oversight, and judicial interaction. It is therefore important that police organisations consider the impact of the organisation on their staff in terms of their health, safety, and well-being. Some research would indicate that this is not the case.

In an organisation where quasi-military structures exist to ensure employee compliance, if not cooperation, administrative and organisational stress may be more significant in negative psychological outcomes for police officers. An explanation for this may lie with the protective effects of the police culture and within the training provided to new recruits. Much of the initial training provided to new officers relates to the legislative powers given to police officers in managing conflict and the protection of persons and property. Other training is provided that allows the officers to successfully negotiate the policing organisation in terms of technology, processes, and protocols, as well as basic investigative skills. The field training that commences upon placement in the community focusses on a specific range of skills, knowledge, and the shaping of police-oriented attitudes. An important part of this field training is the exposure of the recruit to the police culture, which provides a protective, professional barrier to many of the duties undertaken by officers, but may also leave the officer vulnerable to organisational stressors, especially criticism, perceived lack of support, poor management practises, and an overreliance on discipline as a performance management tool (Garcia, Nesbary, & Gu, 2004; Woody, 2005).

Part of this vulnerability is explained by the social exchange relationship between employee and employer (Armeli, Eisenberger, Fasolo, & Lynch, 1998), where officers exchange loyalty and performance to the police organisation for a range of incentives, including salary, status, and opportunities for promotion, approval, affiliation, emotional support, and esteem. For many police officers, there is an expectation that police work will be difficult and at times stressful; this view is supported by media representations of police work and by policing organisations themselves. The proposal that policing organisations may provide more stress to the officers than their work-related duties may be viewed as the officer perceiving that the organisation is not as loyal, supportive, or caring as it is expected to be. A critical factor is the level of engagement (positive or negative) that employees had with their workplace and employing organisation (Richardsen, Burke, & Martinussen, 2006).

A further complication is that the work lives of police officers often affect the family lives of officers. This may be as a direct consequence of duty rotations, shift work, internal complaint investigations, and work-related trauma or management practises. Work–family boundaries appear to be permeable, where work stress often affected family support systems and family distress (e.g., relationship breakdowns), and in many cases directly affected the work performance of police officers (McCreary & Thomson, 2006).

Mental illness has increasingly become a concern for researchers into policing; the difficulty is that there are no sources of data for research in this area. Medical practitioners are appropriately unable to supply information regarding patients; policing organisations are not able to accurately determine the numbers of police officers, at any time, who might be taking prescribed medication for a mental condition—even if such medication may impact upon the officer's ability to drive a motor vehicle or handle machinery (firearms are usually not mentioned in drug warnings to patients). Police officers are usually unwilling to voluntarily declare to the organisation because of their perception—rightly or wrongly—that a declaration might prevent them accessing promotion or a desirable duty location/rotation. Organisations are usually informed when officers are referred by supervisors for support or declare an illness as part of a workers' compensation entitlement (such as hurt on duty).

Clearly, there are no reliable data upon which to base any assertion that mental illness is a significant policing problem, though it has been accepted that if left untreated, sudden and routine exposure to stress can result in psychiatric injury. Inference must be made from literature into nonpolice populations regarding the prevalence of mental illness in the community. Difficulties arise when police recruitment practises and organisational support services tend to screen out those persons who might present with mental illness as part of the officer selection process. In a culture where reliability and dependability are regarded as essential attributes of a police officer, disclosure of any mental condition could lead to early discharge with minimal benefits, unless the mental illness, such as post-traumatic stress disorder or stress, is determined to be as a direct consequence of duties as a police officer. Such determination is usually made only after considerable deliberation by the police organisation and based upon numerous psychiatric and psychological examinations. This process can typically take years, where the officer and his family are left in limbo until a decision is made.

Depression is also a significant risk factor in the suicide of police officers (Martelli, Martelli, & Waters, 1989; Cantor et al., 1994; Violanti, 1996; Marzuk, Nock, Leon, Portera, & Tardiff, 2002; Barron, 2007), but rates of depression among police officers are usually unavailable. Wang (2004) found that work-related stress was a strong risk factor in developing depression, with high psychological work demands, fatigue, work-related physical illnesses, traumatic events, job insecurity, supervisor/co-worker conflict, as well as a range of personal variables being the most reported. Despite depression commonly being associated with a range of sociodemographic, clinical, and psychological factors, poor adaptation to work stress is increasingly prevalent among police officers (Barron, 2007).

Records held by policing agencies do not include those officers who seek assessment, diagnosis, and treatment by general practitioners and allied health professionals within the general community. The figures held by police command are the increasing levels of absenteeism, work-related injuries, detected levels of alcohol and drug-related offending by officers, reported domestic violence incidents, workers' compensation claims, and insurance premiums paid to work cover and related insurers.

The Association of Chief Police Officers of England, Wales and Northern Island in 2002 developed a strategy designed to address the above-mentioned organisational issues surrounding the health and well-being of police officers. The Strategy for a Healthy Police Service was principally developed to reduce absenteeism among officers. Strategies included individual focussed and organisational focussed policies and procedures to identify and support officers with a stated intention of returning them to work as quickly as practicable, and highlighting OHS practises to reduce work-related injuries. An important part of the overall programme was to collate accurate statistics regarding police officer absenteeism and communicating best practise. The responsibility in the strategic management of health and safety matters was left to the chief constables (chiefs of police) in the respective forces and overseen by a government (home office) committee. To date, the strategy has resulted in significant reductions in police officer absenteeism and work-related injuries.

Collins and Gibbs (2003) reported that in two separate studies conducted with UK police officers, 17% to 22% of officers reached significant levels of mental ill health (using a recognised mental health scoring system), and that those officers contributed their ill health to organisational issues. The authors highlighted that these figures were a concern with respect to recent organisational changes in policing, such as "employee assistance programs, improved recruitment selection, better performance recognition, equal opportunities and sexual equality training to try to mitigate the effects of the organisational stress-strain reaction" (p. 257). In their study, they concluded that 41% of the police officers in their sample reported measureable ill health. The principal issues related to mental ill health were work structure and climate. Suggested solutions were to modify the "organisational workload and improving the managerial climate, rather than into further medical or welfare interventions" (p. 262).

Clearly, though the literature is replete with studies indicating that police work is an inherently dangerous occupation, and much effort is undertaken in studies to improve the safety of officers while at work, mortality rates indicate that police officers are more at risk of suicide than by any other means (homicide, motor vehicle collisions, accidents, and cardiovascular problems). Police organisations do not routinely collect information regarding the illness or deaths of officers; as indicated, this is because many officers choose not to inform their employer or avail themselves of support services provided by police organisations for that purpose.

In essence, employers are bound to consider the physical and mental health of employees as part of their obligations under occupational health and safety legislation. While an important part of those obligations relates to the process and environment of work, a growing consideration is on the way the employer relates and engages with its employees. This is particularly important in the occupation of policing, where employees may be directed to certain duties, exposing them—at their employer's discretion—to a range of work-related critical and traumatic events. Notwithstanding that many police organisations provide medical, psychological, and support services to their officers, research tends to indicate that a range of administrative and managerial factors have a greater effect on police officers than duty-related incidents (Barron 2010).

In an Australian study by Hart and Cotton (2002), the authors reported that a number of police officers regarded "organisational aspects of their work (leader and management practices, appraisal and recognition processes, career opportunities, clarity of roles, co-worker relations, goal alignment) to be more stressful than the operational nature of police work" (p. 104). The study suggested that the nature of the stress-strain approach in police research has tended to assume that the adverse work experiences of policing caused psychological and behavioural strain. Many officers found that though aspects of their duties were challenging, these duties often provided an important source of positive feelings regarding the importance of their role and their position in the community. The shift from police stress management to one where the well-being of the officer is important has resulted in a closer examination of the organisation as a source of negative emotional and cognitive outcomes for officers.

Davey, Obst, and Sheehan (2001) found a similar outcome in their study into the demographic and workplace characteristics of police officer stress. The authors reported that "organisational factors emerged as the important predictors of job stress for police officers" (p. 37). Further, the "job content factor of dealing with dangerous and unpredictable duties was not predictive of job stress but in fact led to higher job satisfaction" (p. 29). Winwood et al. (2009) found a similar result in their study: Officers who were indicated by practitioners as having significant psychological injury due to work-related trauma also reported robust emotional health and high work engagement.

The Hart and Cotton study (2002) concluded that "organisational experiences were more important than operational experiences in determining police officers' levels of occupational functioning" (p. 124) and "showed the central role that was played by organisational climate" (p. 128). A strategy that might be useful in improving the well-being of police would be "use regular employee opinion surveys, to build accountability among managers for the development of their people management practices" (p. 131). Further, the trend to increasing work-related claims for compensation was more attributed to low morale than work-related distress.

In a 2007 New Zealand study (Berry, 2010), an employee engagement survey was conducted with a random sample of over 6,700 police employees in New Zealand. The results indicated that many of the issues raised by staff within the survey were not confined to employment status, gender, or rank. Overall, scores on officer engagement (positive affiliation and psychological connectedness) were low, productivity scores were low, and middle management officers tended to be the least engaged of all police employees. The study concluded that a number of areas required addressing: Staff had comparatively low perceptions of the police as a place to work, did not believe that they were resourced effectively, were of the opinion that they did not receive recognition and praise for good work, held little trust in the organisation to provide an environment of fairness for employees, and were not optimistic about the future of the police portrayed by the leadership of the organisation.

Peterson, Park, and Castro (2011) reported that the U.S. military had previously focussed on the "negative indicators of psychosocial well-being, such as suicide, PTSD, drug and alcohol use, child abuse and neglect, domestic violence and divorce" (p. 10), rather than on a more comprehensive "soldier fitness programme," designed to develop psychological fitness among military personnel. The work of the U.S. military has been significant in the area of suicide prevention and promotion of mental health programmes across their 800,000 employees.

A Way Forward

One of the leading agencies to take a broad, organisational approach to suicide prevention and employee well-being has been the U.S. Air Force. Their intervention strategy was designed to target a range of organisational, cultural, and individual risk factors across the entire Air Force community. Its aim was to reduce suicide through early intervention of mental health problems (not specifically self-harming behaviour), strengthening socioenvironmental protective factors such as promoting a sense of belonging, and implementation of policies to reduce stigma and promote help-seeking behaviour. Supervisors were seen as gatekeepers in identification and referral of mental health issues for their staff, and senior management were directed to promote mental health awareness through their operational environments.

In an evaluation of the programme, reductions of 80% of suicide rates were reported (over their highest rate recorded in 1980), and reductions were also noted in incidents of accidental death, homicide, and domestic violence. In 2009, the U.S. Department of Defense (DOD) consolidated the various suicide prevention programmes across their separate military agencies and established a single strategy for all of their armed service and ancillary staff. The final report of the DOD Task Force into suicides by members of the U.S. Armed Forces (U.S. DOD, 2010) identified that the Task Force "knows of no other employer that has focused as much attention and resources on suicide prevention" (p. ES-3).

The report established a centralised set of strategic initiatives, critical to the success of their commitment to improve mental health, safety, and well-being, as well as seeking a permanent and significant reduction in suicides among their Armed Forces. Among these strategic initiatives were procedural standardisation and oversight; leadership responsibility; wellness enhancement and training; access to, and delivery of, quality care—assessment, diagnosis, counselling, and treatment; and surveillance, investigations, and research into suicide prevention. The DOD programme offers a single organisational approach to many of the issues raised in police work-related stress and organisational-level problems. Though the focus remains on the individual, the programme is designed to address organisational structures, management, and effective identification of those personnel who indicate some level of mental health concerns. Importantly, there is a declaration within the language of the 2010 report that the military organisation holds a responsibility to provide the strategies to promote well-being, mental health, and safety among its employees, rather than leaving employees to self-identify, self-refer and access support mechanisms that are provided for them. The work by the DOD represents an important shift in emphasis from the individual view of mental health to a more corporate focus and ownership of the problem.

Mental Illness and Stigma

The literature on mental illness stigma within law enforcement generally agrees that it is an important issue in officers being able to admit they require assistance, and the organisation is willing to provide such assistance without inordinate and negative impact on that officer's career, prospects of promotion, transfer, and entitlements. Unfortunately, this is not always the case. This reinforces the perception that the organisation is unable to manage the issues surrounding suicide and self-harm.

The prevalence of stigma regarding mental illness within the general community is regarded as an issue in providing sufficient support services. Since officers are drawn from the general community, some stigma associated with mental illness is understandable, though not acceptable. Such stigma is usually based on a general lack of education and lack of confidence in officers managing challenging situations with individuals who present with some behaviour associated with mental illness. In policing, many officers demonstrate a reluctance to seek support, for fear that their colleagues will see them as unreliable or weak. Further, the policing culture promotes a sense of competence, professional and personal, as well as the need to be seen as stoic, reliable, and dependable. The study by Griffith University found that stigma associated with mental illness was detected in the suicides of two NSW Police officers (Hawgood, Klieve, Harris, & De Leo, 2008).

Research conducted by the University of South Australia in 2008 found that an unsupportive culture of "mental toughness" combined with ineffective mental health services was "endangering" the psychological well-being and welfare of general duties officers in the NSW Police. The study found that instead of encouraging psychological safety, "police culture tends to promote and endorse emotional control, emotional suppression and mental toughness." The report also criticised the availability of peer support services; officers were expected to self-identify and approach the police force for assistance. The services that are available within NSW Police, well-check (an internally managed health process of workplace sickness-related absence) and counselling, are based on self-referral. Research into men's health has generally demonstrated that men hold more negative attitudes toward seeking psychological assistance than women. Specifically, men demonstrate a negative self-perception that seeking assistance is socially unacceptable; the general avoidance is driven by the necessity of avoiding the label of being weak, resulting in a loss of self-esteem. Male police officers who seek help also face fears over being labelled as unfit for duty because of any resulting diagnosis, or having a history of psychological service made part of their permanent personnel record. Police officers who have the greatest difficulty ignore or deny their symptoms, believing that their fellow officers will shun them to avoid being associated with them because of their own socialised male gender role.

Wester, Arndt, Sedivy, and Arndt (2010) reported that police (law enforcement) officers were often reluctant to seek assistance and support due to a perception that there may be left a permanent record of that assistance, especially where any diagnosis is later made regarding their mental health issue. The authors further suggested that the officer may feel a loss of self-esteem in seeking counselling and engage in a self-risk assessment regarding the benefits of any counselling against the effects of possible stigmatisation that might occur. Typically stigma takes the form of stereotyping the officer, causing mistrust, fear, and avoidance by colleagues, often resulting in the officer not seeking professional intervention and accessing organisational welfare and support. This is not surprising, given that police in the course of their duties often come into contact with members of the general community who have mental health illnesses. Many officers in that contact make assumptions on the appearance, behaviour, and socioeconomic status, and form negative depictions of mental health illnesses and those who present with some form of mental health problem. Generally, individuals with some form of mental illness are stereotyped as dangerous, unpredictable, and weak-willed. Historically, contact between police and the mentally ill is rarely seen as a positive experience for police (who often receive little formal training in management of the mentally ill) or the mentally ill person.

A possible solution is provided by the establishment of a positive obligation on officers and supervisors to provide information in writing when they hold concerns with respect to a possible depressive illness of one of their colleagues. This is not without challenges. First, it may discourage officers discussing their issues or concerns with fellow officers (and peer support officers, where available); second, it may ultimately lead to disciplinary action against an officer or supervisor who fails to make a relevant disclosure or who conceals a disclosure with "good intentions" on the basis of friendship or other relationship with the subject officer. The stigma to mental illness within the many police agencies may be a significant concern to officers seeking promotion, transfer, or redeployment, where their illness may be perceived to impact on their operational capacity or aptitude to perform their new duties, or the health and safety of the officer or their colleagues in the workplace.

Police Officers, Antidepressants, and Firearms

Many police agencies have a range of policies and procedures to address police officer behaviour, health status, and the availability of police issue firearms. Current New South Wales Police policies (Drug and Alcohol Policy, Sick Leave Management Policy) mandate that officers should not work if impaired by general medications or prescription drugs. Further, if the medication carries a warning that it has the potential to impair normal functioning, a supervisor *must* be informed. Similarly, there is an obligation on combining prescription medication with alcohol. The diagnosis of depression (among many other mental health issues that may result in self-harm) is a complex process, with many co-morbid and differentiating co-diagnoses. Depression may be due to some biological cause (endogenous) or related to a situational, transient, or permanent family, personal, occupational, or environmental stressor. The diagnosis can be further complicated with a range of anxiety and other disorders, affected by alcohol or drug use. Further, the range of medications available is generally prescribed with a trial-and-error approach to determine effectiveness, and then dosage is manipulated to determine the most effective therapeutic dose. Side effects vary and may determine moving to an alternate medication if the side effects are undesirable, regardless of medication effectiveness.

The prescription of medication is one consideration, and especially on an operational police officer, where the medication carries a warning "not to use heavy machinery." In cases like this, the effects may be significant if that officer is involved in a high-speed pursuit or an incident where his or her firearm is used within the course of that duty. It is common sense that where an officer is experiencing distress, caused by any number of factors, and exposed to further extreme stressful events (medicated or not), then that officer is working in an unsafe environment—placing himself or herself, his or her colleagues, and members of the community at risk. An officer whose judgement and decision-making processes are impaired by any medication is potentially a danger to himself or herself and others, due to the unpredictable and often unmanageable nature of policing, especially general duties policing. This relationship between medication and operational effectiveness ignores the effects of family, shift work, poor diet, cumulative stress, and any predisposing vulnerability to a range of physiological and psychological impacts that can exponentially increase the range of negative possible outcomes.

With respect to confidentiality, the service (U.S. Air Force) established a policy where communications between service personnel and therapists (medical officers, medical staff, psychologists, and allied health staff) were confidential and was protected from unauthorised disclosure. Confidential communications were disclosed to persons or agencies with a proper and legitimate need—concept of limited privilege (DOD, 2010). This approach could be adopted by the NSW Police in exercising their responsibility to take effective notification measures when confronted by an officer who is suffering a depressive illness or taking antidepressive medication, and therefore at greater risk of self-harm.

Many pharmaceutical companies responsible for the manufacturing, development, evaluation, and marketing of a range of antidepressant medication warn "that in the first month of taking this type of medication there is an increased risk of suicide." Additionally, the American College of Occupational Medicine (ACOEM) recommends that there is a temporary restriction to firearm access at the beginning of treatment and the monitoring of behavioural changes during this period when medications are prescribed for depression (ACOEM, 2011, p. 41).

Many antidepression medications are designed to initiate changes in brain chemistry, causing the reuptake of certain neurochemicals, supplementing neurochemicals, or assisting in the metabolism of those neurochemicals. As such, there is likely to be a period where behaviour, judgement, sleep, intimate functioning, and other aspects of behaviour and performance may be affected. If the diagnosis is correct and the initial medication is correctly prescribed, and if the individual adheres to the suggested dosage and compliance regime, then such restrictions to arms and appointments may be a matter of weeks. Where the depression is caused by some biological or chemical defect, then medication is generally prescribed for a lengthy period of time. Where the medication is prescribed for a personal, family, environmental, or occupational stressor or maladaptive response to a stressor, then psychotherapy or counselling is essential; otherwise, the tendency is to simply increase the dosage as the individual does not seek to reduce or better manage the stressor and relies on the medication for adaptive functioning.

Where antidepression medication at high doses is maintained for a lengthy period of time and then the individual stops taking the medication for any reason, there is likely to be a prompt and significant adverse reaction. Similarly, where one type of medication is changed, for a variety of reasons, then a washout period is usually recommended. During that period, there is likely to be a behavioural adjustment, which could result in unusual behaviour, changes in judgement, and a variety of unanticipated side effects. In summary, the length of time that an officer has restriction to duty type or arms and appointments should be determined on a case-by-case basis. The medication is prescribed to improve the management of the depression; it does not remove or cure the individual of depression. Generally, once a person has a depressive episode, he or she remains vulnerable to further depressive episodes for the duration of his or her life.

The decision to return an officer to operational duty and have access to arms and appointments should made by the PMO, after information is obtained from general practitioners, treating psychiatrists or psychologists, and other allied health practitioners. In terms of public policy and the possibility of civil litigation against a police officer who is involved in a critical incident while affected by prescribed medication, some restrictions are required for an officer who is taking antidepressant medication. These restrictions may only be required until an officer is stabilised by his or her medications, receiving appropriate psychological support, and is under the regular care of his or her medical practitioner. Compliance with antidepressant medication, appropriate medication among many alternatives, and the determination of appropriate therapeutic dosages are all areas of concern with respect to this type of medication. Considering the numbers of police officers worldwide who may be in receipt of prescribed medication for a range of mental health-associated issues—and completing operational duties, driving marked and other police vehicles at high speeds, carrying a police issue firearm (and other appointments), and being exposed to a variety of emotionally charged and difficult duties—antidepressant medications represent a specific concern for police management and officers, as well as the general community.

Final Remarks

Policing as an occupation is a potentially dangerous occupation, notwithstanding the training and operational support that officers receive during the course of their duties. Each officer, from those who have little experience to those with many long years of experience, may be confronted with a situation or experience that may result in some psychological trauma. The traditional view is that policing is an inherently difficult occupation, where the stress is experienced by the individual, and so organisations direct their welfare and support services toward that individual. More effective intervention strategies have focussed on providing support to enhance well-being and psychological health through a mixed portfolio of organisational and individually focussed strategies, such as Employee Assistance Programs, peer support, and training designed to improve officers' emotional resilience and recovery. Recent research has tended to implicate the organisation in the psychological harm experienced by many police officers as opposed to their exposure to operational trauma and stress.

References

Aamodt, M.G., & Werlick, N. (2001). Police officer suicide: Frequency and officer profiles. Paper presented at Suicide and Law Enforcement Conference, FBI Academy, Quantico, VA.

Agerbo, E., Gunnell, D., Bonde, J., Mortenson, P.B., & Nordentoft, M. (2007). Suicide and occupation: The impact of socio-economic, demographic and psychiatric differences. *Psychological Medicine*, 37(8), 1131–1140.

American College of Occupational and Environmental Medicine. (2011). *ACOEM guidelines for the medical evaluation of law enforcement officers—Medications section*. Retrieved July 15, 2011, from www.acoem.org/LEOGuidelines.aspx

Armeli, S., Eisenberger, R., Fasolo, P., & Lynch, P. (1998). Perceived organizational support and police performance: The moderating influence of socioeconomic needs. *Journal of Applied Psychology*, 83(2), 288–297.

Aussant, G. (1984). Police suicide. *Royal Canadian Mounted Police Gazette*, 46(5), 14–21.

Barron, S.W. (2007). Police officer suicide—A review and examination using a psychological autopsy. Doctor of Psychology thesis, Charles Sturt University, Bathurst.

Barron, S.W. (2008a). Occupational stress: The emerging threat to police officers. *Journal of Occupational Health and Safety*, 24(6), 553–561.

Barron, S.W. (2008b, August 14–17). Police suicide in Australia. Paper presented at the 116th Annual Convention of the American Psychological Association, Boston.

Barron. S.W. (2010, August). Police officer suicide within the New South Wales Police Force from 1999 to 2008. *Police Practice and Research: An International Journal*, 11(4).

Beautrais, A.L. (2005). National strategies for the reduction and prevention of suicide. *Crisis: The Journal of Crisis Intervention and Suicide Prevention*, 26(1), 1–3.

Benner, A. (2001). Suicide in San Francisco: Lessons learned and preventions. Paper presented at Suicide and Law Enforcement Conference, FBI Academy, Quantico, VA.

Berry, A.R. (2010, Summer). The engagement of senior sergeants in the New Zealand Police. *Australasian Policing: A Journal of Practice and Research*, 2(2), 2–6.

Brent, D.A., Perper, J.A., Kolko, D.J., & Zelenak, J.P. (1988). The psychological autopsy: Methodological considerations for the study of adolescent suicide. *Journal of the American Academy of Child and Adolescent Psychiatry*, 27, 362–366.

Campbell, J.H. (2001). An FBI perspective on law enforcement suicide. Paper presented at Suicide and Law Enforcement Conference, FBI Academy, Quantico, VA.

Campion, M.A. (2001). Police suicide and small departments: A survey. Paper presented at Suicide and Law Enforcement Conference, FBI Academy, Quantico, VA.

Cantor, C., Tyman, R., & O'Brien, D. (1994). *Report to the commissioner, Queensland Police Service on suicide in Queensland Police, 1843–1992*. Brisbane: Queensland Police Service.

Collins, P.A., & Gibbs, A.C.C. (2003). Stress in police officers: A study of the origins, prevalence and severity of stress-related symptoms within a county police force. *Occupational Medicine, 53*, 256–264.

Cooper, C.L. (2001). *Theories of organizational stress*. New York: Oxford University Press.

Curran, P.S., Findlay, R.J. & McGarry, P.J. (1988). Trends in Suicide. *Irish Journal of Psychological Medicine, 5*, 98–102.

Dash, J., & Reiser, M. (1978). Suicide among police in urban law enforcement agencies. *Journal of Police Science and Administration, 3*, 267–273.

Davey, J.D., Obst, P.L., & Sheehan, M.C. (2001). Demographic and workplace characteristics which add to the prediction of stress and job satisfaction within the police workplace. *Journal of Police and Criminal Psychology, 16*(1), 29–39.

Dear, G.E., Thomson, D.M., Hall, G.J., & Howells, K. (1998). *Self-harm in Western Australian prisons: An examination of situational and psychological factors*. Joondalup: School of Psychology, Edith Cowan University.

Friedman, P. (1968). Suicide among police: A study of ninety-three suicides among New York City Policemen 1934–1940. In E. Shneidman (Ed.), *Essays in self-destruction*. New York: Science House, Inc.

Garcia, L., Nesbary, D.K., & Gu, J. (2004). Perceptual variations of stressors among police officers during an era of decreasing crime. *Journal of Contemporary Criminal Justice, 20*(1), 33–50.

Harris, E.C., & Barraclough, B. (1997). Suicide as an outcome for mental disorders: A meta-analysis. *British Journal of Psychiatry, 170*(3), 205–228.

Hart, P.M., & Cotton, P. (2002). Conventional wisdom is often misleading: Police stress within an organisational framework. In M.F. Dollard, H. Winefiled, & H.R. Winefiled (Eds.), *Occupational stress in the service professions*. London: Taylor & Francis.

Harvey, S.B., Henderson, M., Lelliot, P., & Hotopf, M. (2009). Mental health and employment: Much work still to be done. *British Journal of Psychiatry, 194*, 201–203.

Hawgood, J., Klieve, H., Harris, K., & De Leo, D. (2008). *Investigation into New South Wales Police suicide: A review of the Lake Macquarie Local Area Command*. Brisbane: Australian Institute for Suicide Research and Prevention, Griffith University.

Hawton, K., & van Heeringen, K. (Eds.). (2002). *The international handbook of suicide and attempted suicide*. Chichester, UK: Wiley & Sons Ltd.

Hawton, K., & Vislisel, L. (1999). Suicide in nurses. *Suicide and Life-Threatening Behavior, 29*(1), 86–95.

Health and Safety Executive. (2000). The scale of occupational stress. In *The Bristol Stress and Health at Work Study* (Contract Research Report 265/2000, pp. 212–218).

Heiman, M.F. (1975). The police suicide. *Journal of Police Science and Administration*, 3, 267–273.

Hem, E., Berg, A.M., & Ekeberg, O. (2004). Suicide among police. *American Journal of Psychiatry, 161*, 767–768.

Herndon, J.S. (2001). Law enforcement suicide: Psychological autopsies and psychometric traces. Paper presented at Suicide and Law Enforcement Conference, FBI Academy, Quantico, VA.

Hill, K.Q., & Clawson, M. (1988). The health hazards of 'street level' bureaucracy: Mortality among the police. *Journal of Police Science and Administration, 16*, 243–248.

Ivanoff, A. (1994). *The New York City Police Training Project*. New York: Police Foundation, 5–15.

Janik, J., & Kravitz, H.M. (1994). Linking work and domestic problems with police suicide. *Suicide and Life-Threatening Behavior, 24*, 267–274.

Joseph, P.N., Violanti, J.M., Donahue, R., Andrew, M.E., Trevisan, M., Burchfiel, C.M., & Dorn, J. (2009). Police work and subclinical atherosclerosis. *Journal of Occupational Medicine, 51*, 700–707.

Josephson, R.L., & Reiser, M. (1990). Officer suicide in the Los Angeles police department: A twelve year follow-up. *Journal of Police Science and Administration, 17*, 227–229.

Kapusuta, N.D., Voracek, M., Etzerdorfer, E., Niederkrotenthaler, T., Dervic, K., Plener, P.L., Scneider, E., Stein, C., & Sonneck, G. (2010). Characteristics of police officer suicides in the Federal Austrian Police Corps. *Crisis, 31*(5), 265–271.

Kasperczyk, R. (2010). Corporate responsibility for systematic occupational stress prevention. *Journal of Business Systems, Governance and Ethics, 5*(3), 51–70.

Kinman, G., & Jones, F. (2005). Lay representations of workplace stress: What do people really mean when they say they are stressed? *Work and Stress, 19*(2), 101–120.

Klockars, C.B. (1980). The Dirty Harry problem. *The Annals, 452*, 33–47.

Kposowa, A.J. (1999). Suicide mortality in the United States: Differentials by industrial and occupational groups. *American Journal of Industrial Medicine, 36*, 645–652.

Lennings, C.J. (1995). Suicide ideation and risk factors in police officers and justice students. *Police Studies, 18*(3/4), 39–52.

Lester, D. (1993). A study of police suicide in New York City. *Psychological Reports, 73*(3), 1395–1398.

Linehan, M.M., Rizvi, S., Welch, S.S., & Page, B. (2000). Psychiatric aspects of suicidal behaviour: Personality disorders. In K. Hawton & K. van Heeringen (Eds.), *The international handbook of suicide and attempted suicide*. Chichester, UK: Wiley.

Loo, R. (1986). Suicide among police in a federal force. *Suicide and Life-Threatening Behavior, 16*, 379–388.

Loo, R. (2003). A meta-analysis of police suicide rates: Findings and issues. *Journal of Suicide and Life-Threatening Behavior, 33*(3), 313–325.

Martelli, J., Martelli, T., & Waters, L.K. (1989). The police stress survey. *Psychological Reports, 64*, 267–273.

Marzuk, P.M., Nock, M.K., Leon, A.C., Portera, L., & Tardiff, K. (2002). Suicide among New York City police officers, 1977–1996. *American Journal of Psychiatry, 159*(12), 2069–2071.

McCraty, R., Tomasino, D., Atkinson, M., & Sundram, J. (1999). *Impact of the HealthMath self-management skills program on physiological and psychological stress in police officers* (Publication 99-075). Boulder Creek, CA: HeartMath Research Center, Institute of HeartMath.

McCreary, D.R., & Thompson, M.M. (2006). Development of two reliable and valid measures of stressors in policing: The operational and organizational police stress questionnaires. *International Journal of Stress Management, 13*(4), 494–518.

Nelson, Z.P., & Smith, W.E. (1970). The law enforcement profession: An incidence of high suicide. *Omega, 1,* 293–299.

O'Hara, A. (2011). *Police suicides in New Jersey: A gathering storm.* Badge of Life Police Mental Health. Retrieved July 13, 2011, from www.policesuicidestudy.com/id10.html

Parsons, J.R.L. (2004). Occupational health and safety issues of police officers in Canada, the United States and Europe: A review essay. Unpublished master's thesis.

Peterson, C., Park, N & Castro, C.A. (2011). Assessment for the U.S. Army Comprehensive Soldier Fitness program. The Global Assessment Tool. American Psychologist, 66, 10–8.

Raue, J. (1989). Coping with police stress. Report to the Winston Churchill Memorial Trust, Australia.

Richardsen, A.D., Burke, R.J., & Martinussen, M. (2006). Work and health outcomes among police officers: The mediating role of police cynicism and engagement. *International Journal of Stress Management, 13*(4), 555–574.

Robins, E., Gassner, S., Kayes, J., Wilkinson, R.H., & Murphy, G.E. (1959). The communication of suicidal intent: A study of 134 consecutive cases of successful (completed) suicide. *American Journal of Psychiatry, 115,* 724–733.

Sainsbury Centre for Mental Health. (2007, December). *Mental health at work: Developing the business case* (Policy Paper 8).

Seltzer, J., Croxton, R., & Bartholomew, A. (2001). Psychiatric autopsy: Its use in police suicides. Paper presented at Suicide and Law Enforcement Conference, FBI Academy, Quantico, VA.

Sheehan, D.C., & Warren, J.I. (Eds.). (2001). *Suicide in law enforcement.* A compilation of papers submitted to the Suicide and Law Enforcement Conference, FBI Academy, Quantico, VA, September 1999. Washington, DC: Federal Bureau of Investigation.

Shneidman, E.S. (1994). The psychological autopsy. *American Psychologist, 49*(1), 75–76.

Shneidman, E.S. (1996). Clues to suicide reconsidered. *Suicide and Life-Threatening Behavior, 24,* 395–397.

Shneidman, E.S., & Farberow, N. (1965). *The cry for help.* New York: McGraw-Hill.

Slosar, J.R. (2001). The importance of perfectionism in law enforcement suicide. Paper presented at Suicide and Law Enforcement Conference, FBI Academy, Quantico, VA.

Stack, S. (2000). Suicide: A 15 year review of the sociological literature part II: Modernisation and social integration perspectives. *Suicide and Life-Threatening Behavior, 30,* 163–176.

Stack, S., & Kelley, T. (1994). Police suicide: An analysis. *American Journal of Police, 13,* 73–90.

U.S. Department of Defense. (2010, August). *The challenge and the promise: Strengthening the force, preventing suicide and saving lives. The full report.*

Vena, J.E., Violanti, J.M., Marshall, J.R., & Fiedler, R.C. (1986). Mortality of a municipal worker cohort. III. Police officers. *American Journal of Industrial Medicine, 10,* 383–397.

Violanti, J.M. (1995). Trends in police suicide. *Psychological Reports, 77,* 688–690.

Violanti, J.M. (1996). *Police suicide: Epidemic in blue.* Springfield, IL: Thomas C. Thomas.

Violanti, J.M. (2001). Police suicide: Current perspectives and future considerations. Paper presented at Suicide and Law Enforcement Conference, FBI Academy, Quantico, VA.

Violanti, J.M. (2004). Predictors of police suicide ideation. *Suicide and Life-Threatening Behavior, 34*(3), 277–283.

Violanti, J.M., Vena, J.E., & Petralia, S. (1998). Mortality of a police cohort: 1950–1990. *American Journal of Industrial Medicine, 33,* 366–373.

Wagner, M., & Brzeczek, R.J. (1983). Alcoholism and suicide: A fatal connection. *FBI Law Enforcement Bulletin, 52,* 8–15.

Wang, J. (2004). Work stress as a risk factor for major depressive episode(s). *Psychological Medicine, 35,* 865–871.

Wester, S.R., Arndt, D., Sedivy, S.K., & Arndt, L. (2010). Male police officers and stigma associated with counselling: The role of anticipated risks, anticipated benefits and gender role conflict. *Psychology of Men and Masculinity, 11*(4), 286–302.

Winwood, P.C., Tuckey, M.R., Peters, R., & Dollard, M.F. (2009). Identification and measurement of work-related psychological injury: Piloting the Psychological Injury Risk Indicator among frontline police. *Journal of Occupational and Environmental Medicine, 51,* 1057–1065.

Woody, R.H. (2005). The police culture: Research implications for psychological services. *Professional Psychology: Research and Practice, 36*(5), 525–529.

World Health Organisation. (2006). *Preventing suicide: A resource at work.* Geneva: WHO.

Suggested Reading

Allen, K.S. (1986). Suicide and indirect self-destructive behavior among police. In Reese & Goldstein (Eds.), *Psychological services for law enforcement* (pp. 427–429). Washington, DC: U.S. Government Printing Office.

Amsel, L.V., Placidi, G., Hendin, H., O'Neill, M., & Mann, J.J. (2001). An evidence-based educational intervention to improve evaluation and preventive services for officers at risk for suicidal behaviors. Paper presented at Suicide and Law Enforcement Conference, FBI Academy, Quantico, VA.

Association of Chief Police Officers of England, Wales and Northern Ireland. (2009). *Strategy for a healthy police service*. London.

Barraclough, B., Bunch, J., Nelson, B., & Sainsbury, P. (1974). A hundred cases of suicide: Clinical aspects. *British Journal of Psychiatry, 125*, 355–373.

Barron, S.W. (2011). Psychological autopsy review in NSW Police suicide: Expert report. NSW Crown Solicitors Office, Attorney Generals Department (NSW).

Beautrais, A.L. (1998). Risk factors for suicide and attempted suicide amongst young people. In *Learnings about suicide*. Canberra: Commonwealth Department of Health and Aged Care.

Bennett, A.T., & Collins, K.A. (2000). Suicide: A ten-year retrospective study. *Journal of Forensic Science, 45*(6), 1256–1258.

Bonifacio, P. (1991). *The psychological effects of police work: A psychodynamic approach*. New York: Plenum Press.

Bonner, R.L., & Rich, A.R. (1987). Toward a predictive model of suicide ideation and behavior: Some preliminary data in college students. *Suicide and Life-Threatening Behavior, 17*, 50–63.

Brewster, J.A., & Broadfoot, P.A. (2001). Lessons learned: A suicide in a small police department. Paper presented at Suicide and Law Enforcement Conference, FBI Academy, Quantico, VA.

Brown, L., Bonger, B., & Cleary, K.M. (2004). A profile of psychologists views of critical factors for completed suicide in older adults. *Professional Psychology: Research and Practice, 35*(1), 90–96.

Canapary, D., Bonger, B., & Cleary, K.M. (2002). Assessing risk for completed suicide inpatients with alcohol dependence: Clinician's views of critical factors. *Professional Psychology: Research and Practice, 33*(5), 464–469.

Canter, D., Giles, S., & Nicol, C. (2004). Suicide without explicit precursors: A state of secret despair? *Journal of Investigative Psychology and Offender Profiling, 1*, 227–248.

Cavanagh, J.T.O., Carson, A.J., Sharpe, M., & Lawrie, S.M. (2003). Psychological autopsy studies of suicide: A systematic review. *Psychological Medicine, 33*, 395–405.

Cheng, A.T.A., Chen, T.H., Chen, C.C., & Jenkins, R. (2000). Psychosocial and psychiatric risk factors for suicide. Case-control psychological autopsy study. *British Journal of Psychiatry, 177*, 360–365.

Colman, A.M., & Gorman, P.L. (1982). Conservatism, dogmatism and authoritarianism in police officers. *Sociology, 16*, 1–11.

Coman, G.J., Evans, B.J., & Stanley, R.O. (1992). The police personality: Type A behaviour and trait anxiety. *Journal of Criminal Justice, 20*, 429–441.

Conwell, Y., Duberstein, P.R., Cox, C., Hermann, J., Forbes, N.T., & Caine, E.D. (1996). Relationships of age and axis I diagnosis in victims of completed suicide: A psychological autopsy study. *American Journal of Psychiatry, 153*, 1001–1008.

Curphey, T.J. (1968). The psychological autopsy: The role of the forensic pathologist in the multidisciplinary approach to death. *Bulletin of Suicidology, 4*, 39–45.

Danto, B.L. (1978). Police suicide. *Police Stress, 38*, 32–36.

De Leo, D., & Evans, R. (2002). *Suicide in Queensland, 1996–1998: Mortality rates and relevant data*. Brisbane: Australian Institute for Suicide Research and Prevention.

De Leo, D., Hickey, P.A., Neulinger, K., & Cantor, C.H. (1999). *Aging and suicide: A report to the Commonwealth Department of Health and Aged Care*. Australian Institute for Suicide Research and Prevention, Griffith University.

Gibbs, J.P. (Ed.). (1968). *Suicide*. New York: Harper & Row.

Goldney, R.D. (1998). Variation in suicide rates: "The tipping point." *Crisis, 19*, 136–138.

Goldney, R.D. (2005). Suicide prevention: A pragmatic review of recent studies. *Crisis: The Journal of Crisis Intervention and Suicide Prevention, 26*(3), 128–140.

Golembiewski, R.T., & Byong-Soeb, K. (1990). Burnout in police work: Stressors, strain and the phase model. *Police Studies, 13*(2), 74–80.

Hackett, D.P., & Violanti, J.M. (2003). *Police suicide: Tactics for prevention*. Springfield, IL: Charles C. Thomas.

Hassan, R. (1995). *Suicide explained: The Australian experience*. Melbourne: Melbourne University Press.

Hawton, K. (1987). Assessment of suicide. *Journal of Psychiatry, 150*, 145–153.

Howe, B., Marshal, J.R., & Violanti, J.M. (1985). Stress, coping and alcohol use: The police connection. *Journal of Police Science and Administration, 10*, 302–314.

Isometsa, E.T. (2001). Psychological autopsy studies—A review. *European Psychiatry, 16*, 379–385.

Jobes, D.A., Berman, A.L., & Josselson, A.R. (1986). The impact of psychological autopsies on medical examiner's determination of manner of death. *Journal of Forensic Science, 31*, 177–189.

Litman, R.E. (1966). Police aspects of suicide. *Police, 10*, 14–18.

Malloy, T.E., & Mays, G.L. (1984). The police stress hypothesis: A critical evaluation. *Criminal Justice and Behavior, 11*(2), 197–224.

Maris, R.W., Berman, A.L., & Maltsberger, J.T. (1992). *Assessment and prediction of suicide*. London: Guilford Press.

National Coroners Information Service. (2011, August). *Suicide of police officers 01/07/2000–22/08/2011*. Victorian Institute of Forensic Medicine.

National Institute for Health and Medical Research. (2004). *Suicide: Psychological autopsy, a research tool for prevention*.

Nicoletti, J., & Spencer-Thomas, S. (2001). Contamination of cop: Secondary stress of officers responding to civilian suicide. Paper presented at Suicide and Law Enforcement Conference, FBI Academy, Quantico, VA.

Niedderhoffer, A. (1967). *Behind the shield: The police in urban society*. New York: Doubleday Pub.

Patterson, G.T. (2001). The relationship between demographic variables and exposure to traumatic incidents among police officers. *Australasian Journal of Disaster and Trauma Studies*, 2001/2. Retrieved July 2, 201, from http://massey.ac.nz/~trauma/issues/2001–2/patterson.htm

Robins, E. (1981). *The final months. A study of the lives of 134 persons who committed suicide*. New York: Oxford University Press.

Sankey, M. (2003). Suicide and risk-taking deaths of children and young people. NSW Commission for Children and Young People, NSW Child Death Review Team and NSW Centre for Mental Health.

Shneidman, E.S. (1981). The psychological autopsy. *Suicide and Life-Threatening Behavior, 11*, 325–340.

Skolnick, J.H. (1966). *Justice without trial*. New York: Wiley & Sons.

Stanistreet, D., Taylor, S., Jeffrey, V., & Gabbay, M. (2001). Accident or suicide? Predictors of coroner's decisions in suicide and accident verdicts. *Medicine, Science and Law, 41*, 111–115.

Turvey, B.E. (1995). Police officers: Control, hopelessness and suicide. Retrieved December 7, 2011, from http://www.corpus-delecti.com/suicide.html

U.S. Department of Mental Health. (2006). *Erasing the stigma of mental illness.* Retrieved February 22, 2011, from http://www.state.sc.us/dmh/erasing_stigma. htm

Waters, J.A., & Ussery, W. (2007). Police stress: History, contributing factors, symptoms and interventions. *Policing: An International Journal of Police Strategies and Management*, 30(2), 168–188.

The Developing World III

Community Policing and People With Mental Disorders

14

Responding to Developing World Challenges in Papua New Guinea

DUNCAN CHAPPELL

Contents

Prevalence of Mental Disorders, and Policing

The notion that mental disorders are problems of industrialized and relatively richer parts of the world is simply wrong. The belief that rural communities, relatively unaffected by the fast pace of modern life, have no mental disorders is also incorrect.... Surveys conducted in developed as well as developing countries have shown that, during their entire lifetime, more than 25% of individuals develop one or more mental or behavioural disorders. (World Health Organisation (WHO), 2001, p. 23)

It is now widely recognised, as this quotation from a seminal report of the WHO on global mental health trends illustrates, that mental disorders, including "unipolar depressive disorders, bipolar affective disorder, schizophrenia, epilepsy, alcohol and selected drug use disorders, Alzheimer's and other dementias, post-traumatic stress disorder, obsessive and compulsive disorder, panic disorder, and primary insomnia" (WHO, 2001, p. 23), form a significant part of the world's overall disease burden, affecting the lives of hundreds of millions of people. It is also well established that the like-lihood of persons with a mental disorder receiving adequate treatment for their condition is quite slim, and especially so in less well-developed regions and countries of the world (Kessler et al., 2009). As a result, those members of the community experiencing a mental disorder are often left in a vulnerable state without access to employment, housing, and other basic needs (see, for example, Chapter 10 by Andrews and Baldry). In such circumstances many live a precarious and nomadic existence, frequently as "street people," where they come into frequent contact with the police (see Chapter 11).

Police are also asked on many occasions to provide emergency assis-tance to persons experiencing some form of mental health crisis since they are usually the sole agency available for such service delivery on a 24-hour basis. Research conducted across numbers of countries and jurisdictions suggests that somewhere between 5% and 15% of all police engagements with the community involve some form of mental health issue like these (see, for example, Chapter 4 by Donohue and Andrews).

For police, no matter in which country, region, or local community they may be located, these encounters with persons with a mental disorder not only are likely to be commonplace, but also sensitive and potentially chal-lenging. In those settings where police are operating in a free society, these challenges include balancing the protection of the rights of persons with a mental disorder to be dealt with in a humane and respectful manner with the rights of all citizens, including the police, to remain secure from possible violence or disturbance (see, in general, Goldstein, 1977).

To give effect to these responsibilities, most democratically oriented jurisdictions allow their police widespread discretion to take a person believed to be suffering from a mental disorder, and at risk of harm to self or others, to the nearest mental health facility for assessment and possible treat-ment (see, for instance, Chapter 2 by Cotton and Coleman and Chapter 12 by Bronitt and Gath). Whether or not a mental disorder is subsequently diag-nosed remains a medical decision, as does the question whether any treat-ment offered is provided in a hospital or community setting. In an age when most nations have drastically reduced the number of beds available in secure psychiatric hospitals, most persons who receive treatment for a mental dis-order do so in the community. Those who remain undiagnosed or untreated may become involved in a revolving cycle of interactions with the police and the mental health system before ultimately finding themselves entangled in the criminal justice process and being confined in a prison. There is now substantial evidence to suggest that prisons have become, by default, the new place of detention of the mentally ill following the widespread closures of asylums during the later decades of the twentieth century (see, for instance, Health Sociology Review, 2005).

Focus on the Developing World

Within this broad context, this chapter is concerned with the particular challenges that confront police in the developing world when interacting with persons with a mental disorder. This focus is justified in large part by the knowledge, much of it referred to and summarised in the earlier chapters of this book, that a quite substantial literature now exists regarding the manner in which police in various parts of the developed world seek to meet these challenges. In marked contrast, very little has been said or documented about the subject in less developed nations.

This approach is also justified by the realisation that so much of the dialogue about mental disorders and their diagnosis and treatment is linked to Western concepts and practises when in reality such approaches almost certainly do not reflect a universal view held among the countries and populations that make up the total global community (see, in general, Al-Issa, 1995). Thus, in a comprehensive overview conducted in 2005 by the WHO of the status of mental health legislation around the world, and its protection of human rights, it was determined that only 75% of countries had such legislation (WHO, 2005b). Of these, about one-half had legislation post-1990, and 15% pre-1960. Among the nations without comprehensive mental health legislation was China, the most populace country in the world. As the WHO emphasised:

> The fundamental aim of mental health legislation is to protect, promote and improve the lives and mental well-being of citizens. In the undeniable context that every society needs laws to achieve its objectives, mental health legislation is no different from any other legislation. (WHO, 2005b, p. 3)

Clearly, in nations lacking any mental health legislation, the exercise of police power or that of any other authority over persons with a mental disorder is likely to be both haphazard and arbitrary. Even where such legislation is in place, the way in which it is administered by the authorities, including the police, will almost certainly be influenced by prevailing community attitudes and beliefs regarding mental illness. It is well documented that in many societies, whether developed or not, both stigma and fear are still commonplace reactions toward persons with a mental disorder (Arboleda-Flórez, 2001). Overcoming such attitudes and beliefs represents but one of the significant challenges to be faced by many communities, and especially by the police who serve those communities and are supposed in democratic societies to uphold the rule of law in a neutral and impartial manner.

The balance of this chapter is intended to explore the way in which police interact with persons with a mental disorder in a developing nation, Papua

New Guinea (PNG), which is a vibrant democracy, and which does have mental health legislation in place. The aim is to at least give some glimpses of the challenges, and especially those relating to human rights, which confront police in settings that are quite far removed from those described in the extant policing literature on this topic. The choice of PNG is influenced by its closeness to Australia, where the author is based, and by the ongoing and large-scale involvement of Australian foreign aid agencies, including police, in a country that remained a colony of its southern neighbour until gaining full independence in 1975.

PNG: Context

PNG now has an estimated population of around 7 million persons, most of whom live in scattered and isolated rural areas of the country where access is mainly by air or foot. One of the world's most ethnically diverse nations, with an estimated 800 language groups, PNG is ranked by the World Bank as a lower- to middle-income group country, with recent mineral and related resource developments providing a larger source of revenue than in the past (United Nations PNG, 2010; World Bank, 2012). Even so, it is estimated that 40% of the population live on less than USD $1 per day and 75% of households depend entirely on subsistence agriculture. The country contributes about 4.4% of its gross domestic product (GDP) to the health budget. The proportion of the health budget spent on mental health is 0.7%, with about 0.24 psychiatric bed per 10,000 population, and 0.09 psychiatrist and 1.2 psychiatric nurses per 100,000 population (see WHO, 2005a, pp. 365–367). The country does have a mental health law inherited from the colonial era, but it has not been revised since 1985 (WHO, 2005b).

Impact of Traditional Beliefs and Culture

Traditional remedies based on cultural beliefs concerning the causes of mental illness remain an important part of health care in PNG, as they do in many other developing countries (see Chapter 15 by Beaupert). In PNG these cultural beliefs are widely centred around sorcery, witchcraft, spirit possessions, and supernatural agents (Koka et al., 2004, pp. 29–30). Sorcery and witchcraft beliefs and practises continue to be feared for their power and influence even among certain tertiary educated members of PNG society, including health professionals. For instance, in a survey conducted in 2004 of final year medical students at the University of PNG (Muga & Hagali, 2006), several students indicated that they believed mental illness could be caused by sorcery, or even by spending much time with the mentally ill. As a group, the students had a negative attitude toward close social contact with them as a neighbour or as in-laws. Most students said that they believed mental illness could be cured by prayer, one in five believed in the effectiveness of traditional healers, and one in five believed modern medicine could not treat mental illness. Apart from a reduction in stigma and in prejudice against a mentally ill neighbour, there was also no significant difference in attitude between students who had been rotated in psychiatry and those who had not (Muga & Hagali, 2006).

No similar systematic attitudinal studies appear to have been conducted with PNG police, but it seems reasonable to assume that they too share the cultural beliefs of many of their fellow citizens about the association of sorcery and witchcraft with mental illness. For instance, during a recent programme on sorcery-related killings in a PNG broadcast on Radio Australia, a senior police officer from the West Sepik region of the country acknowledged his belief in the powers of sorcerers to cause the death of individuals. He described these fatal sorcery practises in the following way:

> Something like grass they have grown in their backyard and they have something where they use that's the evil thing and kill the people. When you throw [your rubbish] they pick it up, and then they take it to where they've got their things, and they just put them in a hole or heat it in the fire and then you get sick and you don't have medicine, you pass away. (ABC Radio Australia, 2012, p. 1)

The commission of an act of sorcery remains a criminal offence in PNG, and sorcery's customary influence and widespread practise has been given statutory recognition by the Sorcery Act 1971 (PNG Law Reform Commission, 1977). While there are now moves afoot to repeal this legislation, with a report and recommendation to this effect from PNG's Constitutional Law Reform Commission currently being considered by the PNG Government (ABC Radio Australia, 2012), it at present allows a claim of being affected or influenced by sorcery to be used as a defence or partial excuse to certain criminal offences (see Chalmers, Weisbrot, & Andrew, 2001).

It is acknowledged that the perception of death by sorcery continues to be regarded as one of the principal precipitants of much of the tribal fighting and unrest in a number of areas of PNG (Chalmers et al., 2001, p. 604). Even more disturbing is the suggestion in recent reports by Amnesty International that in certain parts of PNG persons believed to be sorcerers or witches, including some who were suffering from a mental illness, have been brutally killed (Amnesty International, 2009a, 2009b). The PNG police reported that in 2008 there were 50 such murders, a figure that critics claimed seriously underestimated the extent of such killings, the majority of which involved female victims and very few of which were either brought to the attention of police or investigated by them (Kinjap, 2008; *The Age*, 2009).

PNG Police and the Mentally Ill

Policing in PNG is the sole responsibility of the Royal Papua and New Guinea Constabulary (RPNGC), with a sworn personnel of about 5,000 members (see Government of PNG Institute of National Affairs, 2004). There are no known published research and allied studies that provide a direct account of the way in which the RPNGC—a poorly educated, trained, and resourced law enforcement body that is heavily dependent on overseas technical assistance and aid, largely provided by Australia (Australian Government AusAID, 2010)—manages its encounters with mentally ill citizens. Like most of their counterparts in the developed world, the PNG police have extensive powers to apprehend, detain, and refer for treatment persons believed to have a mental illness. Thus, Section 110 of the PNG Public Health Act 1973 provides:

> (1) A commissioned officer of the Police Force shall arrest any person—
>   (a) found wandering at large whom he reasonably suspects of being of unsound mind; or
>   (b) whom he suspects of being dangerous by reason of unsoundness of mind, and bring him without delay before two medical practitioners, one of whom is a Medical Officer.
> (2) The medical practitioners shall separately examine a person brought before them under Subsection (1) and, if satisfied that the person is of unsound mind, shall each make an order in Form 2.
> (3) When orders are made under Subsection (2) by both of the medical practitioners examining a person, the commissioned officer of the Police Force shall send him, in suitable custody, to the mental hospital specified in the orders, and in any other case the person shall be discharged.

There are no statistics available regarding the frequency of use by the RPNGC of these somewhat archaically defined powers, nor of the outcome of assessment referrals to medical practitioners. However, as noted earlier, WHO descriptions of the public health resources devoted to mental health in PNG indicate that the availability of psychiatric and nursing staff to undertake assessment and treatment is extremely limited. Further, in a scathing report released in 2011 by the United Nations Human Rights Council's (UNHRC) special rapporteur on torture, following a mission to PNG, severe criticism was made of the police facilities and practises regarding the detention of persons, including those with disabilities (UNHRC, 2011). In the course of his inspections of police lockups the special rapporteur found a number of mentally ill persons who had been detained for extensive periods in shocking conditions. He concluded that:

Psychiatric support in detention facilities did not comply with international minimum standards. Psychiatric evaluations were not performed on a routine basis or in an independent and professional manner; as a result, many detainees with both physical and mental disabilities in correctional institutions and police lock-ups have no access to adequate medical treatment and rehabilitation. At the Mount Hagen and the Buka police stations, the Special Rapporteur found detainees with mental disabilities locked in police cells. In Buka, one detainee had been held for 18 months, without ever having had access to a psychiatrist or a lawyer. At the Baisu correctional institution, at least five mentally ill detainees were held together with the general population. (UNHRC, 2011, p. 14)

The special rapporteur also visited the sole psychiatric facility in the country for persons with mental disabilities—the Laloki Psychiatric Hospital located in PNG's capital city, Port Moresby. He described the hospital as being very old and in poor condition. Plans were in place to build a new facility, but no funds were available for construction. The hospital had no resident or permanent psychiatrist, relying instead on sporadic visits by local psychiatrists.

Effecting Change

In the current policing and mental health environment in PNG that has been described, albeit in brief, the challenges for those seeking change are clearly enormous. As a result of the special rapporteur's report, the RPNGC has been engaged in an extensive training programme designed to enhance its knowledge of and commitment to basic human rights norms and values (United Nations PNG, 2010). This training appears to be of a general nature and not intended to tackle the specific issues associated with the management of interactions between the police and persons with a mental illness where culturally driven fear, prejudice, and stigma remain confronting issues.

There is also a massive resource gap in the delivery of health services in PNG, including those related to mental health. As health workers have observed, in the absence of adequate public mental health treatment facilities either in hospitals or in the community, the principle burden of care delivery falls upon families (Koka et al., 2004, p. 39). It is families who must maintain and assist a mentally ill relative in the local community without assistance from the government health system. It is only when that relative becomes aggressive or violent that a call for specialist help is likely to be made. Even so, in urban areas the majority of the mentally ill seem left to cope as best they can on the streets, while in rural communities there would seem to be a growing reluctance among families and local residents, driven partly by fear and prejudice, to accept responsibility for caring for the mentally ill (Noble, 1997, p. 115).

The increasing use of police diversion of mentally ill persons into the health system, a practise that has received encouragement in numbers of developed nations, appears to be a remote possibility in PNG with the very thinly spread mental health treatment facilities available throughout the nation seemingly already overwhelmed by the demand for services (Noble, 1997; WHO, 2005a). Instead, there is a risk that increasing reliance will be placed upon potentially unsafe or ineffective traditional treatments, including sorcery, with herbal medicines, animal sacrifices, rituals, and counselling being administered by local healers (Koka et al., 2004). The PNG Health Department is not adverse to promoting traditional medicine but has excluded sorcery and witchcraft-related practises as forms of traditional treatment because they are believed to be inherently dangerous practises and should not be given any legitimacy (PNG Department of Health, 2000). More recently the WHO, in its regional strategy for the Western Pacific region on the recognition of traditional medicine, has set the following five key strategic objectives for the period 2011–2020:

- To include traditional medicine in the national health system
- To promote safe and effective use of traditional medicine
- To increase access to safe and effective traditional medicine
- To promote protection and sustainable use of traditional medicine resources
- To strengthen cooperation in generating and sharing traditional medicine knowledge and skills (WHO, 2012)

It remains to be seen how these objectives will be given effect in the area of mental health in Western Pacific countries like PNG, but some accommodations seem likely between traditional healers and the regular health system, if only to assist in the early identification and referral for treatment of persons in the community who are experiencing the symptoms of a serious mental disorder. At the same time, changing the community beliefs and practises surrounding mental illnesses that have been described in PNG will clearly be a Herculean task in a society where the rule of law is extremely fragile, and the nation is already struggling to cope with other pressing health problems, including an HIV/AIDS epidemic (Australian Government AusAID, 2006). It is also a challenge that is almost certainly not limited to PNG. Similar cultural beliefs and practises have, for example, been reported from certain parts of Africa (see Chapter 15) where superstition, fear, and discrimination continue to surround interactions between the mentally ill and the rest of society.

Some encouragement about the possibility of bringing about positive change may, however, be secured from the knowledge that a belief in witchcraft, and the notion that the mentally ill were possessed by the devil, which dominated European and early American thought several centuries ago and resulted in the persecution and death of tens of thousands of people, did give way eventually to the more humane and acceptable treatment of mental illness sufferers (see, in general, Porter, 2002). We cannot, however, wait for decades to see such improvement in countries like PNG, where there is credible evidence of severe maltreatment of such persons, including their brutal murder. These crimes, which at present seem to go undetected or unpunished, have no place in a country committed to democratic principles and upholding the rule of law.

References

ABC Radio Australia. (2012, January 24). Call for PNG to repeal sorcery act after West Sepik deaths. Retrieved September 22, 2012, from http://www.radioaustralia. net.au/international/radio/onairhighlights/call-for-png-to-repeal-sorcery-act-after-west-sepik-deaths

The Age. (2009, January 12). PNG to toughen laws on sorcery killings. Retrieved September 22, 2012, from http://news.theage.com.au/world/png-to-toughen-laws-on-sorcery-killings-20090112-7f2y.html

Al-Issa, I. (1995). Handbook of culture and mental illness—An international perspective. Madison: International Universities Press.

Amnesty International. (2009a). Amnesty International report 2009—Papua New Guinea. Retrieved September 22, 2012, from http://www.unhcr.org/refworld/docid/4a1fadccc.html

Amnesty International. (2009b, February 11). Increasing sorcery-related killings in Papua New Guinea. Retrieved September 22, 2012, from http://www.amnesty.org/en/news-and-updates/news/increasing-sorcery-related-killings-papua-new-guinea-20090211

Arboleda-Flórez, J. (2001). Stigmatization and human rights violations. In WHO (Ed.), Mental health: A call for action by world health ministers. Geneva: WHO.

Australian Government AusAID. (2006). Impact of HIV/AIDS 2005–2025 in Papua New Guinea, Indonesia and East Timor. Canberra: Australian Government AusAID.

Australian Government AusAID. (2010). Papua New Guinea. Retrieved September 22, 2012, from http://www.ausaid.gov.au/country/papua.cfm

Chalmers, D., Weisbrot, D., & Andrew, W. (2001). Criminal law and practice of Papua New Guinea (3rd ed.). North Ryde, NSW: Law Book Co.

Goldstein, H. (1977). Policing a free society. Cambridge, MA: Ballinger Publishing Company.

Government of PNG Institute of National Affairs. (2004). Report of the Royal Papua New Guinea Constabulary Administrative Review Committee to the Minister for Internal Security Hon. Bire Kimisopa. Retrieved September 22, 2012, from http://www.inapng.com/Police%20Review%20Report%20final.pdf

Health Sociology Review. (2005). Closing asylums for the mentally Ill: Social consequences. Sydney: Content Pty Ltd.

Kessler, R., Haro, J., Huang, Y., Ormel, J., Scott, K., Schoenbaum, M., & Alonso, J. (2009, April 18). The WHO World Mental Health Survey Initiative IFPE Congress, Vienna Austria. Retrieved September 22, 2012, from http://www.hcp.med.harvard.edu/wmh/IFPE_WMH.pdf

Kinjap, P. (2008, January 3). Sorcery and witchcraft beliefs remain prevalent in Papua New Guinea. *The National*. Retrieved September 22, 2012, from http://www.religionnewsblog.com/20258/witchcraft-11

Koka, B. E., Deane, F. P., & Lambert, G. (2004). Health worker confidence in diagnosing and treating mental health problems in Papua New Guinea. *South Pacific Journal of Psychology, 15*, 29–42.

Muga, M., & Hagali, M. (2006). What do final year medical students at the University of Papua New Guinea think about psychiatry? *PNG Medical Journal, 49*(3–4), 126–136.

Noble, F. (1997). Long-term psychiatric care in Papua New Guinea. *Psychiatric Bulletin, 21*, 113–116.

Papua New Guinea Law Reform Commission (PNGLRC). (1977). *Sorcery* (Occasional Paper 4). Port Moresby: PNGLRC.

Papua New Guinea National Department of Health. (2000). *National health plan 2001–2010; Health vision 2010; Program policies and strategies* (Vol. II). Port Moresby: Papua New Guinea National Department of Health.

Porter, R. (2002). *Madness. A brief history.* Oxford: Oxford University Press.

United Nations Human Rights Council (UNHRC). (2011). *Report of the special rapporteur on torture and other cruel, inhuman or degrading treatment or punishment, addendum: Mission to Papua New Guinea* (A/HRC/16/52/Add.5). Retrieved September 22, 2012, from http://www.unhcr.org/refworld/docid/4d8718932.html

United Nations Papua New Guinea. (2010). *United Nations Papua New Guinea annual progress report 2010*. Retrieved September 22, 2012, from mdtf.undp.org/document/download/6821

World Bank. (2012). Papua New Guinea overview. Retrieved September 23, 2012, from http://www.worldbank.org/en/country/png/overview

World Health Organisation (WHO). (2001). *The world health report 2001. Mental health: New understanding, new hope.* Geneva: WHO.

World Health Organisation (WHO). (2005a). *Mental health atlas 2005.* Geneva: WHO.

World Health Organisation (WHO). (2005b). *WHO resource book on mental health, human rights and legislation.* Geneva: WHO.

World Health Organisation (WHO). (2012). *The regional strategy for traditional medicine in the Western Pacific (2011–2020).* Geneva: WHO. Retrieved September 23, 2012, from http://www.wpro.who.int/publications/2012/regionalstrategyfortraditionalmedicine_2012.pdf

Reflections on Policing and Mental Health in Africa

15

Integrating and Regulating Diverse Healing and Policing Systems

FLEUR BEAUPERT

Contents

This chapter will consider challenges relating to mental health and policing in Africa. Although there are dangers when generalising across the African continent, this chapter nonetheless speaks about Africa as a whole, while taking examples from individual countries. As will be seen, there is a paucity of literature dealing directly with the topic of mental health and policing in Africa. Thus, the literature as it relates singularly to mental health and to policing has been examined with a view to identifying relevant issues requiring further attention in moving toward better police responses to people with mental illness.

The first section of the chapter outlines the mental health services and policy context, the second addresses the role of traditional healers in systems of care, and the third turns attention to policing systems. The need to enhance and optimise collaboration between mental health services and the police through proactive policy is increasingly recognised. While it is unclear to what extent such an approach is being implemented in African countries, concrete steps have been taken to this end in South Africa—the focus of the final section. It is suggested that the roles of traditional healers and nonstate police warrant careful consideration within intersectoral collaboration.

Mental Health Services, Policies, and Legislation

Police interactions with people with mental illness pose unique challenges in African countries, where there is still much to be done to develop and deliver effective health services at large, including those relating to mental health. Research is needed to identify the incidence and type of interactions between police officers and people with mental illness in the African context, where policies governing the provision of care at both the institutional level and in community facilities are still in the process of being developed. Insights from literature from other parts of the world provide a starting point when considering how to develop effective policies to regulate how police interact with people with mental illness in Africa. It is evident that mental health crisis situations are dealt with more effectively when there is close formal liaison between police services and mental health systems (Wolff, 1998). In the African context there is a need for reform of general health and connected service systems, incorporating broader mental health policy planning, to ensure that service systems support appropriate police responses to people with mental illness.

Upon encountering a person suspected of having a mental illness, police officers have to make a decision about whether the person is likely to have a mental illness and how best to deal with that person. There are at least two broad categories of situations in which police may deal with people with mental illness: (1) during mental health crises or psychiatric emergencies, and (2) when people with mental health problems are engaged in conflict, violence, or criminal acts (either as offender or victim). Police may try to diffuse the situation using informal tactics. Where this approach does not work, they may decide to intervene by taking the person to a mental health service, and they may have to decide also whether or not to exercise their discretion to deal with the matter as a criminal one (Lamb, Weinberger, & DeCuir, 2002, p. 1267). If it is considered necessary to take the person into custody, there is the question of appropriate assessments being carried out and care being provided. Due to the major shortcomings of mental health services in most African countries, the options available to police may be restricted.

Mental health is increasingly being recognised as a crucial public health and development issue for low- and middle-income countries. Unfortunately, mental health often loses out in competition with other social, economic, and health problems—such as poverty eradication (which is, for example, given priority in Uganda), combatting disadvantage due to apartheid in South Africa, and (in a number of African countries) communicable disease, especially HIV/AIDS (Omar et al., 2010). However, the World Health Organisation (WHO) has recently supported the inclusion of mental health in development strategies, noting that people with mental health conditions have been largely overlooked as a target of development work despite their vulnerability (WHO, 2010). Many of the development problems confronting African countries, such as income poverty (Mental Health and Poverty Project, 2010), poor education, environmental degradation, poor housing, and lack of basic services (Skeen, Lund, Kleintjes, Flisher, & Mental Health and Poverty Research Programme Consortium, 2010, pp. 627–628), also pose an ongoing problem in broader efforts to protect mental health. Many African countries are experiencing or coming out of a stage of conflict or civil war and are home to groups of displaced peoples—situations that may also exacerbate psychological stress and mental illness (Miller & Rassmussen, 2009).

The stigma surrounding mental illness in African countries adds to the burden for people with mental health problems and their carers. Poor levels of understanding of the causes of mental illness and negative attitudes to mental illness were found to be prevalent in Nigeria, for example (Gureje, Lasebikan, Ephraim-Oluwanuga, Olley, & Kola, 2005). Ugandan research has also emphasised the stigma attaching to mental illness in Africa due to associations with disgrace and loss of respect, and even indicated that psychiatric facilities themselves can be a major source of stigma (Nsereko et al., 2011). In Zambia, stigmatising and discriminatory attitudes toward mental illness are common among primary health care providers (Kapungwe et al., 2011). Lack of mental health facilities, especially in rural areas, can mean that families struggle to manage disturbed and sometimes aggressive relatives and resort to abusive management strategies. A number of problematic practises were revealed by research on treatment of people with mental illness in rural Ghana: Almost all those encountered had been chained at home or within healing centres (Read, Adiiboka, & Nyame, 2009).

Part of the complexity surrounding mental illness in African countries relates to community beliefs attributing mental illness to supernatural causes such as sorcery and witchcraft (among others), as established by research in Nigeria (Abiodun, Adewuya, & Makanjuola, 2008, p. 394), and in Ghana, where the view that madness is a punishment for transgressions and moral failings is also common (Read et al., 2009). The way in which police approach and interact with people with mental illness is likely to be influenced by officers' personal attitudes and beliefs (Lamb et al., 2002). The question of the extent to which views of police officers align with such broadly held community beliefs, and how this in turn may affect their treatment of people with mental illness, requires research. Providing the police with training about mental health issues and the mental health system with which they are expected to work may go some way toward counteracting negative stereotypes associated with mental illness, while increasing police officers' confidence in their ability to deal with people with mental illness (Compton, Bahora, Watson, & Oliva, 2006). Such training could potentially be achieved through arrangements between police and mental health services. However, broader community education is equally necessary as a long-term goal and may be the only way to minimise stigma and discrimination, including among police officers (Chappell, 2008, p. 46).

Only 53% of African countries have mental health policies (WHO, 2005), and in those countries that have them, the policies are at different stages of development and are generally poorly implemented (Omar et al., 2010). Where mental health policies or programmes do exist, their execution may be hindered by lack of resources or budget (especially a lack of dedicated budgets for mental health at the district level), lack of relevant guidelines, lack of training for health professionals, and even lack of awareness among health professionals and others as to the existence of these policy guidelines—as found by a review of data relating to mental health services in Uganda, Ghana, and South Africa (Bhana, Peterson, Baillie, Flisher, & Mental Health and Poverty Research Programme Consortium, 2010, pp. 602–603).

South Africa has a fairly well-developed set of policy guidelines for mental health services that has been in place since 1997, but these guidelines are not recognised as national policy, and are rather broad in their approach and intended to inform development of policy in the provinces (Draper et al., 2009). Implementation of these guidelines is uneven across provinces, and provincial and district mental health in particular is very underresourced (Bhana et al., 2010). Uganda has far fewer specialist mental health services than South Africa, but it should be borne in mind that a number of positive steps have been taken to improve its mental health care system in comparison to other developing countries. A national mental health programme was initiated in 1996, and the National Policy and Health Sector Strategic Plan launched in 1999–2000 strengthened this programme (Nsereko et al., 2011). However, mental health services are very poorly funded, and there are few or no guidelines to ensure implementation of the draft national mental health policy; until recently, mental health services were only available at the national mental health hospital (Bhana et al., 2010).

National health budgets in African countries are very low compared to those in developed countries. In many African countries 1% or less of health budgets is spent on mental health (Ghana is a notable exception, devoting 6% of its health budget to mental health in 2010) (Omar et al., 2010), and such budgets mostly support stand-alone custodial psychiatric institutions in urban centres, with little devoted to community mental health services. Lack of specialist mental health professionals is also a significant problem: There is, on average, only 1 psychiatrist per million population, 1 psychiatric nurse per 250,000 population, and psychiatric social workers and psychologists are a rarity (Bartlett, Jenkins, & Kiima, 2011). Moreover, loss of mental health specialists to high-income countries, or "brain drain," is an ongoing dilemma (Bartlett et al., Bhana et al., 2010, p. 608). Uganda has 28 psychiatrists for a population of 33 million people (Kiwawulo, 2010). Kenya has 23 psychiatrists in public service, and only 1 or 2 psychiatric nurses per district of around 150,000 (Jenkins et al., 2010, p. 38).

Given the shortage of mental health care specialists, integration of mental health into primary care is an essential measure. A number of African countries have made systematic efforts to integrate mental health into primary care settings, through training primary care workers to deliver mental health services under the supervision of district-level mental health staff, most usually psychiatric nurses (Bartlett et al., 2011). Kenya ran a successful national primary care training project from 2005 to 2010, which will now be continued on a long-term basis (Jenkins et al., 2010). However, in other African countries primary health care systems do not make adequate provision for the needs of people with mental illness, despite governments endorsing this approach at the policy level (Bhana et al., 2010). The number of psychiatric beds is very low, particularly outside urban centres. Accessing mental health services in rural areas is extremely difficult and generally requires substantial travel, which is not easy due to limited public transport infrastructure. Police in rural areas may therefore not be in a position to easily transport people with mental illness to mental health facilities in urban centres, without detracting from what are considered core police duties.

There should ideally be a legal framework setting out police responsibilities toward people with mental illness in certain situations, such as the responsibility to transport a person meeting certain criteria to mental health services. Many African countries do not, however, have mental health legislation or other laws to clarify police obligations and guide the exercise of their discretion. In those countries that do have such legislation, it is generally what may be described as a colonial inheritance, although some countries, such as South Africa and Tanzania, have enacted modern mental health legislation. South Africa's Mental Health Care Act 2002, which dictates certain police obligations in relation to people with mental illness, came into force on December 15, 2004, and is broadly consistent with international human rights standards and principles. Uganda's Mental Health Act, on the other hand, is very outdated, having been last revised in 1964. Even where new mental health legislation has been passed, such as in Kenya, there remains the problem of incomplete implementation due to lack of funding (Bartlett et al., 2011).

On the positive side, a number of advances in mental health policy and legislation have been made over the last few years, due in part to the work of the Mental Health and Poverty Project (MHaPP) operating in Ghana, South Africa, Uganda, and Zambia, with the object of developing, implementing, and evaluating mental health policy. A new mental health bill was developed in Ghana, a first-draft national mental health policy has been developed and circulated to the provinces for consultation in South Africa, and a new mental health bill and draft national Mental Health Policy and Strategic Plan have been written and are awaiting adoption in Uganda (Mental Health and Poverty Project, 2010, p. 8).

Traditional and Faith Healers: Toward a Collaborative Approach?

In most African countries, ways of healing people with mental health problems are shared between conventional mental health services using a biomedical approach and traditional and faith healing systems (Ae-Ngibise et al., 2010, p. 558). Traditional healers, according to WHO, use

> diverse health practices, approaches, knowledge and beliefs incorporating plant, animal and/or mineral based medicines, spiritual therapies, manual techniques and exercises applied singularly or in combination to maintain well-being, as well as to treat, diagnose or prevent illness. (WHO, 2002, p. 7)

Faith healers attached to churches, who work from "prayer camps" or healing centres, treat diseases through prayer, fasting, and sprinkling of holy waters. Given that traditional and faith healers may be the first port of call for many, one issue for the development of policies regarding how police deal with people with mental illnesses is the extent to which healers do and should form part of a collaborative intersectoral approach, especially given that biomedical services may be particularly difficult to access in rural areas.

Traditional healers bear a large burden of care of patients with mental illness. WHO estimates that up to 80% of the African population uses traditional medicine (WHO, 2002, p. 1). In Ghana traditional healers far outnumber medical doctors and psychiatrists, and 70% of people, especially those living in rural areas, consult one of the 45,000 traditional healers in the country for mental health problems (Ae-Ngibise et al., 2010, pp. 558–559). Many people with mental health problems in Uganda also seek help from traditional healers in the first instance, and interviews with stakeholders found that even where a traditional healer refers clients to conventional health facilities, clients are likely to try another traditional healer—lacking faith in the ability of conventional psychiatric treatment to help them (Nsereko et al., 2011). In many African countries attribution of mental illness to supernatural or spiritual causes (witchcraft or evil forces) is common, and traditional healers are believed to be able to target such causes directly. There are concerns that such beliefs may lead to the development of untreated or chronic illness in the case of individuals where traditional healers are consulted first and there is delay in seeking help from mental health services (Aina, 2004, p. 25), and the efficacy of traditional remedies has not been studied (Kale, 1995).

Interestingly, however, aside from any perceived benefit that may be derived from traditional healing due to a perception that it is better able to target the root cause of the illness, Ugandan research has revealed that traditional healers were also preferred because they were perceived as having better counselling and listening skills. They were also said to treat patients with much more care than conventional mental health services, which were claimed to involve brief and hostile encounters (Nsereko et al., 2001)—a not surprising outcome given the very low clinician-to-client ratio within biomedical health services in most African countries. A number of studies corroborate this finding about the value placed on traditional healers because of the immense psychosocial support they provide (Hewson, 1998; Meissner, 2004; Tanner, 1999; Van der Beest, 1997). Aside from these factors, traditional healers are much more accessible than conventional mental health facilities, especially in rural areas.

Given the prevalence and popularity of traditional healers, there have been initiatives in some African countries to foster collaboration between traditional healers and biomedical services, beginning with an international commitment made by the WHO in 1978 to promote the inclusion of traditional healers in health programmes. More recently the WHO and member states aim to collaborate to support and integrate traditional medicine into national health systems, ensure the use of safe and quality products and practises, and acknowledge traditional medicine as part of primary health care (WHO, 2008). Such measures at the national level have included recognition and regulation of traditional healers under mental health legislation, as in Ghana, although attempts to integrate effectively the workings of traditional and biomedical healing systems have so far been largely unsuccessful in that country (Ae-Ngibise et al., 2010, p. 559). The South African Traditional Health Practitioners Act 2007 provides for setting up of a Traditional Health Practitioners Council to regulate traditional healing. Formalising traditional healing and ensuring oversight by the council is complicated by the plurality of traditional healing associations that may not be linked to the council (Dickinson, 2008, p. 284).

In South Africa the relationships between traditional and Western healing systems are complex. Despite lack of formal structured mechanisms for collaboration, the help-seeking behaviour exhibited by many people suggests that biomedical mental health services and traditional services are largely integrated in people's minds. Interviews with South African service users indicated that while they offer mainly traditional healing explanations for mental illness, two-thirds of those interviewed reported using both systems of healing at different times (Peterson et al., 2009, p. 146). Psychiatric nurses themselves will often be in a position of having to negotiate and reconcile two sets of belief systems—traditional beliefs absorbed from early childhood and those learned through their psychiatric training. Most adopt a position of coexistence (Kahn & Kelly, 2001, p. 37). According to both traditional healers and practitioners from mental health services, however, there is inadequate liaison between their two systems, despite willingness among traditional healers to incorporate Western medicine in their care plans (Peterson et al., 2009, p. 146).

Arguments against collaborative strategies relate to concerns that some traditional healers operate without oversight and may engage in one or all of exploitation vis-à-vis a money-poor and uneducated clientele; abusive practises, including chaining and beating people (Ae-Ngibise et al., 2010, p. 562); or the use of potentially toxic ingredients in medication (Sorsdahl, Flisher, Wilson, & Stein, 2010). Research on the treatment of mental illness in rural Ghana uncovered the common perception among traditional healers that mental illness is a punishment for moral failings as well as the use of beatings for disciplinary purposes, or to rid people of evil spirits (Read et al., 2009). On the other hand, some traditional healers may adopt a more complex position than popular beliefs that mental illness is caused by supernatural phenomena: A small group of traditional healers who participated in South African research revealed that they "saw their role not as witch finders but as healers helping to ease accusations of witchcraft within communities" (Dickinson, 2008, p. 285).

Most commentators agree that the answer is to regulate and foster links between traditional and biomedical services, rather than to suppress or condemn traditional healing altogether, in light of the reality of the coexistence of the two systems of care and management for some time to come. Measures should include exchange of information, developing referral procedures, and generally developing mutually respectful relationships between the two systems (Burns, Jhazbhay, & Emsley, 2011). The interaction between mental health services and traditional and faith healers deserves attention and reflection in the process of developing more appropriate police responses to people with mental illness and enhancing and optimising collaboration between police and mental health services. There is likely great variation in the beliefs and practises of traditional healers, and attempts to integrate them into any such collaborative efforts would need to be developed within individual communities and subject to careful regulation. Research may be needed in particular to examine interactions between police and traditional healers in the many rural areas with few or no mental health services.

Policing, Nonstate Policing, and Training

Effective policing practises depend to a large degree upon the nature of the political and socioeconomic environment prevailing in a country (Hills, 1996). In recent times some African countries, such as Somalia, have lacked a regular police system altogether, owing to the absence of any effective government (Hills, 1997, p. 46). Many countries are at different points in the spectrum of development or reconstruction post-war and civil strife, and the greater the strife, the greater the likelihood that the focus of the police becomes maintenance of civil order—in particular targeting violence seen as threatening political stability—rather than, for example, general crime control and maintenance of justice (Hills, 1996). Given this focus, coupled with scarce resources, the issue of policing and mental health is likely to be given a low priority.

Establishing a sufficient police presence to provide policing services across the whole of each country is of fundamental concern, with rural areas particularly neglected (Baker, 2006, p. 44). As Baker writes, "many African governments have been unable to enforce law because they have struggled to establish order" (Baker, 2006, p. 26). Even so, it is important to consider how police services that do exist in African countries can slowly start to develop more proactive policy and practises in relation to interactions with people with mental illness. The possible role of nonstate police should arguably be factored into such an assessment: Nonstate justice systems often play a prominent role in post-conflict societies where state systems are not functioning properly, and are widespread across the African continent (OECD, 2007, p. 195).

The prevalence of nonstate policing in African countries raises questions about the state's ability to encourage nonstate police to respond more appropriately to people with a mental illness, or possibly to require them to do so. Part of the difficulty with any such enterprise is the diversity of activities comprising nonstate policing, ranging from neighbourhood watch type activity and private security companies to vigilantism (OECD, 2007, p. 169). An attempt to regulate these diverse actors to the extent at least of bringing them under the one banner may not necessarily be helpful, desirable, or even possible, but it should be recognised that they nonetheless share important common ground, being "forces of coercion engaged by groups of society to preserve social order" that are "controlled only poorly or not at all by state institutions" (Baker, 2002, p. 30).

Many people in African countries depend upon nonstate police and security providers for most of their everyday policing. Although state partnerships with these kinds of agents are often dismissed as unacceptable, there are already numerous links between state and non-state security providers, and such links should arguably be strengthened in order to achieve better delivery of justice and security; community and other forms of nonstate policing can assist police services with limited resources to extend order and security (Baker, 2010). Owing to recruitment of nonstate police by state police and other entities, and sharing of information between the sectors, the division between state and nonstate police is not always easy to maintain (Baker,

2010, p. 33). State police are themselves not immune from the criticisms of lawlessness, corruption, and human rights abuses (Baker, 2010, p. 46), which are frequently levelled against nonstate police (OECD, 2007, p. 104).

Collaboration in a number of areas between state police and nonstate police may have implications for police (both state and nonstate) interactions with people with mental health problems. At least four categories of links exist between state and nonstate security providers: intelligence sharing, sharing of equipment and training, sharing of operations, and enrolment— the police may enlist nonstate agents to undertake patrols, trace suspects, or provide intelligence, or may hand over responsibility for handling lesser criminal matters to customary chiefs (Baker, 2010, pp. 602–604). The police may agree to turn a blind eye on the request of vigilantes, so long as stolen goods are recovered, "offenders" disciplined, or information provided that results in successful prosecution—a deal that benefits both parties, as vigilantes maintain control and crime statistics appear to be improved, as in South African townships (Buur, 2006, p. 748). How are suspects or offenders with mental illness dealt with by nonstate police in these situations? This question is particularly vexed in cases where appearances would suggest that police are enlisting nonstate agents to do their "dirty work"—for example, by using community "police" to engage in measures that are illegal for police, such as using the threat of violence.

In terms of the advantages of collaboration, is there scope for the possibility of joint training of state police and nonstate police in the area of mental health and how to respond appropriately to people with mental illness? This is most likely a long-term goal: It may seem that a crucial first step is to develop relevant policies and training for *state* police. However, any initiatives developed in this area should arguably integrate nonstate policing practises from the outset if possible, given the reality of the interdependence of state policing and nonstate policing. Localised informal responses, taking into account the unique state police and nonstate police links within different cities and districts, are likely to be most successful. Although national legislation, policy, and guidelines would assist, responses may need to be tailored to individual urban and rural communities, depending upon the availability of both mental health and police services.

The Organisation for Economic Cooperation and Development (OECD) writes in relation to design of donor programmes:

> Evidence suggesting that in sub-Saharan Africa at least 80% of justice services are delivered by non-state providers should guide donors to take a balanced approach to supporting state and non-state security and justice service provision. Programs that are locked into either state or non-state institutions, one to the exclusion of the other, are unlikely to be effective. (OECD, 2007, p. 11)

The OECD suggests that security system reform programmes should take a multistakeholder approach, which assists state and nonstate security simultaneously (OECD, 2007, p. 11), and development circles are considering the possibility of *conditional* support for nonstate providers (Baker, 2010, p. 608). It may be useful for conditions on which any such support is provided to include requirements in relation to models for dealing with people suspected of having a mental illness.

Training for police officers in mental health issues and how to respond appropriately to people with mental illness is essential. A number of negative outcomes may result from lack of or inadequate training (Browning, Van Hasselt, Tucker, & Vecchi, 2011, p. 235). Police may perceive the person with a mental illness as being more dangerous and aggressive and act or perhaps overreact accordingly, and the person may then respond in an unpredictable manner to police (Browning et al., 2011, p. 236). This may lead police officers to use more force, increasing the risk of injury to either the person with mental illness or officers (Engel & Silver, 2001), and creating a situation where arrest may be the most likely outcome. Research in this area has, however, produced conflicting results. One study found that as symptoms of mental illness increased, police officers became more lenient in dealing with people with mental illness suspected of involvement in minor and summary offences (Godfredson, Ogloff, Thomas, & Luebbers, 2010, p. 1401).

When it comes to training police officers in relation to mental health, there are the alternatives of (1) providing training to all police officers, and (2) specialised responses involving intensive training for select officers who are deployed as a first-line response in mental health crises. Many countries have now developed mobile crisis teams or intervention services of police, mental health services, or both, specifically to respond to situations involving people with mental illness (Lamb et al., 2002, p. 1268). Specifically, specialised responses may be divided into three main categories:

- *Police-based specialised police responses*, where police officers with mental health training are the first to respond to mental health crises
- *Police-based specialised mental health responses*, where mental health professionals employed by police services respond in person to assist police officers and are available for telephone consultation
- *Mental health-based specialised mental health responses*, involving collaborative arrangements between police and mobile mental health crisis teams that are part of community mental health services (Hails & Borum, 2003, p. 54)

When developing strategies to respond to people with mental illness in African countries, it is important to bear these distinctions in mind.

Specialised responses may greatly enhance responses to people with mental illnesses, in addition to overall training of police officers (Hails & Borum, 2003), although more basic training for all police should arguably be the starting point in a context of extremely limited resources for both police and mental health services.

South Africa

Most of the literature that was able to be identified as dealing specifically with the topic of policing and mental health focused on South Africa. The high level of police involvement in interactions involving mental illness in South Africa indicates a need for police to receive training regarding the Mental Health Care Act 2002 (MHCA) and how best to work with people with a mental illness (Lund et al., 2010). Research on pathways to care in a region of South Africa revealed that 51% of a sample of 21 first-episode and 50 multi-episode patients had police escort on admission to the hospital; when it came to the first point of contact on pathways to care, contact rates with police services were high for both those having a first episode (23.8%) and those with a prior history of episodes (26%). Males were much more likely to make first contact with the police than females (Temmingh & Oosthuizen, 2008, p. 730).

The South African Police Service (SAPS) has a number of formal responsibilities and discretions in relation to mental health under the South African MHCA:

- The police are required to apprehend and take to a health establishment any person who they believe is likely to inflict serious harm on himself or herself or others due to a mental illness under s. 40(1).
- They must comply with a request to apprehend assisted or involuntary mental health care users who have absconded from a health establishment and to transfer a person between services under s. 40(4)–(5), and to apprehend state patients who have absconded under s. 44, and if so requested, must be told of the estimated level of dangerousness of the person.
- A person may be held in custody at a police station for a period to effect the return or transfer of a person to a health establishment under s. 40(7).
- When apprehending a person they "may use such constraining measures as may be necessary and proportionate in the circumstances" under s. 40(7).

Mental health sector stakeholders identified a need for police services to develop guidelines for the implementation of s. 40 of the MHCA, and to collaborate in developing guidelines for early identification and the management of forensic and behaviourally disturbed clients in police custody while in transit to, or awaiting, hospitalisation (Skeen et al., 2010, p. 618). Training guidelines prepared by the National Department of Health in 2003 outline how to identify and approach people with mental health problems (including management of violent people or people threatening violence, aiming to calm the situation and use minimum force), list relevant definitions and obligations under the MHCA with commentary on all relevant statutory provisions, and contain training scenarios (National Department of Health and Directorate Mental Health and Substance Abuse, 2003). The SAPS has developed a standing order setting out police roles and responsibilities in relation to mental health, which in 2008 was still in draft form (Skeen et al., 2010, p. 613).

A key finding of the MHaPP referred to earlier is that sectors other than mental health need to be involved in order to effectively address mental health issues in South Africa, including the police service sector, particularly at the district (as opposed to provincial or national) level (Mental Health and Poverty Project, 2008). The MHaPP recommended that the mental health directorate within the Department of Health take the lead in fostering intersectoral collaboration, including between mental health and sectors like the police, education, social development, housing, justice, corrections, labour, local government, and public works.

South Africa has gone further than other African countries in fostering intersectoral collaboration, including between mental health and police services, to implement mental health policy and legislation. A national forum on forensic psychiatry has been convened by the Department of Health, including the SAPS, the Department of Justice, and the Department of Correctional Services, and such intersectoral collaboration is also occurring in some provinces, but is scarce at the district level (Skeen et al., 2010, p. 613). There is some collaboration between the SAPS and the Department of Health in relation to the transportation of psychiatric patients, for example. However, reluctance among police to transport psychiatric patients, due to stigma and fear, emerged as a major problem according to a 2008 MHaPP report (Lund et al., 2008, p. 195), despite the fact that the MHCA requires them to transport patients where necessary, and the existence of specific policy guidelines on how to deal with psychiatric patients.

Part of the police reluctance to engage with psychiatric patients, according to research conducted in a rural district in South Africa in 2007, was a belief that the core role of a police officer was to deal with criminals, and that people with mental illness should rather be dealt with by the health system, as underlined by the following quote from a SAPS member:

"They (health) are shifting the responsibility. They should be taking these people from the community, not unless the person has done something incriminating [sic]. Somebody who has not really done anything criminal is not our case because for them it is all about illness." (Peterson et al., 2009, p. 145)

Despite the existence of laws and policies governing police interactions with people with mental illness in South Africa, more needs to be done to achieve the cultural shift necessary to optimize such interactions. This may be difficult to achieve, however, without dedicated training and programmes aimed at ensuring coordinated responses toward mental health crisis situations.

Conclusion

There are unique features of the mental health and policing landscapes in African countries that need to be negotiated before developing appropriate models for policing and mental health on the continent, taking into account country-specific factors and differences in health/healing and policing systems in urban and rural areas.

First, popular beliefs about the causation of mental illness may shape police responses to people with mental illness and may be in part responsible for the primacy of traditional healers as the first port of call—although it should be acknowledged that this tendency may be exacerbated by the lack of biomedical mental health resources, especially in remote rural areas. It has been suggested in this chapter that, given their pervasiveness and popularity, traditional healers may have a useful role to play in collaborations between police and mental health services.

Second, the variable existence of police services and prevalence of non-state policing across the continent, in the context of civil war and political instability, with the resultant dislocation of infrastructure and displacement of people, has implications for the development of policies and practises regarding mental health and policing.

Third, across the African continent mental health services and policies are at vastly different stages of development. There are numerous shortcomings in mental health service delivery (vast distances, inadequate funding, and the shortage of trained clinical staff) that would inevitably limit the ability of police and communities in general to respond appropriately to people with mental illness. Moreover, and compounding this, with the exception of those few states that have recently enacted mental health laws, most African states lack modern mental health legislation, setting out the responsibilities of the police in their day-to-day interactions with those suspected of having a mental illness. Where formal laws or guidelines are not in place, there may be scope for strengthening informal measures to this end.

Possibilities for training and continuing education programmes designed to guide police in putting into practise their responsibilities toward people with mental illness and helping them interact more effectively with those suspected of having a mental illness, in collaboration with mental health services, require further attention. It has been suggested that the development of any system of collaborative effort between police and mental health services requires that consideration be given to the integration of traditional healers, the engagement of nonstate police, and the establishment of regulatory frameworks designed to accommodate the diversity of healing and policing systems found on the African continent.

References

Abiodun, O., Adewuya, R., & Makanjuola, O.A. (2008). Social distance towards people with mental illness in Nigeria. *Australian and New Zealand Journal of Psychiatry, 42*(5), 389–395.

Ae-Ngibise, K., Cooper, S., Adiibokah, E., Akpalu, R., Lund, C., Doku, V., & Mental Health and Poverty Research Programme Consortium (MHaPP). (2010). "Whether you like it or not people with mental problems are going to go to them": A qualitative exploration into the widespread use of traditional and faith healers in the provision of mental health care in Ghana. *International Review of Psychiatry, 22*(6), 558–567.

Aina, O.F. (2004). Mental illness and cultural issues in West African films: Implications for orthodox psychiatric practice. *Medical Humanities, 30*, 23–26.

Baker, B. (2006). The African post-conflict policing agenda in Sierra Leone. *Conflict, Security and Development, 6*(1), 25–49.

Baker, B. (2010). Linking state and non-state security and justice. *Development Policy Review, 28*(5), 597–616.

Bartlett, P., Jenkins, R., & Kiima, D. (2011). Mental health law in the community: Thinking about Africa. *International Journal of Mental Health Systems, 5*, 21.

Bhana, A., Peterson, I., Baillie, K.L., Flisher, A.J., & Mental Health and Poverty Research Programme Consortium (MHaPP). (2010). Implementing the World Health Report 2001 recommendations for integrating mental health into primary health care: A situation analysis of three African countries: Ghana, South Africa and Uganda. *International Review of Psychiatry, 22*(6), 599–610.

Browning, S.L., Van Hasselt, V.B., Tucker, A.S., & Vecchi, G.M. (2011). Dealing with individuals who have mental illness: The crisis intervention team (CIT) in law enforcement. *British Journal of Forensic Practice, 13*(4), 235–243.

Burns, J.K., Jhazbhay, K., & Emsley, R.A. (2011). Causal attributions, pathway to care and clinical features of first-episode psychosis: A South African perspective. *International Journal of Social Psychiatry, 57*, 538–545.

Buur, L. (2006). Reordering society: Vigilantism and sovereign expressions in Port Elizabeth's townships. *Development and Change, 37*(4), 735–757.

Chappell, D. (2008). Policing and emotionally disturbed persons: Disseminating knowledge, removing stigma and enhancing performance. *Australian Journal of Forensic Services, 40*(1), 37–48.

Compton, M.T., Bahora, M., Watson, A., & Oliva, J.R. (2006). Crisis intervention team training: Changes in knowledge, attitude, and stigma related to schizophrenia. *Psychiatric Services, 57*(8), 1199–1202.

Dickinson, D. (2008). Traditional healers, HIV/AIDS and company programmes in South Africa. *African Journal of AIDS Research, 7*(3), 281–291.

Draper, C.E., Lund, C., Kleintjes, S., Funk, M., Omar, M., Flisher, A.J., & Mental Health and Poverty Research Programme Consortium (MHaPP). (2009). Mental health policy in South Africa: Development process and content. *Health Policy and Planning, 24*(5), 342–356.

Engel, R.S., & Silver, E. 2001. Policing mentally disordered subjects: A reexamination of the criminalization hypothesis. *Criminology, 39*(2), 225–252.

Godfredson, J.W., Ogloff, J.R.P., Thomas, S.D.M., & Luebbers, S. (2010). *Criminal Justice and Behavior, 37*(12), 1392–1405.

Gureje, O., Lasebikan, V.O., Ephraim-Oluwanuga, O., Olley, B.O., & Kola, L. (2005). Community study of knowledge of and attitude to mental illness in Nigeria. *British Journal of Psychiatry, 186*, 436–441.

Hails, J., & Borum, R. (2003). Police training and specialized approaches to respond to people with mental illnesses. *Crime and Delinquency, 49*(1), 52–61.

Hewson, M.G. (1998). Traditional healers in southern Africa. *Annals of Internal Medicine, 128*(12), 1029–1034.

Hills, A. (1996). Towards a critique of policing and national development in Africa. *Journal of Modern African Studies, 34*(2), 271–291.

Hills, A. (1997). Warlords, militia and conflict in contemporary Africa: A re-examination of terms. *Small Wars & Insurgencies, 8*(1), 35–51.

Jenkins, R., Kiima, D., Okonji, M., Njenga, F., Kingora, J., & Lock, S. (2010). Integration of mental health into primary care and community health working in Kenya: Context, rationale, coverage and sustainability. *Mental Health in Family Medicine, 7*(1), 37–47.

Kahn, M.S., & Kelly, K.J. (2001). Cultural tensions in psychiatric nursing: Managing the interface between Western mental health care and Xhosa traditional healing in South Africa. *Transcultural Psychiatry, 38*(1), 35–50.

Kale, R. (1995). South Africa's health: Traditional healers in South Africa: A parallel health care system. *British Medical Journal, 310*(6988), 1182.

Kapungwe, A., Cooper, S., Mayeya, J., Mwape, L., Wikwese, A., Lund, C., & Mental Health and Poverty Research Programme Consortium (MHaPP). (2011). Attitudes of primary health care providers towards people with mental illness: Evidence from two districts in Zambia. *African Journal of Psychiatry, 14*, 290–297.

Kiwawulo, C. (2010). Uganda: Mental health—Over 11.5 million countrymen suffer disorders. Retrieved December 19, 2011, from allafrica.com/stories/201004050547.html

Lamb, H.R., Weinberger, L.E., & DeCuir, W.J. (2002). The police and mental health. *Psychiatric Services, 53*(1), 1266–1271.

Lund, C., Kleintjes, S., Campbell-Hall, V., Mjadu, S., Petersen, I., Bhana, A., Ritsusko, K., Mlanjeni, B., Bird, P., Drew, N., Faydi, E., Funk, E., Green, A., Omar, M., & Flisher, A.J. (2008). Mental health policy development and implementation in South Africa: A situation analysis. Mental Health and Poverty Project. Retrieved December 22, 2011, from http://www.dfid.gov.uk/R4D/Output/177419/Default.aspx

Lund, C., Oosthuizen, P., Flisher, A.J., Emsley, R., Stein, D.J., Botha, U., Koen, L., & Joska, J. (2010). Pathways to inpatient mental health care among people with schizophrenia spectrum disorders in South Africa. *Psychiatric Services, 61*(3), 235–240.

Meissner, O. (2004). The traditional healer as part of the primary health care team? *South African Medical Journal, 94*, 901–902.

Mental Health and Poverty Project. (2008). *Inter-sectoral collaboration for mental health in South Africa* (Policy Brief 6). Retrieved December 22, 2011, from www.who.int/mental_health/policy/development/MHPB_SA6.pdf

Mental Health and Poverty Project. (2010). *The Mental Health and Poverty Project: Mental health policy development and implementation in four African countries* (HD 6, Final report). Retrieved December 19, 2011, from MHaPP_Final_Report_forR4D(2).pdf

Miller, K.E., & Rassmussen, A. (2010). War exposure, daily stressors, and mental health in post-conflict settings: Bridging the divide between trauma-focused and psychosocial frameworks. *Conflict, Violence, and Health, 70*(1), 7–16.

National Department of Health and Directorate Mental Health and Substance Abuse. (2003). *The Mental Health Care Act 2002 training guidelines for the South African Police Services.*

Nsereko, J.R., Kizza, D., Kigozi, F., Ssebunnya, J., Ndyanabangi, S., Flisher, A.J., Cooper, S., & Mental Health and Poverty Research Programme Consortium (MHaPP). (2011). Stakeholder's perceptions of help-seeking behaviour among people with mental health problems in Uganda. *International Journal of Mental Health Systems, 5*, 5.

Omar, M.A., Green, A.T., Bird, P.K., Mirzoev, T., Flisher, A.J., Kigozi, F., Lund, C., Mwanza, J., Ofori-Atta, A.L., & Mental Health and Poverty Research Programme Consortium (MHaPP). (2010). Mental health policy process: A comparative study of Ghana, South Africa, Uganda and Zambia. *International Journal of Mental Health Systems, 4*, 24.

Organisation for Economic Cooperation and Development. (2007). *OECD DAC handbook on security system reform: Supporting security and justice.* Retrieved December 19, 2011, from www.oecd.org/dataoecd/43/25/38406485.pdf

Peterson, I., Bhana, A., Campbell-Hall, V., Mjadu, S., Lund, C., Kleintjies, S., Hosegood, V., Flisher, A.J., & Mental Health and Poverty Research Programme Consortium (MHaPP). (2009). Planning for district mental health services. *Health Policy and Planning, 24*(2), 140–150.

Read, U.M., Adiibokah, E., & Nyame, S. (2009). Local suffering and the global discourse of mental health and human rights: An ethnographic study of responses to mental illness in rural Ghana. *Globalization and Health, 5*, 13.

Skeen, S., Lund, C., Kleintjes, S., Flisher, A., & Mental Health and Poverty Research Programme Consortium (MHaPP). (2010). Meeting the Millennium Development Goals in sub-Saharan Africa: What about mental health? *International Review of Psychiatry, 22*(6), 624–631.

Sorsdahl, K.R., Flisher, A.J., Wilson, Z., & Stein, D.J. (2010). Explanatory models of mental disorders and treatment practices among traditional healers in Mpumulanga, South Africa. *African Journal of Psychiatry, 13*, 284–290.

Tanner, R.E.S. (1999). Concern, cooperation, and coexistence in healing. *British Medical Journal, 319*(7202), 133.

Temmingh, H.S., & Oosthuizen, P.P. (2008). Pathways to care and treatment delays in first and multi episode psychosis: Findings from a developing country. *Social Psychiatry and Psychiatric Epidemiology, 43*(9), 727–735.

Van der Beest, S. (1997). Is there a role for traditional medicine in basic health services in Africa? A plea for community perspective. *Tropical Medicine and International Health, 2*(9), 903–911.

Wolff, N. (1998). Interactions between mental health and law enforcement systems: Problems and prospects for cooperation. *Journal of Health Politics, Policy, and Law, 23*(1), 133–174.

World Health Organisation (WHO). (2002). *WHO traditional medicine strategy 2002–2005*. Retrieved December 19, 2011, from whqlibdoc.who.int/hq/2002/who_edm_trm_2002.1.pdf

World Health Organisation (WHO). (2005). *Mental health atlas*. Geneva: WHO.

World Health Organisation (WHO). (2008, December). *Traditional medicine* (Fact Sheet 134). Retrieved December 19, 2011, from http://www.who.int/mediacentre/factsheets/fs134/en/

World Health Organisation (WHO). (2010). *Mental health and development: Targeting people with mental health conditions as a vulnerable group*. Geneva: WHO.

Policing and Mentally Ill Persons in Hong Kong

16

SHARON INGRID KWOK
T. WING LO
PERCY LEE

Contents

Introduction

Since community-oriented policing was introduced in Hong Kong, interaction between the police and the public has increased significantly. Greater public accessibility to police as a result of decentralisation and the 999 emergency response line, as well as increased police mobility due to more police vehicles and patrols, is also likely to have contributed to the increase in contacts between police and mentally ill persons (MIPs). However, the shift toward community-oriented policing has led to an increase in public expectation of the police and the services they provide. Coupled with the commonly held misperception that MIPs are dangerous, and the lack of alternative on-call assistance, police are typically the first and only community service called to manage situations involving such people (Finn & Sullivan, 1989; Tucker, Van Hasselt, & Russell, 2008).

Recently, MIPs have been attracting considerable attention in Hong Kong, as a number have been involved in violent offences, injuring those around them. One of the more tragic offences concerned a three-year-old child who was killed on May 29, 2009 (Ming Pao, 2009). The attack took place around noon in a park where the victim was playing alone, while the father was at the market across the street. The MIP, who lived on the lower floor of a building near the park, attacked the child with a 10-inch knife. Incidents like this lead to a rise in public awareness of the social problems faced and created by MIPs and to the call for adequate social services to assist them.

Procedures in Handling Mentally Ill Persons in Hong Kong

The police are usually the first contact point in handling MIPs, and their gatekeeping role is crucial to the disposition and consequences for these persons. When police encounter a person suspected of being mentally ill, they first consider if he or she has violent tendencies. If the person is found to be nonviolent, the police officer initiates further investigation, which may lead to informal disposition or referral to the relevant social services. If the person is found to have self-destructive or violent tendencies, police may call the police emergency unit for support, arrange for an ambulance, and forcibly escort the person to the hospital for examination and treatment (see Cap 136, Mental Health Ordinance).

If an MIP is found to have committed an offence or created a serious nuisance for others, police can arrest, or even restrain and escort, the person to an ambulance for examination in the hospital. A relative or friend is notified and asked to come to the hospital to provide information to the medical officer conducting the examination. A report is then sent to the court, possibly resulting in an order by a judge or magistrate for involuntary hospitalisation. Where no violent or self-destructive behaviour has been exhibited or an offence committed, the police have no right to escort MIPs to the hospital against their will, even if they display symptoms of mental illness. Thus, violent and nonviolent MIPs are handled differently by the police. Figure 16.1 summarises how police handle MIPs under the current system.

A violent person suspected of suffering from mental illness would normally be restrained by the police using handcuffs, which may be used on both wrists and ankles if necessary. Rope will not usually be used for this purpose unless handcuffs are not immediately available. Whenever possible, the police officer would first seek assistance before tackling a violent person unless it is necessary to take immediate action to preserve life or property. As soon as the person has been overpowered, any object with which the person may do harm to him- or herself or others is taken away. If the person cannot or will not walk, he or she is carried, preferably strapped to a stretcher.

The first responsibility of the police is to get the person to the hospital as soon as possible for medical observation, which eliminates the possibility of

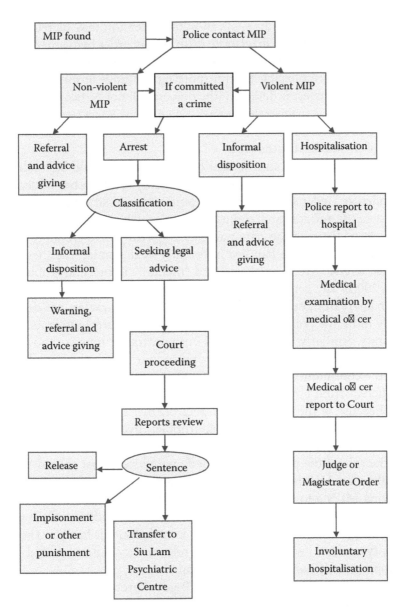

Figure 16.1 How the Hong Kong Police handle MIPs.

a violent or unpleasant scene at either a police station or in a public place. It is the responsibility of the escorting police officer to supply as much information as possible to the medical officer at the hospital, regarding the case and the circumstances in which the person was found. If the medical officer considers that there are grounds for sending the MIP to a mental hospital, he or she will complete a Form 1 or 2 as appropriate and request the escorting police officer to obtain a Form 3 signed by a district court judge or magistrate. The subject of an application for detention may be requested to appear before the judge or magistrate prior to any order being made. If such a request is made, or the judge or magistrate wishes to interview the subject, the police will be responsible for transporting the judge or magistrate to the place where the subject is detained (the person will not be taken to the court or to the judge's or magistrate's home). Once Form 3 has been signed, it is handed to the medical officer and the escorting officer leaves the subject in the care of the medical authorities.

In addition, there is an informal disposition that could be made when the police are confronted with an MIP, especially one who has not committed an offence. Under such disposition, police can classify the person as one who just needs referral and counselling, in which case the person would not have to go through the criminal justice system. There are three types of MIPs that are likely to be handled informally by the police: the "neighbourhood characters," "troublemakers," and "mentally ill but non-troublesome" (Teplin, 2000). The neighbourhood characters are people whose behaviours set them apart from other people. Although these characters are defined as mentally ill by the police, their odd behaviours are largely tolerated by the community. Similarly, the mentally ill but nontroublesome are those whose mental illness does not lead to offensive behaviour; hence, they are also tolerated in the community. The troublemakers are problematic in that they are very different from both the latter and the neighbourhood characters. It is exactly because of the problematic aspect of their character that the police decline to arrest them in order to avoid trouble. Given the option of avoiding the trouble and paperwork involved for hospitalisation via informal disposition, the role of the police is conflicted, as the steps that should be taken in handling an MIP become more complex than is shown in Figure 16.1. Classifying MIPs into different typologies is merely based on police discretion and perspective rather than the actual medical condition of the person. Lacking proper training and appropriate knowledge, it is hard for the police to identify correctly who is suitable for referral to counselling and who is more appropriately handled in the hospital.

Once involved in an offence, an MIP goes through the same due process as a mentally capable suspect, as generally criminal suspects would be arrested and investigated by the police regardless of their mental condition. When MIPs are transferred to the criminal justice system, they are charged and tried in court. If the court cannot identify the MIP's symptoms of mental illness in the hearing process, he or she is sentenced to jail if convicted. However, if symptoms are identified during the hearing process, the judge sentences the offender to the Siu Lam Psychiatric Centre for involuntary treatment. In some situations, the symptoms of mental illness are identified during incarceration by correctional officers, and the MIP is also sent to the

Siu Lam Psychiatric Centre for involuntary treatment. The criminal justice system provides no other alternative than to place the MIP in custody in a secure setting first, and then arrange for psychiatric treatment if necessary. After release from a correctional institution, MIPs are returned to the community where some are monitored by health professionals. However, the monitoring normally lasts for a limited period of time, so it is possible that the person may not be completely cured while living in the community.

Two Case Studies

To demonstrate how police encounter and handle MIPs in reality, two well-known cases in Hong Kong that attracted much public attention are presented below.

The Cheung Case (September 2001)

Cheung, who was first arrested by the police in 1985 due to involvement in an assault at his workplace, was identified as mentally ill. During his arrest Cheung vigorously resisted police, who ultimately forcibly escorted him to the hospital for examination, where it was confirmed he was suffering from mental illness. As a result of this experience, Cheung became antagonistic toward the police.

In May 2001, Cheung was working in a hospital as a cleaner with a monthly salary of around HKD 2,000. The incident began when Cheung was absent from work for three days and his employer tried to call him at home to ask the reason. Irritated and upset by the calls, Cheung began brandishing a chopper and his father called the police.

After the police arrived, emergency unit officers also came to the scene to assist. In view of Cheung's medical history, the police carried armadillo shields and pepper sprays. A number of verbal warnings were given, but when he responded violently and was not making sense, police decided to suppress him and send him to the hospital for medical treatment. However, he resisted arrest, brandishing the chopper and attacking the police. One of the police officers carrying a shield was attacked and his thumb cut off. Three other officers were also injured during the struggle. Pepper spray into Cheung's face did not subdue him and led him to cause further injuries to the police.

Finally, Cheung was restrained and taken by ambulance to the hospital. Upon arrival, a medical officer certified Cheung as dead, although with no apparent lethal wound. However, Cheung's father claimed that the police officers at the scene continued to beat his son even after subduing him. His father also said he saw assault wounds all over his son's body in the mortuary. He blamed the officers and questioned why his son was still being beaten after being subdued.

In this case, Cheung's death was classified by the coroner as an accident. The judge of the coroner's court commented:

- The police should increase communication and contact with an MIP after an incident.
- Further training on how to handle MIPs should be provided to police officers.
- The professional standard of ambulance officers should be enhanced and their performance audited regularly.

The Lee Case (May 2003)

Lee, who had a history of mental illness and a criminal record for assault and fighting, was a 45-year-old, strongly built, unemployed person who lived alone in a flat on a public estate. Prior to this case, the police had summoned Lee twice for illegal cycling. However, since Lee did not receive the summons tickets, which were sent by registered mail, a traffic police officer took the tickets to his home. After receiving the tickets, Lee reacted by tearing the tickets, shaping them into balls, and throwing them at the officer. He then went to the kitchen, picked up a chopper, and brandished it. The officer escaped and immediately called for support. Later the emergency unit officers, in police armour, arrived, and when after an hour the police negotiation cadres failed to negotiate with Lee, they broke into the flat. However, due to the narrowness of the corridor in the flat, despite using pepper spray in Lee's face, he still managed to attack with the chopper four armoured officers, causing serious injuries.

Lee was eventually arrested by the police. However, the incident revealed that the police armour could not protect the officers completely in such a dangerous situation. The armour could protect only a portion of the officer's body, leading them to be hurt.

Review of the Two Cases

In the Cheung Case, his mental illness was not identified following his first arrest for the assault in 1985. Apparently, the officers could not communicate well and failed to detect his symptoms. After the first incident, Mr. Cheung viewed the police as being against him, finally leading to the violent incident that caused his death. Thus, enhancing communication skills in dealing with

MIPs is essential as part of police training. The fact that Cheung earned a low salary working as a cleaner in a hospital, with an ex-wife and son to support, may have contributed to stress and low esteem on his part. The case raises the issue that it is not easy for MIPs to conduct a normal life due to their medical condition and that the mental illness label may make it more difficult for them, than for ordinary people, to find a job that makes a better living.

After the assault incident, Cheung was unwilling to seek help from social workers or medical professionals. His father also did not know how to seek help when Cheung stopped going to work and showed some symptoms of relapse. Owing to a lack of resources in the medical and social welfare systems, Cheung's case was not properly monitored, especially during the period when he relapsed, and his father was not informed regarding how to seek professional help. This eventually worsened the situation, leading to violence and death. If proper follow-up actions had been taken, the outcome might have been avoided.

Furthermore, in this case, the police emergency unit officers carried armadillo shields and pepper spray to prevent them from being attacked by Cheung. This made him agitated, as he felt the police action was offensive. This fit his earlier image of police, as the mentally ill are particularly sensitive to how they are treated by the police (Watson & Angell, 2007). This suggests that the heavy-handedness of the police at the initial stage of interaction with Cheung might have provoked him and led to the violence. A solution might have been to assign a police negotiating cadre team to intervene in the situation or plainclothed officers to approach Cheung in the first instance.

In the Lee case the traffic officer obviously did not obtain enough information about Lee before arriving at the flat, and was therefore not aware of his mental illness. Their miscommunication triggered the violence. The traffic officer informed the police negotiation cadres, who arrived at the scene in plainclothes. After negotiation failed, they let the police emergency unit officers break into the flat. The officers were fully equipped with pepper spray, police armour, and armadillo shields, which they were trained to use. However, due to the awkward layout of the flat, they failed to suppress Lee with the pepper spray. As a result, Lee reacted more violently against them. Similar to the case of Cheung, the pepper spray seemed to have induced negative worse reaction.

Moreover, the gaps in the police armour failed to protect the officers completely, leading to their injuries when arresting Lee. In Cheung's case the police shield also showed it had a crack mark after being used. Both cases revealed that the equipment failed to protect the officers in violent situations. After the Cheung case, the police immediately replaced the old shields with new ones that were more durable and gave sufficient protection. Some procedures were developed to change the shields and test the quality periodically.

Police Encounters With MIPs

Having reviewed the two cases involving MIPs, in the following two sections we further explore the issues of police encounters with MIPs and the availability of community care services. Information is collected through interviews with three police officers, one informant who reported a case to the police, two nurses, and one social worker. The findings are outlined below.

Police Culture

In their daily work, dealing with criminals and protecting citizens' lives and property are the priority of police officers (Lamb, Weinberger, & DeCuir, 2002). In police culture, arresting criminals can help a police officer receive commendation from the management and increase the chance of receiving a good appraisal report, which is essential for promotion. On the other hand, dealing with MIPs is regarded as doing something with low reward. Police officer A said, "If an officer did not handle the case well, it might endanger his/her safety and also impact his/her career prospect. Therefore, my colleagues thought handling MIPs was fruitless work." Many police officers feel uncertain and insecure when dealing with violent MIPs, mainly because of the lack of knowledge about their mental state. When the MIPs exhibit a tendency for violence, many officers tend to overreact. As police officer B said,

> I felt uncertain when I dealt with MIPs. I didn't know what they had in mind so I felt insecure when handling them. I was afraid that they would commit suicide and sometimes I worried if they would attack us and other people. Therefore, I mostly tended to be reactive in dealing with them. I think many of my colleagues have the same kind of feeling.

Because of this thinking, many police officers are not willing to shoulder the responsibility of dealing with MIPs who offend. In many circumstances, the MIPs only commit minor offences and their mental health history is disclosed in the investigation period, but the police are not courageous enough to handle the cases informally due to the offender's medical history. As police officer C stated, "We would not risk releasing the MI offenders because some accidents may occur. This could cause stress to the victims and lead to questions from the mass media." Thus, the police would rather allow the court to handle the cases.

Police Equipment and Tactics

Armadillo shields are always in patrol cars ready for use in dealing with crises. However, the first case study shows that this kind of shield could not provide sufficient protection for the police officers. Although the old shields were changed after the attack, their effectiveness in dealing with violent MIPs is still in doubt. Police officer B said, "It is ridiculous for a modern police force to keep using the same kind of shields after the incident when they broke. Although the shields are now changed and checked periodically, they are still the same type and may crack again in a violent case." On the other hand, in Mr. Lee's case, the inadequate safety of the armour also contributed to police injuries. Commenting on the low quality, police officer C said, "The renewal of armour is more frequent nowadays after the recent MIP attacks. However, I still think the equipment is not sufficient enough to protect us against those violent attacks." Not only is the armour flawed, but during the interviews with other police officers, it was revealed that many were not familiar with the equipment and how to use it appropriately. Moreover, pepper spray may not be a suitable weapon in handling the MIPs. Both case studies show that the ejecting of pepper spray seemed to provoke the MIPs into becoming more violent, and thus worsened the incidents.

The existing tactics seem to be deficient in dealing with violent MIPs. The officers sometimes underestimate the environmental factors of the scene, which may contribute to their injuries. Serious consequences were seen from time to time, for example, an officer's thumb being cut off in the first case, and many officers injured seriously in both cases. In fact, the officers should be more alert when handling violent MIPs to prevent tragedy from happening. Police officer A mentioned, "The tactic of fast break-in at the scene may not be suitable in handling such cases. It may aggravate the MIP and provoke more vigorous reactions." The uncertainty and reluctance in having contact with MIPs further creates a hostile relationship between the two parties.

Informal Disposition

If the MIPs are violent, the officers may make an easy decision to arrest them. However, most officers would rather ignore nonviolent MIPs who are only causing a minor nuisance to the public than handle them provocatively. Police officer A said, "It is really hard to control the circumstances when dealing with MIPs because they do not always obey our instructions, or may react crazily. It is really a tedious and annoying task and we sometimes just choose to ignore them if the issue is minor."

Moreover, since there is no formal referral system for the nonviolent MIPs between the police and social services, the police tend to handle most MIPs with informal dispositions and do not make further social welfare and health referrals. Thus, the nonviolent MIPs are required to return to the community without proper follow-ups, and their mental illness may worsen, leading to further violence and self-destructive acts. The above two case studies highlighted such serious consequences. An informant, who reported his mentally ill brother who had relapsed at home, said:

My brother has been suffering from mental illness for several years. He was always suspicious that we would do something to harm him. Once my brother quarrelled with us when he became suspicious. He attempted to attack me and my parents called the police immediately. The police arrived and classified my brother as having no violent tendency. They only convinced my brother to consult a doctor. However, my brother refused to go to receive treatment and finally the police left without further action. I felt angry about the approach of the police. They did nothing to help my brother in the incident. I was helpless and disappointed that they didn't take any constructive action to help admit my brother to a hospital.

Somehow, the police would not take action in a case involving mental illness simply based on the information provided by witnesses (Watson, Corrigan, & Ottati, 2004). The issue of informal disposition of MIPs is significant in understanding the interaction between the police and MIPs, since it is the predominant means of police resolution. As police officer A revealed, "Nearly seventy percent of all MIPs are handled by the police via informal means." During another interview, police officer C expressed his opinion on the issue concerning informal disposition:

There are guidelines for dealing with MIPs, but usually the guidelines would only be followed if the incident asks for it. It really depends on the police officers' perspective on the issue. If the MIPs are not violent nor show violent tendency, the police will often consider the issue as minor when recording the incident. The police officers judge the situation, and if the MIPs do not pose immediate threat, the officers usually cannot do anything even if later on the MIPs cause other trouble. The police may only arrest the MIPs if they did something harmful or illegal. Very often, unless the situation is immediate and negative consequences are obvious, the police would just settle the issue quickly.

In the issue of informal disposition, police discretion is the core element (Patch & Arrigo, 1999; Teplin, 2000). Without proper training and clear instructions to follow when dealing with MIPs, police discretion is influenced by many factors, one of which is the typology of police officers—the role and identification taken by the police. According to Pursley (1977), the typology of the police can be classified into four types: the enforcer, the social service agent, the zealot, and the watchman. These different types directly influence and complicate the role of a police officer in the interaction with MIPs because, based on such characteristics, law enforcement can vary. For instance, the enforcer generally places low value on individual rights and a higher value on social order. The social service agent is more idealistic and ensures the well-being of MIPs. Similarly, the other typologies have their own distinctive values and priorities, such as the zealot who treats all offenders equally and the watchman who generally ignores minor violations. This suggests that the same MIP may receive different treatment when confronted by police officers of different typology. This factor complicates the role of the police and allows them much discretion. Pursley's (1977) concept of typology is also observed in the context of Hong Kong. Police officer C talked about the main disposition of Hong Kong police when dealing with MIPs: "Usually police officers in the Emergency Unit are more eager to solve the problems caused by the MIPs. But generally, other ordinary police officers don't really care about mental illness issues unless there is violence or injury. They would try not to make a big deal out of the issues in order to avoid writing reports." Indeed, as they require neither paperwork nor unwanted "downtime" (time off the street), informal dispositions are undoubtedly the best option for many police officers.

Insufficient Mental Health Training and Support

Similar to their overseas counterparts, the Hong Kong police are not given sufficient training on mental illness and how to handle MIPs (Ruiz & Miller, 2004). Police bias and prejudice against MIPs are inevitable, especially when mental health training and knowledge are limited. Police officer C remarked, "There are training programmes but the content is very shallow. The guidelines are broad. Police officers generally don't learn much from them." Insufficient training further induces MIP stereotypes by the police, which may affect their objective judgement. Although police guidelines and procedures are there, they do not cover most circumstances in handling MIPs. For instance, there are no clear instructions on handling nonviolent MIPs. Guidelines are provided only when strong evidence of destructive intent and violent behaviour of the MIPs exists. Hence, the officers usually suggest that the family of the MIP seek help from the Social Welfare Department or Hospital Authority. If the MIP and his or her family refuse to cooperate, many police officers would not take further action due to insufficient mental health knowledge. This may endanger the well-being of the MIP and probably the safety of the community, leading to a vicious cycle of MI-induced violence and self-destructive behaviour.

Moreover, the lack of collaboration between the police and other mental health institutions leaves the police with insufficient professional backup. In relation to this issue, police officer C said, "The police usually don't collaborate with the mental health organisations. We would have meetings but only on rare occasions when police injuries have occurred due to MI incidents." Without sufficient training, assistance, and support from professional mental health experts, the police are facing great challenges.

Community Support Services for MIPs

Similarly to the experiences of other countries (Lamb & Weinberger, 2001), mental health services tend to be deinstitutionalised in Hong Kong. This means that many MIPs need strong support in the community. However, the current community mental health services can only provide limited support to MIPs because of the heavy service demand. Nurse A stated,

> I need to conduct home visits to monitor 120 patients monthly. For the new cases, I need to see the patient for one hour at the first time. For the repeated cases, I need to spend half an hour with a patient and I will visit each patient monthly. I think the resources are really insufficient for monitoring the progress of the patients. Also, many patients are good at pretending and it is impossible to guarantee their mental state is being well monitored.

Apart from the problems in the monitoring of MIPs, there are other operational difficulties in community rehabilitation. Nurse A said, "Some patients flee from the registered address. It is really a problem for us to monitor their progress. Although we can recall them back to the hospital when we locate them again, it may be dangerous to the community if their medication is not taken on time." In addition, even if the community psychiatric nurses can locate the MIPs at home, their personal security is another matter. When discussing home visits, nurse B stated,

> I remember on one occasion, I entered an MIP's flat but he locked the door after I got in. I asked him not to lock the door but he insisted to lock it for security. I finally let him lock the door because I was afraid of ruining our relationship if I insisted. Then I started to talk with him but he picked up a pole-like object and suddenly became emotional. I was very frightened at that moment. Luckily, I could finally end the visit safely. However, that incident really scared me.

Without sufficient safety measures, the frontline nurses may be put in a dangerous position. Another operational constraint concerns medication, which is crucial for the recovery of MIPs. The cost of effective treatment is expensive and the Hospital Authority cannot provide the best medications to the MIPs due to budget constraint. As Nurse B mentioned, "Many good treatments are expensive and many psychiatrists would only dispense these medicines to some younger, treatable patients. They are thought to be more deserving of these medicines because they are more beneficial to the society in the long-run. Unfortunately, many older and seriously ill patients would not receive the best treatments." This differential handling might have slowed down the recovery of some MIPs.

In social welfare organisations, social workers also play an important role in helping MIPs (Yip, 1995), such as cooperating with mental health professionals, and applying for different types of allowances and social benefits. A social worker who worked in a public hospital said,

> Social workers mainly help MIPs to access the resources available in the community. Very few of them would really have time to provide counselling and follow up their progress closely. We usually leave it to the psychiatric nurses to do the job. They play the key role in following up the cases and detecting any relapse. In my social work training, I didn't learn sufficiently about mental illness. I think it is more suitable for psychiatric nurses to handle them. I think I help solve their problems except mental illness. We do not pay too much attention to their illness and we cannot prescribe them medications. Unless their symptoms are apparent, it's hard for us to notice their MI, and we will mostly let the psychiatric professionals deal with their MI problems.

Social workers face tremendous constraints in helping MIPs in the community due to heavy workload and limited resources (Yip, 2000). Many of them do not have sufficient time to provide counselling to the MIPs, or fail to make timely referrals so they can receive sufficient mental health service.

Conclusions

Owing to the increasing service orientation of the police, they are regarded as the only recourse for the citizens to seek immediate help with MIPs. Doubtlessly, managing MIPs in the community has now become an essential part of police work (Sced, 2006). Ironically, police training does not provide much knowledge about mental illness, and the legal structure establishes no guidelines for dealing with nonviolent MIPs. Whether an MIP is defined by the police as bad or mad is really a matter of discretion (Patch & Arrigo, 1999; Teplin, 2000) rather than the rule of law (Watson & Angell, 2007). However, police officers have different characteristics, so different typologies (Pursley, 1977) will result in different dispositions. Moreover, the decision-making process of police officers in dealing with MIPs is complicated intervention, which is affected by various factors, including knowledge about mental illness, normal deviance, community and organisational characteristics of the society, workload of the handling officers, substance abuse involvement, the severity of the offence, immediate behaviour, and time and efficiency concerns (Morabito, 2007).

Generally, police officers around the world have a set of MIP beliefs or stereotypes, which may include the perceptions that they are dangerous, troublesome, and unreliable due to their mental illnesses (Ruiz & Miller,

2004; Watson et al., 2004). The Hong Kong police are no exception. Moreover, insufficient knowledge about mental illness means that many officers fail to identify related symptoms. Frontline officers predominantly choose informal disposition in dealing with MIPs because this resolution requires neither paperwork nor unwanted downtime. This practise reduces the need to refer MIPs to hospital or welfare departments to receive continuous psychiatric treatment and counselling.

Police training is crucial if we are to provide effective and responsive intervention programmes to help MIPs (Hails & Borum, 2003; Lamb, Weinberger, & Gross, 2004; Wells & Schafer, 2006). Our findings suggest that in Hong Kong police training concerning the psychological state of officers and MIPs and how to deal with MIPs in different circumstances is insufficient. The current training content mainly focusses on the procedures and handling guidelines. In fact, the psychological state, workload, knowledge of mental illness, police decision to arrest, safety worries, and so on, also affect the police officers when dealing with MIPs. The lack of sufficient training may lead to criminalisation (Teplin, 2000; Lo & Wang, 2012) and stigmatisation of MIPs (Chappell, 2008) in frontline police work. Hence, it is recommended that all of these factors are covered in police training. The training should be provided periodically and not only limited to newly recruited officers, so as to enhance the self-confidence of the frontline police when dealing with MIPs in real cases. It helps them to treat the MIPs as clients instead of troublemakers. Police training should cultivate understanding that dealing with MIPs is meaningful work rather than a fruitless endeavour. The training should convey the message that this type of work is a valuable part of service-oriented police culture, which can motivate the frontline officers to provide quality services.

In terms of the police equipment, it is suggested that the police should be equipped comprehensively, since many cases (including the two discussed in this chapter) have revealed the weaknesses and insufficient maintenance of the equipment. It is worth considering the upgrade of the current equipment and the introduction of more advanced alternatives. It is also necessary to provide regular and comprehensive training to the officers on using the equipment. This will mean that frontline officers are better protected and the injuries caused by MIPs reduced.

Community mental health care can be costly, but it is far cheaper than incarceration or institutionalisation (Steverman & Lubin, 2007). MIPs in Hong Kong are living in an environment with limited community mental health resources. Such an environment creates a vicious cycle: Many MIPs are not given sufficient support in the community; rather, they are labelled, discriminated, victimised, or eventually reinstitutionalised (Fitzgerald et al., 2005; Goodman et al., 2001; Hiday, Swartz, Swanson, Borum, & Wagner, 1999; Priebe et al., 2005, 2008; Teplin, McClelland, Abram, & Weiner, 2005).

They are handled by the police repeatedly, but informal dispositions are preferred, and this delays referring the nonviolent MIPs to appropriate social welfare and health services. Consequently, the MIPs remain in the community without quality professional support (Wang et al., 2007).

In fact, the police cannot handle the issue of MIPs alone; they have to be assisted and supported by other mental health professionals (Finn & Sullivan, 1989). Western countries have many years of experience of deinstitutionalisation and community care of MIPs (Lamb & Weinberger, 2001), which could serve as reference for authorities in Hong Kong. For example, some community schemes, such as crisis intervention teams (Compton & Chien, 2008), mental health courts (Steadman, Davidson, & Brown, 2001), and the police-based diversion programme (Reuland, 2004), are innovative approaches to keep MIPs from jail or court. In Hong Kong no effective cross-disciplinary collaboration mechanism exists among mental health care, social welfare, and the police regarding this issue. There is no comprehensive system for the referral of MIPs to the psychiatry centres of the Hospital Authority. In the current system, MIPs may only be sent to the psychiatry centres for involuntary treatment after they are judged in a court hearing. If the cross-departmental system for dealing with MIPs were set up, it would be beneficial to both MIPs and society, as it would help stop the aforementioned vicious cycle. The police can also consider employing mental health professionals in police stations to assess the arrested MIPs, so that the most relevant intervention could be made to help them. To preserve privacy and family life (Kinderman & Tai, 2008), the MIPs should live in a community that focusses on recovery rather than suffering. Government and health and welfare organisations should think rigorously about how multidisciplinary collaboration can improve the well-being of MIPs in the community.

References

Chappell, D. (2008). Commentary. Policing and emotionally disturbed persons: Disseminating knowledge, removing stigma and enhancing performance. *Australian Journal of Forensic Sciences, 40*(1), 37–48.

Compton, M.T., & Chien, V.H. (2008). Factors related to knowledge retention after crisis intervention team training for police officers. *Psychiatry Services, 59*, 1049–1051.

Finn, P., & Sullivan, M. (1989). Police handling of the mentally ill: Sharing responsibility with the mental health system. *Journal of Criminal Justice, 17*(1), 1–14.

Fitzgerald, P.B., de Castella, A.R., Filia, K.M., Filia, S.L., Benitez, J., & Kulkarni, J. (2005). Victimization of patients with schizophrenia and related disorder. *Australian and New Zealand Journal of Psychiatry, 39*(3), 169–174.

Goodman, L.A., Salyers, M.P., Mueser, K.T., Rosenberg, S.D., Swartz, M., Essock, S.M., Osher, F.C., Butterfield, M.I., & Swanson, J. (2001). Recent victimization in women and men with severe mental illness: Prevalence and correlates. *Journal of Traumatic Stress*, *14*(4), 615–632.

Hails, J., & Borum, R. (2003). Police training and specialized approaches to respond to people with mental illnesses. *Crime and Delinquency*, *49*, 52–61.

Hiday, V.A., Swartz, M.S., Swanson, J.W., Borum, R., & Wagner, H.R. (1999). Criminal victimization of persons with severe mental illness. *Psychiatric Services*, *50*(1), 62–68.

Kinderman, P., & Tai, S. (2008). Psychological models of mental disorder, human rights, and compulsory mental healthcare in the community. *International Journal of Law and Psychiatry*, *31*, 479–486.

Lamb, H.R., & Weinberger, L.E. (2001). *Deinstitutionalization: Promise and problems. New direction for mental health service.* San Francisco, CA: Jossey-Bass.

Lamb, H.R., Weinberger, L.E., & DeCuir Jr., W.J. (2002). The police and mental health. *Psychiatric Services*, *53*, 1266–1271.

Lamb, H.R., Weinberger, L.E., & Gross, B.H. (2004). Mentally ill persons in the criminal justice system: Some perspectives. *Psychiatric Quarterly*, *75*(2), 107–126.

Lo, T.W. & Wang, X. (2012). Policing and the mentally ill in China: Challenges and prospects. In Duncan Chappell (Ed.), *Police Responses to People with Mental Illnesses* (pp. 54–65). New York: Routledge.

Ming Pao. (2009, May 30). Mentally ill person chopped 3-year old boy. *Ming Pao*, p. A02.

Morabito, M.S. (2007). Horizons of context: Understanding the police decision to arrest people with mental illness. *Psychiatric Services*, *58*, 1582–1587.

Patch, P.C., & Arrigo, B.A. (1999). Police officer attitudes and use of discretion in situations involving the mentally ill: The need to narrow the focus. *International Journal of Law and Psychiatry*, *22*, 23–35.

Priebe, S., Badesconyi, A., Fioritti, A., Hansson, L., Kilian, R., Torres-Gonzales, F., et al. (2005). Reinstitutionalization in mental health care: Comparison of data on service provision from six European countries. *British Medical Journal*, *330*, 123–126.

Priebe, S., Frottier, P., Gaddini, A., Kilian, R., Lauber, C., Martinez-Leal, R., et al. (2008). Mental health care institutions in nine European countries, 2002–2006. *Psychiatric Services*, *59*, 570–573.

Pursley, R.D. (1977). *Introduction to criminal justice* (2nd ed.). Encino, CA: Glencoe.

Reuland, M. (2004). *A guide to implementing police-based diversion programs for people with mental illness.* Delmar, NY: Technical Assistance and Policy Analysis Center for Jail Diversion.

Ruiz, J., & Miller, C. (2004). An exploratory study of Pennsylvania police officers' perceptions of dangerousness and their ability to manage persons with mental illness. *Police Quarterly*, *7*, 359–371.

Sced, M. (2006). *Mental illness in the community: The role of police.* Australia: Australasian Centre for Policing Research.

Steadman, H.J., Davidson, S., & Brown, C. (2001). Mental health courts: Their promise and unanswered questions. *Psychiatric Services*, *52*, 457–458.

Steverman, S., & Lubin, T. (2007). *Avoiding jail pays off.* Washington, DC: National Conference of State Legislatures.

Teplin, L.A. (2000). Keeping the peace: Police discretion and mentally ill persons. *National Institute of Justice Journal, 244*, 8–15.

Teplin, L.A., McClelland, G.M., Abram, K.M., & Weiner, D.A. (2005). Crime victimization in adults with severe mental illness: Comparison with the national crime victimization survey. *Archives of General Psychiatry, 62*(8), 911–921.

Tucker, A.S., Van Hasselt, V.B., & Russell, S.A. (2008). Law enforcement response to the mentally ill: An evaluative review. *Brief Treatment and Crisis Intervention, 8*, 236–250.

Wang, X., Zhang, D., Jiang, S., Bai, Y., Cucolo, H.E., & Perlin, M.L. (2007). Reassessing the aftercare treatment of individuals found not guilty due to a mental disability in Hunan, China: Supplemental study into the disposition of mentally ill offenders after forensic psychiatric assessment. *Australian and New Zealand Journal of Psychiatry, 41*, 337–342.

Watson, A.C., & Angell, B. (2007). Applying procedural justice theory to law enforcement's response to persons with mental illness. *Psychiatric Services, 58*, 787–793.

Watson, A.C., Corrigan, P.W., & Ottati, V. (2004). Police responses to persons with mental illness: Does the label matter? *Journal of the American Academy of Psychiatry and the Law, 32*(4), 378–385.

Wells, W., & Schafer, J.A. (2006). Officer perceptions of police responses to persons with a mental illness. *Policing: An International Journal of Police Strategies and Management, 29*, 578–601.

Yip, K.S. (1995). The role institutionalization of social workers plays in psychiatric case management in Hong Kong. Unpublished doctoral dissertation, University of New South Wales, Sydney, Australia.

Yip, K.S. (2000). Have psychiatric services in Hong Kong been impacted by the deinstitutionalization and community care movements? *Administration and Policy in Mental Health, 27*(6), 443–449.

Index

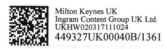

Milton Keynes UK
Ingram Content Group UK Ltd.
UKHW020317111024
449327UK00040B/1361